Practicing Primary Palliative Care

Editor

PRINGL MILLER

SURGICAL CLINICS OF NORTH AMERICA

www.surgical.theclinics.com

Consulting Editor
RONALD F. MARTIN

October 2019 • Volume 99 • Number 5

ELSEVIER

1600 John F. Kennedy Boulevard • Suite 1800 • Philadelphia, Pennsylvania, 19103-2899

http://www.surgical.theclinics.com

SURGICAL CLINICS OF NORTH AMERICA Volume 99, Number 5
October 2019 ISSN 0039–6109, ISBN-13: 978-0-323-70890-6

Editor: John Vassallo, j.vassallo@elsevier.com
Developmental Editor: Casey Potter

Surgical Clinics of North America (ISSN 0039–6109) is published bimonthly by Elsevier Inc., 360 Park Avenue South, New York, NY 10010-1710. Months of publication are February, April, June, August, October, and December. Business and Editorial Offices: 1600 John F. Kennedy Blvd., Suite 1800, Philadelphia, PA 19103-2899. Periodicals postage paid at New York, NY and additional mailing offices. Subscription prices are $417.00 per year for US individuals, $845.00 per year for US institutions, $100.00 per year for US students and residents, $507.00 per year for Canadian individuals, $1071.00 per year for Canadian institutions, $536.00 for international individuals, $1071.00 per year for international institutions and $250.00 per year for Canadian and foreign students/residents. To receive student/resident rate, orders must be accompanied by name of affiliated institution, date of term, and the *signature* of program/residency coordinator on institution letterhead. Orders will be billed at individual rate until proof of status is received. Foreign air speed delivery is included in all *Clinics* subscription prices. All prices are subject to change without notice. POSTMASTER: Send address changes to *Surgical Clinics*, Elsevier Health Sciences Division, Subscription Customer Service, 3251 Riverport Lane, Maryland Heights, MO 63043. **Customer Service (orders, claims, online, change of address): Telephone: 1-800-654-2452 (U.S. and Canada); 314-447-8871 (outside U.S. and Canada). Fax: 314-447-8029. E-mail: journalscustomerservice-usa@elsevier.com (for print support); journalsonline support-usa@elsevier.com (for online support).**

Reprints. For copies of 100 or more, of articles in this publication, please contact the Commercial Reprints Department, Elsevier Inc., 360 Park Avenue South, New York, New York 10010-1710. Tel. 212-633-3874, Fax: 212-633-3820, E-mail: reprints@elsevier.com.

The Surgical Clinics of North America is also published in Spanish by McGraw-Hill Interamericana Editores S.A., P.O. Box 5-237 06500 Mexico D.F. Mexico; and in Portuguese by Interlivros Edicoes Ltda., Rua Comandante Coelho 1085, CEP 21250, Rio de Janeiro, Brazil; and in Greek by Paschalidis Medical Publications, Athens Greece.

The Surgical Clinics of North America is covered in *MEDLINE/PubMed (Index Medicus), EMBASE/Excerpta Medica, Current Contents/Clinical Medicine, Current Contents/Life Sciences, Science Citation Index*, and *ISI/BIOMED*.

Contributors

CONSULTING EDITOR

RONALD F. MARTIN, MD, FACS
Colonel (retired), United States Army Reserve, Department of Surgery, York Hospital, York, Maine

EDITOR

PRINGL MILLER, MD, FACS
Assistant Professor, Surgery and Medicine, Rush University Medical Center, Chicago, Illinois

AUTHORS

JESSICA H. BALLOU, MD, MPH
Division of Trauma, Acute Care, and Emergency General Surgery, Department of Surgery, Oregon Health & Science University, Portland, Oregon

EMILY H. BEERS, MD
Clinical Assistant Professor of Medicine, Division of Geriatric, Hospital, Palliative and General Internal Medicine, Keck Hospital and Norris Cancer Center, University of Southern California, Los Angeles, California

ANA BERLIN, MD, MPH, FACS
Assistant Professor, Department of Surgery, Division of General Surgery, Department of Medicine, Division of Hematology/Oncology, Adult Palliative Medicine Service, Columbia University Medical Center, New York, New York

KAREN J. BRASEL, MD, MPH, FACS
Division of Trauma, Acute Care, and Emergency General Surgery, Department of Surgery, Oregon Health & Science University, Portland, Oregon

BENJAMIN P. BROWN, MD, MS
Assistant Professor of Obstetrics and Gynecology, Clinician Educator, The Warren Alpert Medical School of Brown University, Division of Emergency Obstetrics and Gynecology, Women and Infants Hospital of Rhode Island, Providence, Rhode Island

TOBY CAMPBELL, MD
Department of Medicine, Division of Hematology, Oncology, and Palliative Care, School of Nursing, University of Wisconsin-Madison, Madison, Wisconsin

TERESA JOHELEN CARLETON, MD, FACS
Medical Director of Palliative Care, Tucson Medical Center Palliative Care, Tucson Medical Center, Tucson, Arizona; Clinical Assistant Professor of Surgery, University of Arizona Phoenix, Phoenix, Arizona

KRISTEL CLAYVILLE, MA, PhD
Acting Director, Zygon Center for Religion and Science, Senior Fellow, MacLean Center for Clinical Medical Ethics, Chicago, Illinois

MACKENZIE R. COOK, MD
Assistant Professor of Surgery, Division of Trauma, Critical Care and Acute Care Surgery, Oregon Health & Science University, Portland, Oregon

JAMES GERHART, PhD
Department of Psychology, Central Michigan University, Mount Pleasant, Michigan

CALISTA M. HARBAUGH, MD
Department of Surgery, University of Michigan Medical School, Ann Arbor, Michigan

MELISSA RED HOFFMAN, MD, ND
Attending Acute Care Surgeon, Department of Surgery, Mission Hospital, Asheville, North Carolina

ROXANE HOLT, MD
Assistant Professor of Obstetrics and Gynecology, Section of Maternal-Fetal Medicine, The University of Chicago, The University of Chicago Medicine, Chicago, Illinois

ANN WILBORN JACKSON, PT, DPT, MPH
Senior Fellow, MacLean Center for Clinical Medical Ethics, The University of Chicago, Owner of Legacy Healthcare Solutions, Flossmoor, Illinois

ERIKA R. KETTELER, MD, MA, RPVI, FSVS, FACS
Chief, Vascular Surgery and Endovascular Therapy, Albuquerque Raymond G. Murphy VAMC, Albuquerque, New Mexico

KIMBERLY E. KOPECKY, MD, MSCI
Department of Surgery, Stanford University, Stanford, California

BUDDY MARTERRE, MD, MDiv
Assistant Professor, Surgical Palliative Care, Departments of General Surgery and Internal Medicine, Wake Forest Baptist Health, Winston-Salem, North Carolina

MARLENE McHUGH, DNP
Department of Family and Social Medicine, Montefiore Medical Center, New York, New York

PRINGL MILLER, MD, FACS
Assistant Professor, Surgery and Medicine, Rush University Medical Center, Chicago, Illinois

ANDREA K. NAGENGAST, MD
Fellow, Trauma, Critical Care and Acute Care Surgery, Department of Surgery, Oregon Health & Science University, Portland, Oregon

SEAN O'MAHONY, MD
Section of Palliative Medicine, Rush Medical College, Chicago, Illinois

JAY A. REQUARTH, MD, FACS
Retired, Winston-Salem, North Carolina

CHARLES RHEE, MD
Section of Geriatrics and Palliative Medicine, The University of Chicago, The University of Chicago Medicine, Chicago, Illinois

EMILY B. RIVET, MD, MBA, FACS, FASCRS
Assistant Professor of Surgery and Internal Medicine, Virginia Commonwealth University Health System, Richmond, Virginia

MICHAEL E. SHAPIRO, MD, FACS
Associate Professor of Surgery, Department of Surgery, Rutgers New Jersey Medical School, Newark, New Jersey

TIMOTHY R. SIEGEL, MD
Assistant Professor, Departments of Surgery and Medicine, Oregon Health & Science University, Portland, Oregon

ERIC A. SINGER, MD, MA, MS, FACS
Assistant Professor of Surgery, Section of Urologic Oncology, Division of Urology, Department of Surgery, Rutgers Robert Wood Johnson Medical School, Rutgers Cancer Institute of New Jersey, New Brunswick, New Jersey

JOSHUA SOMMOVILLA, MD
General Surgeon, Division of Hospice and Palliative Medicine, University of Wisconsin-Madison, Madison, Wisconsin

PASITHORN A. SUWANABOL, MD, MS
Department of Surgery, University of Michigan Medical School, Ann Arbor, Michigan

CHRISTINE C. TOEVS, MD, MA (Bioethics)
Trauma Medical Director, Terre Haute Regional Hospital, Clinical Faculty, Indiana University School of Medicine, Terre Haute, Indiana

SANDY TUN, MD
Section of Geriatrics and Palliative Medicine, The University of Chicago, Chicago, Illinois

Contents

Foreword: Palliative Care xiii

Ronald F. Martin

With Gratitude xv

Pringl Miller

Dedication: Honoring Balfour Michael Morgan Mount, OC, OQ, MD, FRCSC, LLD - The Father of North American Palliative Care xvii

Pringl Miller

Preface: The Time Is Always Right to Do What Is Right for Our Patients xix

Pringl Miller

Advantages and Challenges of an Interdisciplinary Palliative Care Team Approach to Surgical Care 815

Charles Rhee, Marlene McHugh, Sandy Tun, James Gerhart, and Sean O'Mahony

Palliative care is an interdisciplinary field that focuses on optimizing quality of life for patients with serious, life-limiting illnesses and includes aggressive management of pain and symptoms; psychological, social, and spiritual support; and discussions of advance care planning, including treatment decision making and complex care coordination. Early palliative care is associated with increased quality of life, decreased symptom burden, decreased health care expenditures, and improved caregiver outcomes. This article discusses integrating interdisciplinary palliative care into surgical practice, and some current models of using and expanding palliative care skill sets in surgery, including training initiatives for both physicians and nurses.

Concurrent Palliative Care for Surgical Patients 823

Ana Berlin and Teresa Johelen Carleton

A common fallacy prevalent in surgical culture is for surgical intervention and palliation to be regarded as mutually exclusive or sequential strategies in the trajectory of surgical illness. Modern surgeons play a complex role as both providers and gatekeepers in meeting the palliative needs of their patients. Surgical palliative care is ideally delivered by surgical teams as a component of routine surgical care, and includes management of physical and psychosocial symptoms, basic communication about prognosis and treatment options, and identification of patient goals and values. Specialty palliative care services may be accessed through a through a variety of models.

assessment and naloxone coprescribing for high-risk patients are addressed.

Ostomy Management: A Model of Interdisciplinary Care **885**

Emily B. Rivet

This article provides an overview of key palliative care considerations for management of patients with wounds and ostomies. Ostomy formation is indicated for a variety of intestinal conditions. Specifics of ostomy management, impact on quality of life, and patient perspectives can be complicated. Wound ostomy and continence nursing professionals play a central role in the successful management of this patient population.

Palliative Wound Care: Less Is More **899**

Emily H. Beers

Palliative wound care is a philosophy of wound management that prioritizes comfort over healing and attends to the emotional distress these wounds can cause. Intervention strategies focus on management of symptoms such as pain, odor, bleeding, and exudate. Historic treatments such as honey, chlorine, and vinegar have gained renewed interest, and although well suited to the palliative setting, there is an increasing amount of research exploring their efficacy in other contexts. The lived experience of patients and caregivers facing these wounds is often stressful and isolating, and any treatment plan must address these issues along with the physical aspects of care.

Image-Guided Palliative Interventions **921**

Jay A. Requarth

This article reviews a few surgical palliative care procedures that can be performed by surgeons and interventional radiologists using image-guided techniques. Treatment of recurrent pleural effusions, gastrostomy feeding tube maintenance, percutaneous cholecystostomy, and transjugular intrahepatic portosystemic shunts (TIPS) with embolotherapy of bleeding stomal varices is discussed.

Palliative Care and the Pregnant Surgical Patient: Epidemiology, Ethics, and Clinical Guidance **941**

Benjamin P. Brown and Roxane Holt

Obstetricians and general surgeons frequently navigate the challenges of providing surgical care that is mindful of the unique circumstances of pregnancy. Ensuring pregnant patients have high-quality surgical care is an ethical imperative. Providers should maintain a high index of suspicion for surgical disease to ensure that surgical diagnoses are not missed or inadequately treated. A variety of imaging modalities are used in pregnancy. Surgical management includes laparoscopic and open approaches. Perioperative fetal monitoring should be the subject of multidisciplinary discussion. Symptomatic control in pregnancy should have the same goals as for nonpregnant patients. Enhanced recovery after surgery pathways frequently are appropriate.

Tracheostomies and PEGs: When Are They Really Indicated? 955

Melissa Red Hoffman

Surgeons are often asked to perform tracheostomies and percutaneous endoscopic gastrostomies for a wide variety of patients. As consultants, surgeons are tasked with honoring the relationship between the referring provider and the patient while also assessing whether the consult is appropriate given the patient's prognosis and goals of care. This article discusses the most common conditions for which these procedures are requested and reviews the evidence supporting either the placement or avoidance of these tubes in each condition. It provides a framework for surgeons to use when discussing these procedures in the context of goals of care.

Beyond the Technical: Determining Real Indications for Vascular Access and Hemodialysis Initiation in End-Stage Renal Disease 967

Erika R. Ketteler

Determining valid indications for vascular access creation and hemodialysis initiation in end-stage renal disease requires utilization of verified prognostication tools and recognition of triggers to initiate serious conversations, and implementation of concurrent palliative care and/or hospice care is recommended. Establishment of a multi-disciplinary team that includes consideration of interventionalists in the pre-dialysis medical situation is important. A "catheter best" approach may be the most appropriate for some patients to meet goals of care.

Postoperative Recovery and Survivorship After Acute Hospitalization for Serious Life-Limiting Illness 977

Ann Wilborn Jackson

This article provides a road map for discharge planning of adult patients with serious life-limiting illnesses. The need for early and guided conversations with specific prompts is offered to assist in the transition of care process. Transparent, patient-centered interactions are emphasized throughout with an acknowledgment that this type of direct, interpersonal communication may challenge a clinical team's typical mode of operation. Nevertheless, when done well, this approach can lead to better outcomes for everyone involved. This framework for discharge planning has led to greater patient and family satisfaction, lower mortality, reduced societal costs, and fewer instances of hospital readmission.

Navigating the Murky Waters of Hope, Fear, and Spiritual Suffering: An Expert Co-Captain's Guide 991

Buddy Marterre and Kristel Clayville

How can surgeons deliver compassionate, holistic care to patients who are beyond cure? Interacting emotionally and understanding hope, fear, and spiritual suffering is key. Responsibly reframing hope to underlying meanings, and away from specific outcomes, is critical. Facilitating moves from cure to comfort to a peaceful dying process requires some retooling of the surgical toolbox. Surgeons possess a unique set of skills, including imagination and an undying sense of hope. Surgeons who have the courage to delve into their emotions and sustain realistic hope for their patients, all the way to the end, will reap deep personal and professional rewards.

Transitioning to Comfort-Focused Care at the End of Life **1019**

Christine C. Toevs

Shared decision making requires the exchange of information from the patient and the surgeon (and ideally involves the expertise of the entire multidisciplinary team) to determine the medical and/or surgical treatment that best aligns with the patient's goals and values. Should the surgical patient wish to transition to end-of-life care, the transition to comfort-focused care is within the scope of practice for surgeons. Incorporating the expertise of other health care professionals is an important consideration for whole-patient care. Integrating primary palliative care into surgical practice can help mitigate unnecessary suffering and allow a smoother transition to comfort-focused care.

Mitigating Burnout **1029**

Timothy R. Siegel and Andrea K. Nagengast

Burnout is characterized by emotional exhaustion, depersonalization, and a reduced sense of personal accomplishment. All physicians, and especially surgeons, are at risk for developing burnout. The best strategies for mitigating burnout mimic a modern approach to medicine: the development of preventive practices to protect, promote, and maintain health and well-being. Job satisfaction, job engagement, and compassion satisfaction help protect from burnout. Individual commitment to self-care in conjunction with support from within health care organizations create the optimal framework in which burnout can be mitigated.

Surgical Palliative Care Education **1037**

Jessica H. Ballou and Karen J. Brasel

Surgical palliative care education is in increasing demand to meet the needs of a growing geriatric population. Multiple accrediting agencies for undergraduate and graduate medical education require that students be trained in end-of-life care. These requirements, however, have resulted in didactic curricula that are implemented in various degrees with uncertain levels of success. Reviews of physician communication on palliative care topics find that skilled feedback has the best evidence for generating improvements. Once graduated, there is little to no requirement that practicing providers seek out opportunities to improve their palliative care skills.

SURGICAL CLINICS OF NORTH AMERICA

FORTHCOMING ISSUES

December 2019
Inflammatory Bowel Disease
Sean J. Langenfeld, *Editor*

February 2020
Melanoma
Rohit Sharma, *Editor*

April 2020
Robotic Surgery
Julio A. Teixeira, *Editor*

RECENT ISSUES

August 2019
Surgical Management of Endocrine Disease
Rebecca S. Sippel and David F. Schneider, *Editors*

June 2019
Management of the Foregut
Sushanth Reddy, *Editor*

April 2019
Diseases of the Biliary
Tract J. Bart Rose, *Editor*

Foreword
Palliative Care

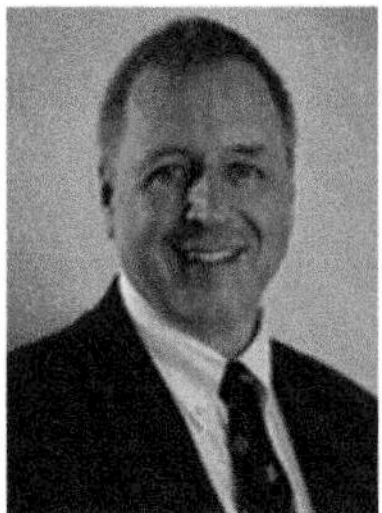

Ronald F. Martin, MD, FACS
Consulting Editor

There was a time when we were in the profession of patient care. Now, it may be that we are in the health care business. Perhaps those 2 constructs are similar or perhaps not. In the evolution of health care delivery, I was taught that in the beginning there were people: some of those people got sick (we call them patients); some people learn ways to help them (the various providers); and to make things more efficient, we created hospitals to have a common place and tools to take care of people. Now, it seems like the monthly and quarterly margins of health care business units are more the determinative forces that cause us to see how we can convince people that they need to more greatly utilize our billable services—as long as they can pay.

Palliative care as a concept brings us to the core of what we do. In some respects, it should be very difficult to define because everything we do should be aimed at palliating some concern. Yet, we separate the field of palliative medicine apart from "other" medicine. I am not sure why. Clearly, we all know when the goals of care are to reduce symptoms without necessarily changing the other trajectory attributes of the underlying disease; that is one way to define palliative care. In reality, though, that construct is true for all of medicine: we all know where the human health trajectory intercepts the x-axis for all of us, we just don't know when. We never really change the endpoint; we just move it around and deflect the path that will take us there. Sometimes we deflect it for better, sometimes for worse.

The tools that we have to "definitively" treat patients or "treat with intent to cure" are not inherently different from the tools we use to palliate. We should all be using the entirety of available tools to provide for patients what they need and, when possible, what they want. To do that, we have to be honest with our patients and ourselves about what we can do—we have to be even more honest with patients about what we should do. The final decision about what we will do, of course, is a decision that the patient (and family) has to make with us.

Surg Clin N Am 99 (2019) xiii–xiv
https://doi.org/10.1016/j.suc.2019.07.001

Taking a step back from the idea that we know what patients need and moving forward with the perspective of the patient telling us what they need after they have been informed and educated requires a shift in mindset for some. It occasionally requires us to suspend our preconceptions and sometimes it requires us, particularly surgeons, to share our authority and dilute our autonomy. None of this should be construed as surgeons taking a backseat; in fact, it probably makes us have to step up our game in terms of leadership and advocacy.

The articles that Dr Miller and her colleagues have compiled for us should help all of us improve our understanding of how to approach problems for patients in ways that some of us don't always have to on a daily basis. They provide us with new ways to use the tools that many of us already have as well as give us other tools with which to work.

One of my mentors use to say that the most important part of patient care is to remember to care for the patient. It sounds simple. It should be simple. In reality, though, there are a lot of forces at play within us and external to us that can make that a challenge to always do as well as we should.

Many of us like to claim that we want to treat our patients the way we would want our families treated. To really do that requires great effort. A great effort to know what can be done by the larger system and not just what we all do individually. It also requires taking time with patients and families to help them tell us what truly matters to them. Our current system does not always value time spent doing that as it does not reimburse well. Yet, we must. It is the essential commitment of our profession. We hope that these articles help anyone to help patients get what will make their life, even if it is near the end of their life, easier.

Ronald F. Martin, MD, FACS
Colonel (retired), United States Army Reserve
Department of Surgery
York Hospital
16 Hospital Drive, Suite A
York, ME 03909, USA

E-mail address:
rfmcescna@gmail.com

With Gratitude

I owe Geoffrey P. Dunn, MD, FACS a debt of gratitude for his inspiration, dedication, and pioneering work in Surgical Palliative Care *and* Palliative Medicine. For me personally, Dr. Dunn has been a mentor, invaluable role-model and has entrusted me with the honor of guest editor of this edition as his successor. I would also like to thank Ronald F. Martin, MD, John G. Vassallo, Meredith Madeira, and Casey Potter for their support during this project.

To all the authors, and the authors helpers, for this first edition of *Surgical Clinics of North America - Practicing Primary Care*, your work is much appreciated and needed, it will change the care of surgical patients. Many of you are also trail blazers in the effort to integrate palliative care into standard surgical practice and the future holds great promise with your individual talents, diverse areas of expertise and commitment to excellence.

> *Gratitude makes sense of your past, brings peace for today, and creates a vision for tomorrow.*
>
> —*Melody Beattie*

Sincerely,

Pringl Miller, MD, FACS
Rush University Medical Center
Kellogg Building–Suite 1126
1717 West Congress Parkway
Chicago, IL 60612, USA

E-mail address:
pringlmillermd@gmail.com

Surg Clin N Am 99 (2019) xv
https://doi.org/10.1016/j.suc.2019.06.017
0039-6109/19/© 2019 Published by Elsevier Inc.

Dedication: Honoring Balfour Michael Morgan Mount, OC, OQ, MD, FRCSC, LLD - The Father of North American Palliative Care

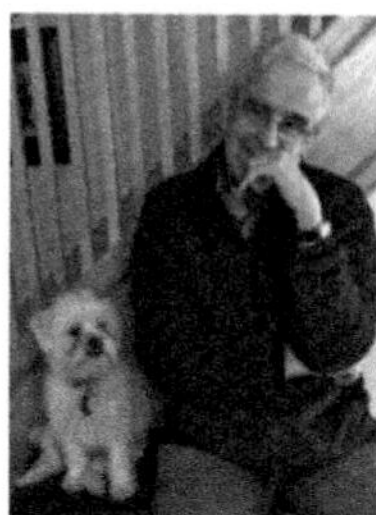

Balfour Mount

This issue of *Surgical Clinics of North America* is dedicated to the father of Palliative Care in North America, Balfour Michael Morgan Mount, OC, OQ, MD, FRCSC, LLD, also described as the "compassionate vanguard of Palliative Care." Dr Mount was named "Balfour" by his father, a neurosurgeon, in honor of his colleague and mentor, Donald Church Balfour, who is famous for his many contributions to surgery, including the abdominal *Balfour retractor*, which we all know of today.

A medical graduate of Queen's University, Dr Mount (who generally is referred to simply as "Bal") completed his postgraduate training at McGill and New York's Memorial Sloan Kettering Cancer Center prior to returning to Montreal as a Urologic Oncologist with clinical, research, and teaching activities at McGill and the Royal Victoria Hospital (RVH). Then, during the early 1970s, Bal carried out a landmark study of the needs of patients dying at their widely respected center of academic excellence. Documentation of previously unrecognized suffering and deficient care of both dying patients and their families led him to visit Dr Cicely Saunders at St. Christopher's Hospice, London, which had opened in 1967. Noting, as a result, that vastly improved end-of-life care was possible, he proposed an RVH pilot project that included (1) an inpatient ward, (2) a home care program, (3) a consultation service to the active treatment services of their teaching hospital as well as (4) a research program, and (5) teaching initiatives to be integrated into the McGill Medical School curriculum. The Board of the Royal Victoria Hospital accepted these proposals with funding to be limited to 2 years. Thus, the design and development of all programs, their staffing, ongoing evaluation, and decision regarding their continuation had to be completed within 24 months.

Surg Clin N Am 99 (2019) xvii–xviii
https://doi.org/10.1016/j.suc.2019.05.003

Because of the pejorative implications of the term "Hospice" in Quebec, a new name for this revised approach to care was needed. Dr Mount decided on "*Palliative Care*" based on its etymology "*to improve the quality of*"; thus, the resulting medical discipline would come to be known internationally as *Palliative Care*.

Dr Mount and his colleagues have made an indelible mark on medical history by integrating research-based Palliative Care in academic medicine, thus opening the door for similar programs at other medical schools and fostering the inclusion of the lessons learned in the medical curriculum.

Dr Mount became the founding Director of the Royal Victoria Hospital Palliative Care Service, the McGill Programs Integrated Whole Person Care, and the biennial McGill International Congresses on Palliative Care. He is the Emeritus Eric M. Flanders Professor of Palliative Medicine at McGill and has been honored with the Degree of Doctor of Laws, *honoris causa*. He is currently writing a memoir and lives in Montreal with his wife Linda, their youngest daughter, Bethany, and their 2 dogs, Paddy and Holly.

The work they did can be accessed in The R.V.H. Manual on Palliative/Hospice Care, *published by The Ayer Company, Salem, New Hampshire, 1982 and through his publications in the medical literature.*

Pringl Miller, MD, FACS
Rush University Medical Center
Kellogg Building-Suite 1126
1717 West Congress Parkway
Chicago, IL 60612, USA

E-mail address:
pringlmillermd@gmail.com

Preface
The Time Is Always Right to Do What Is Right for Our Patients

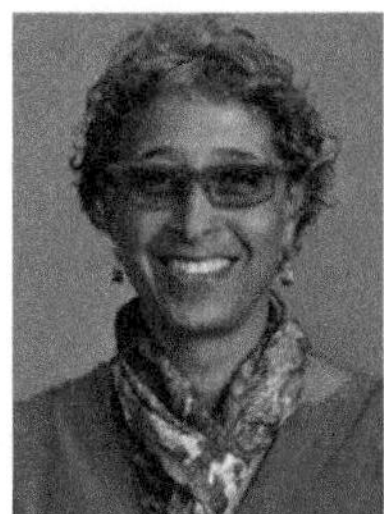

Pringl Miller, MD, FACS
Editor

As the operative repertoire and our professional status become increasingly transient, we will be compelled to ground our identities in something more fulfilling and enduring.

—Geoffrey Dunn, MD, FACS

Surgeons have been engaged in surgical palliation since antiquity. Trepanation was first described in 3000 BC to rid the body of spirits … and later to relieve pressure on the brain.[1] Paré, a sixteenth century French surgeon, stated that to perform surgery is "to eliminate that which is superfluous, restore that which has been dislocated, separate that which has been united, join that which has been divided and repair the defects of nature."[2] Billroth performed the Billroth I (B-I) for the first time in 1881 on a 43-year-old woman with pyloric cancer presumably suffering from gastric outlet obstruction.[3] Today, the B-I is considered one of the first palliative operations recorded in modern history. Subsequent to 1881, many other surgical, endoscopic, and interventional procedures have been popularized because of their palliative benefit and quality of life enhancement.

Surgical palliative care is defined by the treatment of suffering and the promotion of quality of life for seriously or terminally ill patients under surgical care. Palliative surgery refers to operative interventions performed for the purpose of relieving distressing symptoms and improving quality of life. Some operations will yield both palliative and curative outcomes, while others will only offer a palliative benefit. Surgical patients with life-limiting illness will also benefit from integrating primary or specialty palliative medicine into their care plans because identified gaps exist in addressing the totality

Surg Clin N Am 99 (2019) xix–xxiii
https://doi.org/10.1016/j.suc.2019.07.002

of needs many surgical patients have. The advantage of providing concurrent palliative care for patients with serious life-limiting illness or at the end of life is based on the interdisciplinary, multimodal, less-invasive, and generally better-tolerated patient-concordant care plans established. While surgical palliative care and palliative procedural interventions have obvious value, not all patients with life-limiting illnesses want to embark on invasive interventions, particularly when such interventions are not aligned with their goals of care and don't ultimately seek to improve their quality of life.[4]

Dr Balfour Mount, a retired urologic surgeon and the Eric M. Flanders Emeritus Professor of Palliative Care at McGill University, is considered the father of North American Palliative Care.[5] In 1975, he coined the phrase "palliative care" as a way to distinguish the practice of palliative care from hospice. Today, the World Health Organization defines palliative care "as an approach that improves quality of life of patients and their families facing the problem associated with life-threatening illness, through prevention and relief of suffering by means of early identification and impeccable assessment and treatment of pain and other problems, physical, psychosocial and spiritual."[6]

While both surgical palliative care and palliative medicine practitioners seek to relieve suffering and improve the quality of life of their patients, contemporary surgical practice patterns, surgical culture, attitudes, care fragmentation, and published research suggest that these common clinical aims infrequently converge in meaningful clinical collaborations to better patient care at the bedside.

Because patients with life-limiting illnesses are complex and have a plethora of needs that often extend beyond the scope, practice, and expertise of any one medical discipline, early identification and impeccable assessment of a patient's palliative care needs require awareness and in some cases multispecialty and interdisciplinary expertise for identification and optimal management. Proper integration of palliative care approaches has been shown to optimize patient and family well-being and best outcomes.[7–11] Therefore, as surgeons, acquiring primary palliative care skills and, when desired, specialty palliative care training is being presented as an adjunctive skill set that has the potential to improve value-based patient-concordant care.

Primary palliative care (also known as generalist palliative care) is best characterized by core practice elements, such as aligning treatment with patient goals and values by engaging in discussions about suffering, prognosis, care goals, and end-of-life preferences, as well as the management of symptoms, such as pain, nausea, constipation, dyspnea, anxiety, and depression. Specialty palliative care skills are more complex and include negotiating difficult family meetings, addressing existential distress, and managing refractory symptoms, which often require fellowship training and practice to learn and apply most effectively.[12] The clinical and economic value of palliative care is increasingly recognized within the health care industry as emerging data and societal benefits are understood. As the population continues to age, the existing and impending palliative care needs of patients have and will continue to exceed the number of palliative care specialists available, thus mandating more surgeon-specific application and ownership of primary palliative care skills.

Palliative care has more recently been associated with whole-person care because of 8 equally important domains outlined by the National Consensus Project (NCP) in the 2018 National Guidelines for Quality Palliative Care and include: Structure and Process of Care, Physical, Psychological/Psychiatric, Social, Spiritual/Religious/Existential, Cultural, Ethical and Legal aspects of care, and End of Life care.[13] For a pdf of the NCP 2018 Clinical Practice Guidelines for Quality Palliative Care, visit this site: https://www.nationalcoalitionhpc.org/ncp/.

The next major practice innovation that will impact many lives and improve value-based patient-concordant care and satisfaction will be the integration of primary palliative care into standard surgical practice and to seek specialty palliative care consultation when the patient's care needs merit it. Greater than 2.5 million people die in the United States annually, 60% in hospitals. Preventable harm is defined by The Institute for Healthcare Improvement as "unintended physical injury resulting from or contributed to by medical care that requires additional monitoring, treatment or hospitalization, or that results in death."[14] One of the most common types of preventable harm is surgical error, which may start with the decision to recommend a nonbeneficial operation. The Centers for Medicare and Medicaid Services and *Scientific American* reported that 30% of Medicare recipients undergo surgery within the last year of life and were more likely to be harmed than benefited.[15] The anticipated silver Tsunami will increase these numbers unless we change our "do-everything-rescue" culture. It is no longer ethical nor forgivable, and it will be remembered if our conduct continues to emulate that which is exemplified in Charles Bosk's book, *Forgive and Remember.* Bosk writes, "The claim that he did everything possible is basically a claim to ethical conduct. When he claims that he did everything possible, the professional claims that he acted in good faith. Although the results are open to debate, his conduct is not." Bosk exposes the underlying ethical dilemma of why doing everything possible may appeal to the surgeon. If he or she operated and gave the case their all, they cannot be faulted; however, contemporary practice paradigms, including the model of shared decision making, reflect on what outcomes really matter and what therapeutic interventions patients want relative to their goals and values. Surgeons should partner with their patients, learn from them what aligns with their preferences, and then formulate recommendations that can best meet those objectives: American College of Surgeons Statement of principles of palliative care #4.[16] John L. Cameron, MD, FACS wrote in his foreword for the Oxford University Press book, *Surgical Palliative Care*, "For far too long surgeons have been considered non-caring technicians, interested only in the surgical procedure itself, and the immediate outcome. Surgeons have a much broader role in being certain that all of the bothersome and disabling symptoms that the patient has are appropriately addressed."[17]

The practice of surgical palliative care alone, given the complexity of patients and emerging evidence-based practices of palliative medicine, will fail to meet the needs of our aged and infirm patient population. Therefore, moving forward, it will be incumbent upon all practicing surgeons to integrate primary palliative care skills into their practices by aiding patients in clarifying their goals of care and then providing them with comprehensive whole-person care, which may or may not include operative intervention.[16] Wielding the scalpel should become one among many vital skills the surgeon can offer their patients, especially when it becomes clear that deployment is nonbeneficial and/or discordant with the patient's goals and values. Learning how to look beyond our operative skills and discern what treatment options best suit each individual patient will undoubtedly confer better patient outcomes and possibly even enhance our professional satisfaction by promoting a richer, more meaningful surgeon-patient relationship across the care continuum.

This issue of *Surgical Clinics of North America* entitled, *Practicing Primary Palliative Care*, is presented as a call to action. It has been 20 years since an innovative group of surgeons, Fellows of the American College of Surgeons, gathered together to compose the first Statement of Principles Guiding Care at the End of Life, which was revised in 2005 as the Statement of Principles of Palliative Care.[16] Let us not wait another 20 years to act upon them.

> *Although the world is full of suffering, it is also full of the overcoming of it.*
> *—Helen Keller*

Pringl Miller, MD, FACS
Rush University Medical Center
Kellogg Building–Suite 1126
1717 West Congress Parkway
Chicago, IL 60612, USA

E-mail address:
pringlmillermd@gmail.com

REFERENCES

1. Whitlock, Jennifer, RN, MSN, FN. The Evolution of Surgery: A Historical Timeline. A History of Surgery. Verywell health. Available at: https://www.verywellhealth.com/the-history-of-surgery-timeline-3157332. Accessed July 1, 2019.
2. Wikipedia. History of Surgery. Available at: https://en.wikipedia.org/wiki/History_of_surgery. Accessed July 1, 2019.
3. Whonamedit? - A dictionary of medical eponyms. Available at: http://www.whonamedit.com/synd.cfm/2730.html. Accessed July 1, 2019.
4. Miner TJ, Brennan MF, Jaques DP. A prospective, symptom related, outcomes analysis of 1022 palliative procedures for advanced cancer. Ann Surg 2004; 240(4):719–26 [discussion: 726–7].
5. Wikipedia. Balfour Mount. Available at: https://en.wikipedia.org/wiki/Balfour_Mount. Accessed July 1, 2019.
6. WHO definition of palliative care. Available at: https://www.who.int/cancer/palliative/definition/en/. Accessed July 1, 2019.
7. Ernst KF, Hall DE, Schmid KK, et al. Surgical palliative care consultations over time in relationship to systemwide frailty screening. JAMA Surg 2014;149(11): 1121–6.
8. Mosenthal AC, Weissman DE, Curtis JR, et al. Integrating palliative care in the surgical and trauma intensive care unit: a report from the Improving Palliative Care in the Intensive Care Unit (IPAL-ICU) Project Advisory Board and the Center to Advance Palliative Care. Crit Care Med 2012;40(4):1199–206.
9. Temel JS, Greer JA, Muzikansky A, et al. Early palliative care for patients with metastatic non-small-cell lung cancer. N Engl J Med 2010;363(8):733–42.
10. Bakitas M, Lyons KD, Hegel MT, et al. Effects of a palliative care intervention on clinical outcomes in patients with advanced cancer: the Project ENABLE II randomized controlled trial. JAMA 2009;302(7):741–9.
11. Gade G, Venohr I, Conner D, et al. Impact of an inpatient palliative care team: a randomized control trial. J Palliat Med 2008;11(2):180–90.
12. Quill TE, Abernethy AP. Generalist plus specialist palliative care–creating a more sustainable model. N Engl J Med 2013;368(13):1173–5.
13. Clinical Practice Guidelines for Quality Palliative Care 4th Edition. National Consensus Project. National Coalition for Hospice and Palliative Care. 2018. Available at: https://www.nationalcoalitionhpc.org/ncp/. Accessed July 1, 2019.

14. Bernazzani S. Tallying the high cost of preventable harm. Costs of Care; 2017. Available at: https://costsofcare.org/tallying-the-high-cost-of-preventable-harm/. Accessed July 1, 2019.
15. Szabo L. Surgery near end of life is common, costly. Scientific American 2018. Available at: https://www.scientificamerican.com/article/surgery-near-end-of-life-is-common-costly/. Accessed July 1, 2019.
16. American College of Surgeons. Statement of principles of palliative care. 2005. Available at: https://www.facs.org/about-acs/statements/50-palliative-care. Accessed July 1, 2019.
17. Dunn GP, Johnson AG. Surgical palliative care. Available at: https://global.oup.com/academic/product/surgical-palliative-care-9780198510000?cc=us&lang=en& ;https://books.google.com/books/about/Surgical_Palliative_Care.html?id=ydt1DwAAQBAJ&printsec=frontcover&source=kp_read_button#v=onepage&q&f=false. Accessed July 1, 2019.

Advantages and Challenges of an Interdisciplinary Palliative Care Team Approach to Surgical Care

Charles Rhee, MD[a,*], Marlene McHugh, DNP[b], Sandy Tun, MD[c], James Gerhart, PhD[d], Sean O'Mahony, MD[e]

KEYWORDS

• Palliative care • Primary palliative care • Surgery • Training • Nursing

KEY POINTS

- The growing complexity of perioperative patient care for seriously ill surgical patients has created an ideal opportunity for the early integration of palliative care into the care continuum given the emphasis on optimizing quality of life and the discussion about each patient's overall goals of care.
- Working collaboratively with surgical colleagues to identify patients with palliative care needs, as well as exposure to and development of primary palliative care principles within the surgical workforce, is imperative.
- Development of novel approaches to improve palliative care integration into standard surgical care continues to be a priority for both physicians and nurses, and there are numerous initiatives in progress to examine the ideal methodology of training, as well as to examine the clinical outcomes from such collaborations.

INTRODUCTION

Palliative care is an interdisciplinary field that focuses on optimizing quality of life for patients with serious, life-limiting illnesses.[1] Palliative care includes aggressive management of pain and symptoms; psychological, social, and spiritual support; as well as discussions of advance care planning, which may include treatment decision making and complex care coordination.

[a] Section of Geriatrics & Palliative Medicine, University of Chicago, The University of Chicago Medicine, 5841 South Maryland Avenue, MC 6098, Chicago, IL 60637, USA; [b] Department of Family and Social Medicine, Montefiore Medical Center, New York, NY, USA; [c] Section of Geriatrics & Palliative Medicine, University of Chicago, Chicago, IL, USA; [d] Department of Psychology, Central Michigan University, Mount Pleasant, MI, USA; [e] Section of Palliative Medicine, Rush Medical College, Chicago, IL, USA
* Corresponding author.
E-mail address: crhee1@medicine.bsd.uchicago.edu

Surg Clin N Am 99 (2019) 815–821
https://doi.org/10.1016/j.suc.2019.05.004 surgical.theclinics.com

The landmark study by Temel and colleagues[2] examined the role and benefits of early involvement of palliative care in advanced lung cancer; before this study, palliative care focused primarily on end-of-life and hospice care, which remains the perception among many health care practitioners. Since this time, the field has expanded tremendously and numerous subsequent studies have shown the association of early concurrent palliative care with increased quality of life, decreased symptom burden, decreased health care expenditures, as well as improved caregiver outcomes.[3] Although most of these studies have been conducted in the oncology population, a growing body of literature examining the role of palliative care within other life-limiting illnesses, including heart failure, end-stage renal disease, advanced pulmonary disease, and progressive neurologic diseases, has shown similar benefits regarding improved quality of life and reduced symptom burden. This article discusses the benefits and challenges of integrating interdisciplinary palliative care into surgical services, as well as some current models of using and expanding palliative care skill sets within the field.

THE GROWING NEEDS OF CHRONICALLY ILL PATIENTS FACING LIFE-LIMITING ILLNESS

According to the Centers for Disease Control and Prevention (CDC), 1 in 2 adults in the United States has a chronic illness, and 1 in 4 adults has 2 or more diseases,[4] with recent trends showing an overall increase in chronic diseases. Care for these complex and often multimorbid patients is complex and fragmented. The nation's aging population, coupled with existing risk factors (eg, tobacco use, poor nutrition, lack of physical activity) and medical advances that extend longevity (if not also improve overall health), have led to the conclusion that these problems are only going to magnify if not effectively addressed now.[5]

In the 2014 Institute of Medicine (IOM) report, *Dying in America: Improving Quality and Honoring Individual Preferences Near the End of Life*,[6] the changing demographics and medical issues that Americans are facing make the IOM study particularly timely, including the rapidly increasing number of older Americans with some combination of frailty, physical and cognitive disabilities, chronic illness, and functional limitations. The US population is becoming more culturally diverse, heightening the need for responsive, patient-centered care. In addition, the nation's health care system is increasingly burdened by factors that hamper delivery of high-quality care near the end of life, including barriers in access to care that disadvantage certain groups, a mismatch between the services patients and families need and the services they can obtain, inadequate numbers of palliative care specialists, and too little palliative care knowledge among other clinicians who care for individuals with serious advanced illness.

Many seriously ill patients enter the health care system without advance care planning conversations. Goals of care are infrequently discussed between the health care team and patients/families, resulting in burdens of treatment and care that often outweigh the benefits. Often patients access expert pain and symptom management or palliative care during their last few days of life, rather than earlier in the disease trajectory, when these services may have a greater impact on their quality of life. In addition, there are currently too few palliative care specialists and limited primary palliative care knowledge among other clinicians who care for people with serious advanced illness.

PALLIATIVE CARE NEEDS OF SERIOUSLY ILL PATIENTS PERIOPERATIVELY

Although operative mortality has declined over time, many elderly patients, in particular those with chronic medical conditions, remain at risk of in-hospital morbidity and mortality.[7] As a result, the American College of Surgeons recommends preoperative advance care planning conversations with older adults.[8] Despite these guidelines, only a minority of patients are reported as having completed advance directives such as a power of attorney for health care decisions documents in advance of surgery. In some studies, less than one-quarter of patients have a surrogate decision maker identified with a health care power of attorney document in the medical record before undergoing elective surgery.[9]

More than 500,000 older adults, many with frailty and cognitive impairment, undergo high-risk surgery annually, and nearly 20% of Medicare decedents undergo an inpatient surgical procedure in the last month of life.[10] Older and seriously ill patients invariably have higher rates of mortality and morbidity after elective and emergency surgery compared with their younger counterparts.[11] Every year, 100,000 patients die after inpatient surgery in the United States, and most never receive palliative care services. In addition, many older patients experience distressing physical and psychosocial symptoms, functional impairments, and reduced quality of life after surgery. As such, these patients are also at a high risk of dissatisfaction with care and receiving care discordant with their overall healthcare goals. Less than one-third of patients who undergo surgery in the last year of life are referred to palliative care.[12,13] In addition, most patients who undergo surgery receive palliative care consultations only within the last 24 to 48 hours of life, typically in the tumultuous period immediately preceding death.[14,15] Much of the surgical community may be reluctant to entertain consultation by palliative care clinicians preoperatively to assess risk tolerance or preferences for end-of-life care because they may view palliative care consultations as being incompatible with life-prolonging or potentially curative surgical care.[16]

However, given palliative care's emphasis on quality of life coupled with growing awareness of the benefits of early involvement of palliative care, one arena in which palliative care is beginning to gain traction is in the preoperative evaluation and optimization of seriously ill patients. Many patients being evaluated for major life-prolonging, or even curative, surgical procedures are initially deemed high-risk surgical candidates because of their poor functional status. Typically, these patients undergo rigorous attempts to improve their surgical eligibility, including aggressive nutritional support (eg, parenteral nutrition or percutaneous endoscopic gastrostomy tube) as well as rehabilitation and physical therapy. This period provides an ideal time to involve the interdisciplinary palliative care team for a comprehensive palliative care assessment which can identify symptoms that may impede patient progress, such as low mood or poorly treated pain, which is often one of the greatest barriers to physical rehabilitation. In addition, the care team can assist in identifying psychosocial barriers or supports that may affect both preoperative and postoperative outcomes and suggest resources to optimize these factors. During this time, the palliative care team can introduce basic advance care planning, starting with fundamentals such as identification of a health care surrogate, in a steady and controlled environment, rather than in extremis during the chaotic, immediate end-of-life period. In addition, for those patients who remain ineligible for surgical interventions despite best efforts at optimizing them, palliative care is already involved in the patients' care and can help guide discussions about further treatment options and goals, which may involve end-of-life discussions.

As an example of how this model of integrated care has been translated into practice, in October of 2014, the Joint Commission on Accreditation of Healthcare Organizations issued a firm mandate that all centers that perform destination left ventricular assist device (LVAD) implantations must have a palliative care representative as part of the interdisciplinary care team in order to maintain their certifications[17]; this requirement was reiterated by the Centers for Medicaid and Medicare Services (CMS), who issued a similar memo mandating palliative care involvement with destination LVADs.[18] Since these mandates, there have been studies examining the optimal role and timing of palliative care involvement with these patients, with further studies in progress.[19] Presently, numerous professional societies have issued guidelines recommending the integration of early palliative care for patients undergoing major procedures, including transplant candidates, patients on extracorporeal membrane oxygenation and other temporizing mechanical circulatory support, and surgical oncology patients.

THE EMBEDDED PALLIATIVE CARE CLINIC: AN EXAMPLE OF AN INTEGRATED CARE MODEL

One model of palliative care involvement that has been used successfully is the embedded palliative care clinic, in which the palliative care practitioner (eg, physician or nurse practitioner) has an outpatient presence within a specialty clinic allowing direct, same-day referrals from the consulting physicians. This model is currently used in many oncology clinics and has been growing within other specialties, notably cardiology and surgical oncology.[20,21] The embedded palliative care clinic model involves colocation within the specialty clinic and allows the referrer and palliative care provider to actively discuss patients, their clinical picture, and agree on a mutual care of plan that can be presented to the patient in a unified message. Reports from these clinics have shown that this collaborative effort ultimately helps normalize palliative medicine, particularly in those fields in which palliative care involvement is still uncommon. Over time, the reciprocal exchange of knowledge and perspectives between primary specialists and the palliative care providers allows a more holistic approach to dealing with the patients' illnesses, which translates to greater patient satisfaction in their care.

CHALLENGES TO PALLIATIVE CARE SERVICE DELIVERY AND THE ROLE OF PRIMARY PALLIATIVE CARE

Many organizations, including the IOM and American College of Surgeons, support the incorporation of palliative medicine into the care of any patient living with serious illness regardless of age, stage of disease, or diagnosis. In 2016, approximately 75% of US hospitals were estimated to have a palliative care team; however, the size and scope of these specialty services vary greatly from institution to institution and often lack true interdisciplinary elements, such as a dedicated social worker or chaplain.[22] In addition, these services are often unavailable in rural areas and community hospitals. Ironically, as acceptance and demand for palliative care increases annually, the number of palliative care physicians remains limited and unable to keep up with the growing demand. At present, there is 1 palliative care physician for every 1300 people diagnosed with a life-threatening illness and 1 for every 20,000 patients with severe chronic illness. There are only about 300 physicians graduating from hospice and palliative care fellowship programs each year entering the workforce and approximately 5000 current HPM board-certified physicians, and many of these only work part time in palliative care[23,24]; these numbers do not keep pace with the number of physicians in the field who are at retirement age. These fellowship programs often lack formal curricula on care of surgical patients, with wide variability in the exposure to complex surgical patients depending on the size and acuity of the teaching institution.

A major initiative that is being actively developed to address the workforce shortage in palliative care is the creation of a primary palliative care curriculum. Briefly, primary palliative care can be defined as a set of fundamental palliative care skills, such as noncomplicated pain/symptom management and basic discussions regarding overall goals of care, including the delivery of bad news, which are taught to other physicians, as well as advanced practice providers. Ideally, these skills allow primary clinicians to deal with basic palliative care needs until these needs become intractable, at which time referral to a palliative care specialist is indicated (eg, symptom burden refractory to basic management or complicated goals of care or family dynamics).[25] One of the key aspects of primary palliative care education should be identification of these more complicated issues and the proper use of specialist palliative care. There are efforts to incorporate these concepts earlier in training, such as during residency or fellowship; however, the training opportunities for surgical residents remain sparse at this time.

When surveyed, most surgeons report not having received formal palliative care curricula during their training, and close to half report deficits in their training in pain and symptom management and communication with seriously ill patients and their families.[26] Residents and faculty are reported to recognize that trainees would benefit from a surgical palliative care curriculum, that surgical palliative care curricula should include a focus on preoperative counseling, and that surgical palliative care education may lead to improvement in comfort care practices.[27]

Immersion training courses for surgical residents have been shown to improve participants' confidence in discussion of palliative care, end-of-life preferences, withdrawal of life-prolonging treatments, and prognosis.[28] A 2-hour training and subsequent individual coaching for attending surgeons for presentation of best-case/worst-case scenarios with standardized patients and actual hospitalized patients for acute surgical problems in high-risk patients was endorsed by patients, families, and surgeons as an effective strategy to support complex decision making.[29] Greater access to conversations about patients' values and risk threshold tolerance may be achieved through incorporation of palliative care curricula for surgical residents and advanced practice providers who care for surgical patients through existing palliative care communication training curricula, such as Vital Talk, that have been adapted for surgical populations. In conjunction with mentorship of surgeons on having such conversations, this will increase the provision of primary palliative care to a greater number of patients undergoing high-risk procedures,[30] thus allowing palliative care specialists to be better used in more complex cases.

Regional Mentoring and Educational Communities

Other efforts to develop a primary palliative care workforce have included regional mentoring communities provided by an interprofessional faculty that includes doctors, chaplains, social workers, advance practice providers, and nurses, which help interprofessional learners to implement new initiatives and expand existing palliative care programs within their organizations and target clinical disciplines that have had few options for advanced training including advance practice providers, social workers, and chaplains.[31] Given the limited potential for workforce development to advance through Accreditation Council for Graduate Medical Education physician fellowship training, these initiatives have focused on educating advance practice providers through immersion training approaches. The program includes face-to-face biannual conferences, monthly webinars, experiential training, and on-line learning. This program has provided education to clinicians working in more than half of the area's hospitals. The program has been associated with growth in the numbers of patients receiving palliative medicine consultations and increased use of hospice by patients at the end of life among participating institutions.

SUMMARY

The growing complexity of perioperative patient care for seriously ill surgical patients has created an ideal opportunity for the early integration of palliative care into the care continuum given the emphasis on optimizing quality of life and the discussion about patients' overall goals of care. Working collaboratively with surgical colleagues to identify patients with palliative care needs, as well as exposure to and development of primary palliative care principles within the surgical workforce, is imperative. Development of novel approaches to improve palliative care integration into standard surgical care continues to be a priority for both physicians and nurses, and there are numerous initiatives in progress to examine the ideal methodology of training, as well as examining the clinical outcomes from such collaborations.

REFERENCES

1. Morrison R, Meier DE. Clinical practice: palliative care. N Engl J Med 2004; 350(25):1755–9.
2. Temel J, Greer JA, Muzikansky A, et al. Early palliative care for patients with metastatic non-small cell-lung cancer. N Engl J Med 2010;363(8):420–3.
3. Gillick M. Rethinking the central dogma of palliative care. J Palliat Med 2005;8(5): 909–13.
4. Centers for Disease Control and Prevention (CDC). Deaths and mortality. Hyattsville (MD): National Center for Health Statistics; 2017. Available at: https://www.cdc.gov/nchs/fastats/deaths.htm.
5. Raghupathi W, Raghupathi V. An empirical study of chronic diseases in the United States: a visual analytics approach. Int J Environ Res Public Health 2018;15(3) [pii:E431].
6. Institute of Medicine (IOM). Dying in America: improving quality and honoring individual preferences near the end of life. Washington, DC: National Academies Press (US); 2015.
7. Lawrence VA, Hazuda HP, Cornell JE, et al. Functional independence after major abdominal surgery in the elderly. J Am Coll Surg 2004;199(5):762–72.
8. Mohanty S, Rosenthal RA, Russell MM, et al. Optimal perioperative management of the geriatric patient: a best practices guideline from the American College of Surgeons NSQIP and the American Geriatrics Society. J Am Coll Surg 2016; 222(5):930–47.
9. Marks S, Wanner JP, Cobb AS, et al. Surgery without a surrogate: the low prevalence of health care power of attorney documents among preoperative patients. Hosp Pract 2019;47(1):28–31.
10. Cooper Z, Scott JW, Rosenthal RA, et al. Emergency major abdominal surgical procedures in older adults: a systematic review of mortality and functional outcomes. J Am Geriatr Soc 2015;63:2563–71.
11. Finlayson E, Fan Z, Birkmeyer JD. Outcomes in octogenarians undergoing high-risk cancer operation: a national study. J Am Coll Surg 2007;205:729–34.
12. Olmsted CL, Johnson AM, Kaboli P, et al. Use of palliative care and hospice among surgical and medical specialties in the Veterans Health Administration. JAMA Surg 2014;149:1169–75.
13. Wilson DG, Harris SK, Peck H, et al. Patterns of care in hospitalized vascular surgery patients at end of life. JAMA Surg 2017;152:183–90.
14. Kross EK, Engelberg RA, Downey L, et al. Differences in end-of-life care in the ICU across patients cared for by medicine, surgery, neurology, and neurosurgery physicians. Chest 2014;145:313–21.

15. Rodriguez R, Marr L, Rajput A, et al. Utilization of palliative care consultation service by surgical services. Ann Palliat Med 2015;4:194–9.
16. Suwanabol PA, Kanters AE, Reichstein AC, et al. Characterizing the role of U.S. surgeons in the provision of palliative care: a systematic review and mixed-methods meta-synthesis. J Pain Symptom Manage 2018;55:1196–215.e5.
17. Available at: https://www.jointcommission.org/assets/1/18/Ventricular_Assist_Device_Destination_ Therapy_Requirements.pdf. Accessed October 1, 2018.
18. Available at: https://www.cms.gov/medicare-coverage-database/details/nca-proposed-decision-memo.aspx?NCAId=268. Accessed October 1, 2018.
19. Wordingham SE, McIlvennan CK, Fendler TJ, et al. Palliative care clinician caring for patient before and after continuous flow left ventricular assist device. J Pain Symptom Manage 2017;54(4):601–8.
20. Walling AM, D'Ambruoso SF, Malin JL, et al. Effect and efficacy of an embedded palliative care nurse practitioner in an oncology clinic. J Oncol Pract 2017;13(9): e792–9.
21. Finlay E, Newport K, Sivendran S, et al. Models of outpatient palliative care clinics for patients with cancer. J Oncol Pract 2019;15(4):187–93.
22. O'Mahony S, Levine S, Baron A, et al. Palliative workforce development and a regional training program. Am J Hosp Palliat Care 2018;35(1):138–43.
23. Kamal AH, Bull JH, Swetz KM, et al. Future of the palliative care workforce: preview to an impending crisis. Am J Med 2017;130(2):113–4.
24. Lupu D. Estimate of current hospice and palliative medicine physician workforce shortage. J Pain Symptom Manage 2010;40(6):899–911.
25. Kavaliertatos D, Gelfman L, Tycon LE, et al. Palliative care in heart failure: rationale, evidence, and future priorities. J Am Coll Cardiol 2017;70(15):1919–30.
26. Dillon BR, Healy MA, Lee CW, et al. Surgeon perspectives regarding death and dying. J Palliat Med 2019;22(2):132–7.
27. Bonanno AM, Kiraly LN, Siegal TR, et al. Surgical palliative care training in general surgery residency: an education needs assessment. Am J Surg 2019;217(5): 928–31.
28. Raoof M, O'Neill L, Neumayer L, et al. Prospective evaluation of surgical palliative care immersion training for general surgery residents. Am J Surg 2017;214(2): 378–83.
29. Kuser JM, Taylor LJ, Campbell TC, et al. "Best Case/Worse Case": training surgeons using a novel communication tool for high risk acute surgical problems. J Pain Symptom Manag 2017;53(4):711–9.
30. Nakagawa S, Berlin A, Blinderman CD. End-of-life preferences should be discussed routinely before high risk surgery. J Palliat Med 2019;22(1):9.
31. Levine S, O'Mahony S, Baron A, et al. Training the workforce: description of a longitudinal interdisciplinary education and mentoring program in palliative care. J Pain Symptom Manage 2017;53(4):728–37.

Concurrent Palliative Care for Surgical Patients

Ana Berlin, MD, MPH[a,b,*], Teresa Johelen Carleton, MD[c,d]

KEYWORDS

- Surgical patients • Surgical palliative care • Palliative surgery
- Concurrent palliative care • Palliative care models of integration

KEY POINTS

- Modern surgeons play a complex role as both providers and gatekeepers when it comes to meeting the palliative needs of their patients.
- Surgical palliative care is delivered by surgical teams as a component of routine surgical care, and includes management of physical and psychosocial symptoms, as well as basic communication about prognosis and treatment options and identification of patient goals and values; in addition, specialty palliative care for surgical patients may be provided through a range of consultative or integrative models.
- A common fallacy in surgical culture is for surgical intervention and palliation to be regarded as mutually exclusive or sequential strategies in the trajectory of a patient's care.
- Because it is difficult to measure palliative care provided by surgeons as a component of routine surgical practice, the evidence base for concurrent palliative care in surgery is sparse.
- Reconceptualizing opportunities to offer palliative care to surgical patients in terms of the phases of the perioperative continuum may help integrate palliative care throughout the clinical trajectory.

CONCEPTUAL FRAMEWORK FOR CONCURRENT PALLIATIVE CARE IN SURGERY

As medical fields go, surgery is hardly a stranger to suffering. Given this, palliative care principles have always been, and will always be, core tenets of high-quality surgical care. Although surgeons are in the business of saving lives (and it takes some amount

Disclosure: The authors have nothing to disclose.

[a] Department of Surgery, Division of General Surgery, Columbia University Medical Center, Herbert Irving Pavilion, 161 Fort Washington Avenue, 5-562, New York, NY 10032, USA; [b] Department of Medicine, Division of Hematology/Oncology, Adult Palliative Medicine Service, Columbia University Medical Center, New York, NY, USA; [c] Tucson Medical Center Palliative Care, Tucson Medical Center, 5301 E. Grant Road, Tucson, AZ 85712, USA; [d] University of Arizona Phoenix, Phoenix, AZ, USA

* Corresponding author. Department of Surgery, Division of General Surgery, Columbia University Medical Center, Herbert Irving Pavilion, 161 Fort Washington Avenue, 5-562, New York, NY 10032.

E-mail address: Ab1254@cumc.columbia.edu

Surg Clin N Am 99 (2019) 823–831
https://doi.org/10.1016/j.suc.2019.06.001
0039-6109/19/

of that mentality to operate on ruptured aortas, massive trauma, or even acute gastrointestinal catastrophes), survival is an imprecise ruler against which to measure the outcome of a carefully considered operation. In addition, the relief of suffering is the primary objective of many common surgical interventions. Whether the intent is curative, restorative, or palliative, a good surgical decision takes into account the ramifications of operative intervention. What will survival look like? Will saving someone's life mean they live bedbound in a nursing home? Will the patient be able to return to work? Does the patient live close enough to the hospital for reasonable postoperative care? Will the patient's elderly spouse be required to drive 200 miles each way for adjuvant chemoradiation? These are the types of questions comprehensive surgical decision making has always encompassed, and good surgical training has always demanded attention to the answers. The personal consequences of surgery are standard considerations in the calculus of benefits versus burdens. For this reason, surgeons are naturally engaged in the everyday practice of palliative care.

Despite a long history at the forefront of palliation, modern surgeons play a complex role as both providers and gatekeepers when it comes to meeting the palliative needs of their patients. Investigations into the role of surgeons in the provision of palliative care are limited by the lack of a uniform definition of palliative care in surgery. Surgical palliative care is delivered by surgical teams as a component of routine surgical care, and includes management of physical and psychosocial symptoms, as well as basic communication about prognosis and treatment options and identification of patient goals and values. Specialist palliative care for surgical patients provided by specialized interdisciplinary palliative care teams can aid in managing complex symptoms, providing an added layer of support for families, resolving conflicts over treatment goals and approaches, and assisting with transitions in care. Although numerous studies have documented the striking levels of underuse of palliative care for surgical patient populations, most of this literature focuses on specialty palliative care, because it is difficult to measure palliative care provided by surgeons as a component of routine surgical practice.

Whether in reference to primary palliative care or specialty palliative care use, surgical culture has been characterized by "the pervasive sense that recovery and palliation are sequential rather than parallel elements of an individual's medical trajectory."[1] Surgical intervention and palliation are often seen as mutually exclusive options, with the latter becoming relevant only after the former has been either ruled out or attempted without success. Because surgeons, along with the lay public and other medical providers, often conflate palliative care with end-of-life care in general and hospice in particular, it is not surprising that palliative care is often introduced late or because of expected mortality.[2] However, this view of palliative care "fails to include the life-affirming quality of active, symptomatic efforts to relieve the pain and suffering of individuals with chronic illness and injury"[3] that form the basis of treatment of patients with a range of surgical problems and prognoses. Nevertheless, in reality, surgeons struggle with prognostication and identifying the right time to introduce palliative care to their patients,[4] as if palliative care were a highly burdensome second-line or third-line zero-sum option, as opposed to a beneficial adjunct at any stage of serious surgical illness.

BENEFITS OF CONCURRENT PALLIATIVE CARE: EVIDENCE BASE FOR IMPROVED CLINICAL OUTCOMES IN ONCOLOGY AND TRAUMA POPULATIONS

In their struggles with prognostication, their focus on maintaining hope and balancing realism with optimism, and their concern over contributing to a sense of failure or abandonment,[4] surgeons share many similarities with oncologists when it comes to beliefs and attitudes that affect the integration of palliative care. In oncology, published data regarding the benefits of early concurrent palliative care alongside usual cancer care have been instrumental in overcoming some of these cultural barriers and promoting uptake of palliative care.[5–7] Reduced symptom burden, improved quality of life, improved survival, improved patient and family satisfaction, improved physician satisfaction and reduced levels of professional burnout, improved survival, and reduced costs of care are all outcomes that have been observed in settings ranging from pulmonary and gastrointestinal malignancy[8–10] to hip fracture.[11]

However, the evidence for concurrent palliative care in the surgical setting is sparse. Evidence for concurrent primary palliative care in surgery is even more limited. For example, a recent evidence-based review of routine palliative care processes in trauma was unable to draw precise and consistent conclusions about the role of early palliative care consultation in the trauma setting, although improved secondary outcomes, such as length of stay, were observed.[12] In view of the rapidity with which palliative care has been adopted as a standard of best-practice care for seriously ill patients, it is fair to question whether and how to continue to attempt to build an evidence base for this in the surgical setting. Although there is an imperative, given the shortage of specialty palliative care clinicians, to pursue research with the potential to inform and justify workforce expansion and use of specialty palliative care, the ethical dilemmas, imperfect metrics, and daunting methodologies that pose challenges for building the palliative care evidence base in surgery are even more formidable for primary palliative care than they are for specialty palliative care.

BARRIERS AND STRATEGIES FOR IMPLEMENTATION

Challenges to concurrent surgery and palliative care arise from insufficient recognition of the potential benefits. Despite the growing body of literature supporting concomitant palliative care, medical culture has the strangely persistent, and hopefully diminishing, misconception that palliative care is hospice. However, hospice is a small subset of palliative care focused only on end of life. A palliative care service in the hospital or the community may not even have an association with a specific hospice agency. An evolved palliative care program offers meaningful support for sick patients, their families, and even their providers, regardless of the anticipated outcome. Although palliative surgical indications may exist in hospice patients, a decision for hospice affords clarity that the patient accepts end-of-life care and the purpose of interventions is comfort. Specialty palliative involvement has a great deal to offer if end-of-life care is not yet appropriate or not yet desired. The best collaborative work can be done when none of the treatment options are ideal or when a surgical solution may have benefit but may also have devastating repercussions. Many patients are not afraid to die in the operating room, but are afraid to be alive months after an operation, still on mechanical life support or bedbound in a nursing home.

The personal consequences of surgery are standard considerations in risk and benefit, which makes surgeons naturally engaged in palliative care. Because surgeons consistently perform surgical palliative care, the involvement of a specialist should be carefully coordinated. The sudden or poorly communicated involvement of a palliative care specialist can undermine the work already done toward defining and achieving the goals of treatment. Planned, thoughtful collaboration is particularly advantageous because palliative care specialists have sophisticated communication skills and the time to use them, but only surgeons fully understand the indications and complications for a given operation. Ernst and colleagues[13] provide an elegant example of systematic and constructive interaction between surgery and palliative care. The investigators report decreased mortality by identification of frail elective surgical patients for suggested preoperative palliative care consultation. Improvements in outcomes were attributable to a combination of patient selection through preoperative administrative review and contingency planning. In the modern health care environment, with the "tsunami" of an aging population, the complex and often formidable consequences of surgery represent the best potential for work at the intersection of surgery and palliative care.

Systematic approaches to specialty palliative care for elective operation have the advantages of planning and preparation. Emergent surgical indications pose even more challenges to cohesive collaboration. Although palliative programs are increasingly available at all hours, surgeons face acute and complicated situations without the availability of specialty palliative support. A systematic approach can still be achieved. For example, Cooper and colleagues[14] developed a structured communication framework to facilitate goal-concordant care for seriously ill older patients with emergency surgical conditions. The recommendations are intended to be implemented by surgical teams and, as an example of communication and decision making in serious illness, constitute primary palliative care by surgeons.

Increasingly, surgical training programs and palliative care programs are both offering educational opportunities for surgeons and surgical trainees to refine their communication skills and direct them toward the burgeoning palliative resources specific to surgery.[15] Ariadne Labs and the Center to Advance Palliative Care have well-established tools applicable to surgical practice. Taylor and colleagues[16] outline a surgery-specific communication framework for improving communication in high-stakes surgical decisions. The Education in Palliative and End-of-Life Care (EPEC) project is developing a surgery-specific palliative care curriculum, led by Joshua Hauser and Pringl Miller.

Although surgeons may be frustrated by limited specialty palliative support in off hours, it may be helpful to fully understand some of the financial barriers. Surgery and palliative care have opposing economic incentives. Although reimbursement structures are evolving with the advent of value-based care, surgeons are financially rewarded to operate. Palliative care programs cannot cover their costs with the evaluation and management codes assigned to their billing and their worth is measured in the costs saved. In essence, surgeons are financially incentivized to operate, which may pose a conflict of interest if patients, once asked, prefer no invasive life-prolonging interventions. It is hoped that these divergent agendas may be reconciled in future health care payment models. Even without the financial incentives, surgeons have an intrinsic bias for action because so much of their training and expertise are directed toward operative intervention. The inability of surgeons to offer a surgical solution can seem defeating because of their investment in technical skill. However, surgeons are not just technicians and nonoperative decisions have the potential to reflect their best clinical judgment.

OPPORTUNITIES AND DELIVERY MODELS FOR CONCURRENT PALLIATIVE CARE IN SURGERY

As described earlier, models of palliative care delivery for surgical patients are typically characterized in terms of primary and specialty palliative care, with specialty services being accessed through a variety of models. Integrative models embed palliative care specialists within surgical teams (eg, a trauma service) to proactively screen patients for palliative care needs and concurrent care integrated with the rest of the team.

Because they are not targeted, integrative models may spread palliative care resources thinly among patients with variable levels of need, reducing the per-provider level of impact on patient outcomes. Consultative models, whereby palliative care specialists are brought in as consultants to assist a primary team in meeting patients' palliative care needs, may rely on voluntary requests for consultation or systems-based triggers (e, prolonged length of stay, readmission to the intensive care unit postoperatively, or referral for advanced device-based heart failure).[17,18] Consultative models risk undertreatment and are associated with delays in introducing palliative care for surgical patients; additionally, depending on the triggers used, the consultative model may reinforce erroneous notions equating palliative care with end-of-life care, and augment artificial distinctions between surgical care and palliative care.[13]

Reconceptualizing opportunities to offer palliative care to surgical patients in terms of the phases of the perioperative continuum so familiar to surgeons may help integrate palliative care, whether primary or specialty, throughout the patient care trajectory. Preoperative, intraoperative, and postoperative considerations for acute care surgeons have been described previously.[19] Defining triggers that move palliative care "upstream" in the course of surgical illness and treatment has been a major focus of efforts to integrate the two. Ensuring access to palliative care upstream enhances the value of surgical care through improved patient selection and optimization, and avoidance of goal discordant or nonbeneficial treatment. For example, a model of early palliative care consultation triggered by a recommendation for *nil per os* on speech therapy evaluation in patients with acute stroke was associated with improved documentation of goals of care.[20] By moving palliative care well upstream of surgical consultation, patients received necessary attention to their goals before surgical systems engagement, such that surgical decision making could proceed in a more goal-concordant fashion without the pressure of surgical momentum. In addition, highlighting preoperative opportunities for improved prognostication and risk assessment, communication, decision making, and symptom assessment and management will help to destigmatize palliative care in the eyes of surgeons as pertaining only to the end of life.

The most obvious opportunities for concurrent surgery and palliative care are operative. In the words of Anne C. Mosenthal, a foundational leader in surgical palliative care, "Sometimes the best palliative care is an operation" (Personal communication, October 24, 2018). Tracheostomy and percutaneous endoscopic gastrostomy are conventional treatment modalities that often lead to palliation for esophageal cancer, head and neck cancers, and amyotrophic lateral sclerosis. Enteric bypasses are performed for relief of malignant bowel obstruction.[21–23] Considerable literature supports biliary drainage to improve survival and quality of life in patients with malignant biliary obstruction.[24,25] Cytoreductive surgery is routinely offered for incurable cancers, particularly ovarian.[26] Vascular surgeons perform palliative amputation[27] and orthopedic surgeons perform palliative repair of hip fractures.[28] In carefully selected patients, these palliative interventions may have a dramatic impact on quality of life and even survival. Defining the parameters of success is especially important; a patient mortality shortly after a palliative operation may not constitute a failure if the goals of the operation were to relieve burdensome symptoms in the setting of a short prognosis. However, patient-centric outcomes are challenging methodologically in the palliative setting, in part because of limited time to gather these data in terminally ill patients and difficulty following up with distressed survivors. Lee and colleagues[29] explore meaningful measures of palliative care delivery in surgical patients, and highlight the paucity of metrics uniquely applicable to surgical patients. For example, there are

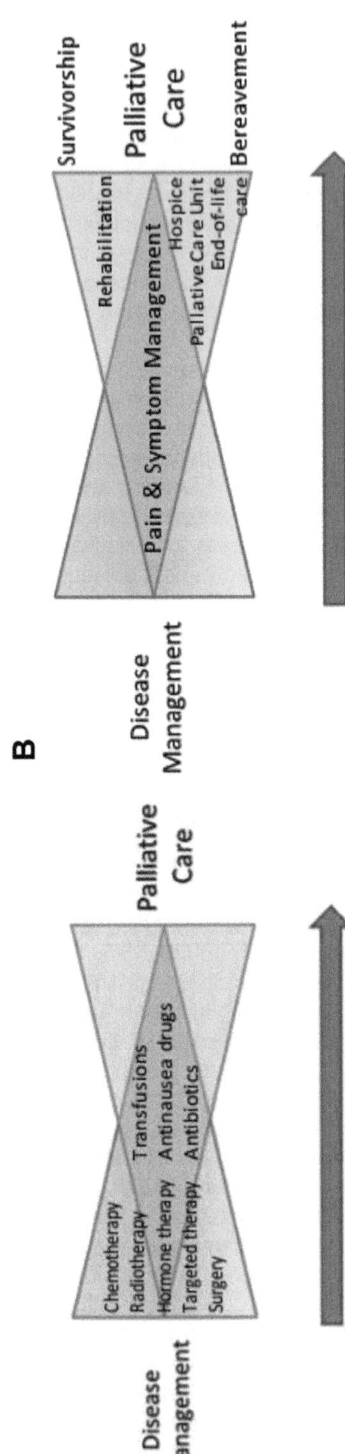

Fig. 1. The bow tie model of palliative care visually depicts how palliative care can be integrated concurrently with disease-directed surgical care. Depending on the patient's needs and goals, different aspects of care can be emphasized accordingly. (*A*) Disease management–enhanced model. (*B*) Palliative care–enhanced model. (*From* Hawley PH. The bow tie model of 21st century palliative care. J Pain Symptom Manage. 2014 Jan;47(1):e2-5. https://doi.org/10.1016/j.jpainsymman.2013.10.009. Epub 2013 Dec 8; with permission.)

currently no standardized quality metrics that capture rates of documentation of preoperative life-sustaining treatment preferences or preoperative palliative symptom assessment for palliative operations. Badgwell and colleagues[30,31] also propose patient-centered alternatives to traditional outcome measures.

The so-called bowtie model of palliative care popularized in oncology by Pippa Hawley[32] provides a powerful visual anchor for communicating about the integration of palliative care with disease management. This model is applicable both preoperatively and postoperatively. By depicting survivorship and rehabilitation on an equal footing with death and bereavement, the bowtie model reassures patients and clinicians that palliative and disease-modifying therapies are not mutually exclusive. This point is important for patients, families, and health care providers who are struggling to accept a role for palliative care in their routine treatment, often based on misconceptions about palliative care (**Fig. 1**).

In conclusion, a sense of conviction about the importance of providing early concurrent palliative care for patients with surgical illness is necessary but not sufficient in the current health care environment. However, there is a robust surgical palliative care research agenda that in part aims to address gaps in evidence about concurrent surgical and palliative care.[33] Just as the past decade has seen interest in surgical palliative care flourish, so is it reasonable to hope that the next decade will usher in a new era of evidence for the value and optimal modes of delivery of concurrent palliative care in surgery, particularly in the form of primary palliative care delivered by surgeons and surgical teams.

REFERENCES

1. Rivet EB, Del Fabbro E, Ferrada P. Palliative care assessment in the surgical and trauma intensive care unit. JAMA Surg 2018;153(3):280–1.
2. Suwanabol PA, Reichstein AC, Suzer-Gurtekin ZT, et al. Surgeons' perceived barriers to palliative and end-of-life care: a mixed methods study of a surgical society. J Palliat Med 2018;21(6):780–8.
3. American College of Surgeons. Statement of principles of palliative care. Available at: https://www.facs.org/about-acs/statements/50-palliative-care. Accessed June 17, 2019.
4. Suwanabol PA, Kanters AE, Reichstein AC, et al. Characterizing the role of U.S. surgeons in the provision of palliative care: a systematic review and mixed-methods meta-synthesis. J Pain Symptom Manage 2018;55(4):1215.e5.
5. Haun MW, Estel S, Rucker G, et al. Early palliative care for adults with advanced cancer. Cochrane Database Syst Rev 2017;(6):CD011129.
6. Hui D, Bruera E. Integrating palliative care into the trajectory of cancer care. Nat Rev Clin Oncol 2016;13(3):159–71.
7. Salins N, Ramanjulu R, Patra L, et al. Integration of early specialist palliative care in cancer care and patient related outcomes: a critical review of evidence. Indian J Palliat Care 2016;22(3):252–7.
8. Parikh RB, Kirch RA, Smith TJ, et al. Early specialty palliative care–translating data in oncology into practice. N Engl J Med 2013;369(24):2347–51.
9. Sadler EM, Hawley PH, Easson AM. Palliative care and active disease management are synergistic in modern surgical oncology. Surgery 2018;163(4):950–3.
10. Temel JS, Greer JA, El-Jawahri A, et al. Effects of early integrated palliative care in patients with lung and GI cancer: a randomized clinical trial. J Clin Oncol 2017;35(8):834–41.

11. Davies A, Tilston T, Walsh K, et al. Is there a role for early palliative intervention in frail older patients with a neck of femur fracture? Geriatr Orthop Surg Rehabil 2018;9. 2151459318782232.
12. Aziz HA, Lunde J, Barraco R, et al. Evidence-based review of trauma center care and routine palliative care processes for geriatric trauma patients; a collaboration from the american association for the surgery of trauma (AAST) patient assessment committee, the AAST geriatric trauma committee, and the eastern association for the surgery of trauma guidelines committee. J Trauma Acute Care Surg 2019;86(4):737–43.
13. Ernst KF, Hall DE, Schmid KK, et al. Surgical palliative care consultations over time in relationship to systemwide frailty screening. JAMA Surg 2014;149(11): 1121–6.
14. Cooper Z, Koritsanszky LA, Cauley CE, et al. Recommendations for best communication practices to facilitate goal-concordant care for seriously ill older patients with emergency surgical conditions. Ann Surg 2016;263(1):1–6.
15. Nakagawa S, Fischkoff K, Berlin A, et al. Communication skills training for general surgery residents. J Surg Educ 2019. https://doi.org/10.1016/j.jsurg.2019.04.001.
16. Taylor LJ, Nabozny MJ, Steffens NM, et al. A framework to improve surgeon communication in high-stakes surgical decisions: Best case/worst case. JAMA Surg 2017;152(6):531–8.
17. Nakagawa S, Yuzefpolskaya M, Colombo PC, et al. Palliative care interventions before left ventricular assist device implantation in both bridge to transplant and destination therapy. J Palliat Med 2017;20(9):977–83.
18. Finkelstein M, Goldstein NE, Horton JR, et al. Developing triggers for the surgical intensive care unit for palliative care integration. J Crit Care 2016;35:7–11.
19. Berlin A, Cooper Z. Palliative care. In: Britt LD, Peitzman AB, Barie PS, et al, editors. Acute care surgery. 2nd edition. Philadelphia: Lippincott, Williams, and Wilkins; 2018. p. 293–311 [Chapter 25].
20. Hwang F, Boardingham C, Walther S, et al. Establishing goals of care for patients with stroke and feeding problems: an interdisciplinary trigger-based continuous quality improvement project. J Pain Symptom Manage 2018;56(4):588–93.
21. Krouse RS, You YN. Prospective comparative effectiveness trial for malignant bowel obstruction: SWOG S1316. Bull Am Coll Surg 2015;100(12):49–50.
22. Pujara D, Chiang YJ, Cormier JN, et al. Selective approach for patients with advanced malignancy and gastrointestinal obstruction. J Am Coll Surg 2017; 225(1):53–9.
23. Roses RE, Folkert IW, Krouse RS. Malignant bowel obstruction: reappraising the value of surgery. Surg Oncol Clin N Am 2018;27(4):705–15.
24. Kuhlmann KF, van Poll D, de Castro SM, et al. Initial and long-term outcome after palliative surgical drainage of 269 patients with malignant biliary obstruction. Eur J Surg Oncol 2007;33(6):757–62.
25. Ueda J, Kayashima T, Mori Y, et al. Hepaticocholecystojejunostomy as effective palliative biliary bypass for unresectable pancreatic cancer. Hepatogastroenterology 2014;61(129):197–202.
26. Narasimhulu DM, Khoury-Collado F, Chi DS. Radical surgery in ovarian cancer. Curr Oncol Rep 2015;17(4):16.
27. Butler CR, Schwarze ML, Katz R, et al. Lower extremity amputation and health care utilization in the last year of life among medicare beneficiaries with ESRD. J Am Soc Nephrol 2019 [pii:ASN.2018101002].

28. Johnston CB, Holleran A, Ong T, et al. Hip fracture in the setting of limited life expectancy: the importance of considering goals of care and prognosis. J Palliat Med 2018;21(8):1069–73.
29. Lee KC, Senglaub SS, Walling AM, et al. Quality measures in surgical palliative care: adapting existing palliative care measures to improve care for seriously ill surgical patients. Ann Surg 2019;269(4):607–9.
30. Badgwell B, Krouse R, Klimberg SV, et al. Outcome measures other than morbidity and mortality for patients with incurable cancer and gastrointestinal obstruction. J Palliat Med 2014;17(1):18–26.
31. Badgwell B, Bruera E, Klimberg SV. Can patient reported outcomes help identify the optimal outcome in palliative surgery? J Surg Oncol 2014;109(2):145–50.
32. Hawley PH. The bow tie model of 21st century palliative care. J Pain Symptom Manage 2014;47(1):e2–5.
33. Lilley EJ, Cooper Z, Schwarze ML, et al. Palliative care in surgery: defining the research priorities. Ann Surg 2018;267(1):66–72.

Goals of Care

Understanding the Outcomes that Matter Most

Mackenzie R. Cook, MD

KEYWORDS

• Goals of care • Advanced care planning • Palliative care

KEY POINTS

- Advanced care planning is the responsibility of all physicians who care for critically and seriously ill patients.
- The right time to start advanced care planning is now!
- When talking about advanced care planning, it is more than just code status and includes an understanding of patient values and goals, and includes their surrogates from an early stage.

INTRODUCTION

Provided in parallel to therapies focused on treating the underlying disease, integration of high-quality palliative care is appropriate for any stage of illness and a responsibility of all clinicians caring for the seriously and critically ill.[1] The National Coalition for Hospice and Palliative Medicine reinforces this point, emphasizing the importance of addressing therapeutic goals as part of primary palliative care.[2–4] Provided by clinicians not subspecialty trained in palliative care, primary palliative care promotes stronger clinician-patient relationships, reduces fragmentation of care, and can easily be integrated with other therapies.[3,5]

Although highly individualized, the seriously ill often value quality of life over extending quantity of life.[2,6,7] Unfortunately, the patient's focus on preserving quality of life does not appear to be reliably honored by the medical system.[8] The skills necessary to clearly elucidate a patient's goals, values, and hopes can be learned, although not all clinicians have this training.[9,10]

This article focusses on defining patient goals as a key component of primary palliative care, a critical skill for all clinicians caring for the critically and seriously ill.

NOT JUST CODE STATUS

Modern medical care is filled with a myriad of medical choices for patients who influence quality and quantity of life. A patient's decision-making experience can be a

Disclosure: The author has nothing to disclose.
Division of Trauma, Critical Care and Acute Care Surgery, Oregon Health and Science University, Mail Code L611, 3181 Southwest Sam Jackson Park Road, Portland, OR 97239, USA
E-mail address: cookmac@ohsu.edu

Surg Clin N Am 99 (2019) 833–847
https://doi.org/10.1016/j.suc.2019.06.005

complex combination of factors, including disease prognosis, expectations for the future, preexisting comorbidities, disease burden, individual values, individual goals, cultural conception of disease, family preferences, and relationships.

Although often used as a shorthand for a discussion about code status or transition to comfort-focused care should the patient find themselves in the position of facing presumed or actual nonbeneficial treatments and interventions, “goals of care discussions” are far broader, more nuanced, and appropriate far earlier in a patient’s clinical course. Best characterized as advanced care planning, frank, honest, and open discussions about a patient’s wishes in the face of a serious illness promotes communication and understanding across the spectrum of care.[2] Advanced care planning that begins as an outpatient improves the likelihood that clinicians comply with their patient’s wishes, reduces hospitalization near the end of life, increases hospice use, increases the chance that a patient will die in their preferred place, and is associated with a higher satisfaction with the quality of care.[11–16]

A reframing of discussions surrounding patient goals is necessary to transition away from a narrow focus on the time of death to a broader focus about the way a patient would like to live given the medical realities. Health care professionals tend to conceptualize goals of care discussions in medical terms, and focus the discussion on medical interventions, assuming that the patient’s goals and preferences exist with a similar medical focus. It is likely that a patient’s goals are far more individualized and less medically oriented than most clinicians assume. Any discussion about goals and advanced care planning must take into account a patient’s desire to maintain and support relationships, to attend family events, and to avoide suffering. Balancing quality of life values along with quantity of life can help guide how the patient understand medical interventions.

WHEN TO START ADVANCED CARE PLANNING

It is common that patients are referred to subspecialty palliative care providers at a relatively late stage, reflecting the reluctance to involve a formal palliative care consultant, a lack of palliative care specialists, or a combination of the 2.[5] With this in mind, it is critical for the advanced care planning process to begin with the primary treating clinicians. Those who work in high-risk/high-acuity fields are encouraged to develop skills to provide advanced care planning as part of providing primary palliative care. Holding advanced care planning discussions and filling out advanced directives when a patient is still able to meaningfully participate in the conversation and has the capacity to make medical decisions is ideal. This allows the discussion to be free of time pressure, longitudinal, and focused on guiding surrogate decision makers. The right time to start advanced care planning is… NOW!

A common concern raised is the stability of patient preferences over time. Data are limited, although a systematic review of 17 studies found that stable patient choices were associated with having a single advanced directive (as opposed to several iterations with different wishes), an expressed preference to forgo high-intensity/low-reward treatments, and the extremes of pathologic conditions, either facing a very serious diagnosis or being essentially completely healthy.[17] Patients admitted to the hospital, however, do seem to change their preferences for life-sustaining treatment with some degree of regularity. Approximately 8% of patients admitted without limitations on care added new limitations to their care plan, and a roughly comparable number removed limitations to their care while in the hospital.[18] The oldest patients were the most likely to add new limitations and the least likely to reverse previous limitation. These data suggest that patient goals elucidated through an advanced care planning process do have a degree of stability over time, but are fundamentally dynamic with some flexibility based on a patient's changing clinical situation.

Although not always possible given the vagaries of sudden illness and injury, a longitudinal discussion about goals of care in the setting of a supportive therapeutic relationship may be the ideal. Wishes should be revisited over time, particularly at times of significant changes in health status or hospital admission. This potential evolution of patient wishes should not be used as an excuse to forgo advanced care planning.

WHO SHOULD START THE ADVANCED CARE PLANNING PROCESS?

Once the "when" is decided, the next question is: Who should start an advanced care planning discussion? This is perhaps best done by a clinician-patient dyad within the setting of a longitudinal clinical relationship and does *not* need to be deferred to a specialist in palliative care. Although classically conceptualized as part of the primary care provider relationship, a specialist working with a patient over a period of time may be equally or more able to undertake an advanced care planning discussion. There is an associated logistical challenge, as an advanced care planning discussion with a full elucidation of patient goals of care requires time, sensitivity, and likely multiple visits.[19] These elective discussions often take a backseat to pressing clinical decisions. The more common setting for goals of care discussions in the current medical system is within the framework of an acute medical deterioration and with a physician who is meeting the patient and the family at the time of an abrupt deterioration. Although emergency physicians, hospitalists, intensivists, palliative care physicians, and acute care surgeons are all compassionate, thoughtful, and invested in the well-being of their patients, they may lack the longitudinal patient relationship and perspective that primary care physicians and long-term outpatient specialists can draw on.[20]

The challenges of goals of care discussions in these 2 settings are related, although somewhat different. In the acute setting, the communication is typically focused on communication surrounding serious, unexpected illness and limitations on high-intensity/low-reward maneuvers. Communicating bad news, efficiently eliciting patient preferences in the setting of questionable patient competence, making time-pressured decisions to proceed with a high-risk/low-reward intervention, and identifying a surrogate decision maker are all key parts of care planning in the acute setting.[21] A proactive discussion regarding a patient's wishes early in the course of a serious medical illness is far more appropriate than an urgent discussion in the middle of the night following acute decompensations.[19,22]

CAPACITY ASSESSMENT IN THE SETTING OF ADVANCED CARE PLANNING

When undertaking an advanced care planning conversation, an obligatory first step is to assess the capacity of a patient or their surrogate. Although this can be a simple decision in the profoundly debilitated patient, the challenge becomes greater in a patient with the ability to speak but an unclear ability to make medical decisions.

An assessment of decision-making capacity can be carried out by the clinician undertaking the advanced care planning with the patient and does not require any special psychiatric or legal expertise. This is in comparison with the more formal legal term, decisional competence, which involves the rigorous evaluations of decision-making capacity in medical and nonmedical endeavors and is determined by the judiciary. Capacity itself is task specific and the inability to live independently or manage one's finances, for example, does not necessarily make one unable to participate in and have capacity for advanced care planning discussions. Similarly, the ability to carry on a superficial conversation does not necessarily indicate that a patient is able to understand the pros and cons of complex medical interventions.

When determining capacity there is no single test that will either confirm or refute decision-making capacity. Outside of cases of extreme impairment, the mini-mental status examination and other cognitive measures applied to assess dementia and delirium do not predict the capacity to make medical decisions.[23] Assessment of capacity is best done in an interview with open-ended questions and generally involves 4 criteria, with the starting assumption that a person *does* have capacity. The 4 components of decision-making capacity are:

1. Understanding: the patient (or their surrogate) must have the ability to understand the information being presented. This often comes down to a patient understanding their diagnosis and prognosis, as well as the risks and benefits associated with the treatment options.
2. Expressing a choice: the patient (or their surrogate) needs to be able to express a choice when presented with options. Although that choice can vary over time, frequent reversals in the setting of an underlying neuropsychiatric condition may suggest an inability to reliably express a choice.
3. Appreciation: the patient (or their surrogate) must be able to appreciate how facts of their medical condition and implication of their choices are relevant to them, and express insight into their medical condition. If a person refuses to accept that they have a metastatic cancer, despite irrefutable evidence, they do not appreciate the nature of their diagnosis and may not have capacity.
4. Reasoning: the patient (or their surrogate) must have the ability to compare and contrast options, drawing on the patient's values and beliefs. In practice, this is tested by being able to explain their rationale and that it is reasoned and reasonable. This does *NOT* mean that the physician needs to agree with their rationale, only that the patient can compare and contrast within the framework of their own belief system and that that comparison is based in the reality of the medical situation.

When caring for patients who may not satisfy all the conditions for capacity but who are still able to communicate, their input should be valued and sought with the assistance of a surrogate decision maker. This situation primarily applies to patients with intellectual impairments, but they are often not included in studies on advanced care planning, and information on this topic is limited.[24] Additional thought should be given when interacting with patients from cultures where decision making is customarily deferred to the family unit and those with strong religious beliefs.[25,26] Physicians should seek to understand the diversity of attitudes within their patient's cultures and be sensitive to and respect the patient's autonomy, even if that means they would defer to their family or church. The astute clinician should not assume a patient's preferences from their apparent ethnic background, but rather ask the patient with whom and how the advanced care planning process should proceed.

If a patient has capacity, they should be directly involved in their own advanced care planning. The only limitation on this recommendation may be patients with coexisting decompensated mood disorders, such as major depressive disorder, whereby they may have adequate decision-making capacity but their preferences and choice may be clouded by the mood disorder.[27] Whereas psychiatric expertise is not necessary for routine evaluation of capacity, assessment of capacity in the setting of a decompensated mood disorder may require psychiatric or legal input. Psychiatric assistance should certainly be sought before over-ruling the choices of a patient with established capacity and a concomitant mood disorder and, if possible, routine advanced care planning should be deferred until the mood disorder has been effectively treated. In an urgent situation, when available, involving a surrogate decision maker may be a reasonable option.

WHEN A PATIENT LACKS CAPACITY: THE SURROGATE

When a patient is unable to speak for themselves or does not have decision-making capacity, a surrogate decision maker is identified. Medical ethics demand that clinicians do not take on the surrogate decision-maker role in isolation, as they do not necessarily know what their patient's wishes are and tend to systematically underestimate quality of life in favor of life-sustaining treatments.[28,29] In an ideal setting, the surrogate is chosen by the patient while they retain decisional capacity. This designee, when properly memorialized on institutional or state documents, is called a health care power of attorney. Legal documentation is not an absolute requirement for a patient to designate their surrogate and, in the absence of a formally designated surrogate decision maker, the next of kin have been typically viewed as the default surrogates—with order of priority determined by local law and institutional policy. Patient-designated surrogates who are outside of this legal progression and without institutional or state legal backing may be more easily challenged by other surrogates in the event of a disagreement. The expectation is that the surrogate should use substituted judgment standard to consider what the patient would want if they could speak for themselves. If a clear decision cannot be reached then the decision can be made by applying the best interests standard, as guided by "what would most people want in this situation" may reasonably be used to guide medical care.[30]

Just because a surrogate decision maker is identified, one cannot necessarily assume that this surrogate decision maker is a valid patient representative. In a large systematic review, surrogates incorrectly predicted patient preferences more than 30% of the time, a rate that was not improved if the patient designated the surrogate and if they had discussions before the decision point.[31] Despite this, a surrogate decision maker is often the best option available.

A formal legal guardian, as appointed through the judiciary, is rarely needed and often only applicable when a patient is deemed incompetent by the legal system or in the setting where a patient is unable to speak for themselves and is without friends or family. The patient without family, friends, or surrogates is a complex problem, and although urgent/emergent care can often be progressed under presumed or 2-physician consent, guardianship is often needed. In a clinical setting, these legal proceedings are triggered when there is a major treatment dilemma, the patient is unable to speak for themselves, and either no surrogate is available or multiple surrogates with equivalent claim to surrogacy are unable to come to consensus. A guardian may also be necessary if the surrogate is thought to be acting in their own interest, or contrary to the interests of the patient.[32] In such a nuanced legal and ethical terrain, treating clinicians are strongly advised to seek available ethics and legal advice when faced with this dilemma. In practice, legal guardianship proceedings can be extremely time consuming and may only be applicable in the most extreme circumstances when longer-term decisions need to be considered. In the emergent, urgent, or semielective setting, guardianship may not be an efficient way to proceed. In this setting, care may reasonably be progressed according to institutional guidelines, potentially including 2-physician consent, presumed consent, or in consultation with the ethics committee.

ADVANCED CARE PLANNING: DISCUSSIONS

An advance care planning discussion typically takes place in the setting of an established clinical relationship, in a semistructured fashion. More rapid conversations following an unexpected injury or decompensation require a slightly different approach, although many principles are the same as detailed later. Although multiple approaches in the elective, nonurgent setting with a seriously ill patient could be appropriate, there are key themes.

Although described here within the framework of a single visit, this process typically progresses over the course of multiple visits. The importance of starting advanced care planning discussions before the moment of crisis cannot be overemphasized because preparation of the surrogate decision maker to participate in these conversations takes some of the pressure off urgent decisions, should a patient's course go awry.[33] The exact order and conduct of an advanced care planning conversation will vary based on the patient and clinician, their relationship, and the urgency of the clinical situation.

1. Obtain permission: an emotional warning shot, asking permission is critical before delivering emotionally charged news and contemplating difficult options. Opening a discussion with a patient about their future care wishes, anticipated prognosis, and current condition should only occur with their permission. In the nonurgent setting, a warning shot at an initial visit followed by a scheduled follow-up may be prudent. Part of this phase is assuring that the people pertinent to the discussion (eg, spouse, partner, children) are present and appropriately prepared. If a formal surrogate decision maker has been established, it is critical for this person to be involved.
2. Establish their understanding of the clinical situation and future prognosis: open-ended questions, teach-backs, and active listening will allow clinicians to meet patients and surrogates at their current level of understanding and neither repeat known information nor presume understanding.
3. Provide specific information about prognosis and anticipated future clinical course: this must be provided in a culturally sensitive way, with attention to the patient's and family's health literacy, keeping their current understanding of prognosis and anticipated course in mind.
4. Introduce the decision(s) to be made (if any): this is typically conceptualized as a decision regarding the provision of high-intensity or life-prolonging measures (eg, mechanical ventilation, salvage chemotherapy). Although a decision is not necessary at an early stage of the discussion, it is often helpful for the patient and their surrogate/family to frame the rest of the conversation in light of these choices.
5. Explore a patient's values, goals, and beliefs: this is an opportunity to understand a patient's understanding of a "good" outcome and focus on the goals that they seek to reach with further treatment.[34] In many situations, most patients have only thought about this in the abstract and may not have a prepared answer. If answering in generalities, they can be redirected by focusing on their interests, values, and relationships. The key framework to keep in mind is that the patient is the expert on their own life, and trying to understand their values, goals, and relationships will allow a physician to target medical interventions to help them reach those goals or provide the guidance that those goals are not feasible.
6. Make a decision (if appropriate): a degree of nuance and sensitivity is required at this point and the urgency of the decision should be informed by the urgency of the clinical situation. A decision to proceed with an emergency operation versus the decision to proceed with salvage chemotherapy, although both challenging, have different time courses. Pushing a patient or a family to make a decision that they are not ready to make is likely to fracture a carefully constructed therapeutic alliance. If a decision is appropriate, the more specifically wishes are clarified, the

better. It may also be reasonable at this point to select a surrogate decision maker. It may also be helpful to understand the amount of understanding and flexibility that a surrogate has. Preparing the patient and the surrogate for the weight of the decisions that they may face is critically important.

7. Document and disseminate their choices: the multiple documents designed to carry advanced care planning decisions forward are detailed in a subsequent section. It is also important for a patient to disseminate their choices among their family and friends. This helps to lighten the load of the surrogate decision maker and avoids conflict should an untoward or fatal event occur.
8. Review regularly: patients can and do change their minds, particularly as an illness progresses, and especially after experiences in the hospital. In this light, advanced care planning is an ongoing process and therapeutic preferences should be reviewed regularly and with each major clinical change.

ADVANCED CARE PLANNING: DISCUSSIONS WHEN TIME IS SHORT

One of the most common questions clinicians caring for seriously ill patients' field while discussing prognosis is some variation of "how much time do I have?" Although commonly conceptualized by clinicians within a discussion of medical interventions, patients commonly cite interpersonal relationships as the driving factor for wanting to know their prognosis. A large fraction of elderly adults would want to know if their treating physician thought they had less than a year left—in order to say goodbyes, make their spiritual peace, and put their earthly affairs in order.[35] Clinician understanding of a patient's prognosis is critical to being able to communicate it effectively and this is doubly important when time is growing short. A clear understanding of a limited prognosis is critical for advanced care planning and limiting additional medical interventions—both therapeutic and diagnostic.

A shared decision-making model in the face of a prognosis with limited time obligates a physician to give patients as much information as possible to help them make decisions to accept or decline treatments. A bidirectional flow of information facilitates collaborative discussion and it is not uncommon for patients to make decisions in light of limited prognostic information.[36–39] Despite clinician fears, prognostic disclosure does not harm the patient-physician relationship, and actually contributes to improved patient satisfaction, reduces incidence of anxiety and depression, supports a more realistic expectation of the future, reduces use of "alternative" treatment strategies, and potentially creates a stronger therapeutic alliance.[40–43] Delivering an unexpectedly poor prognosis requires a thoughtful approach and the following steps help frame the discussion.

1. Put the prognosis in context: it is rare that a discussion of the anticipated course of a disease happens in isolation and often occurs in the setting of at least some history of cure-focused therapy. Discussions about prognosis are irrevocably tied to discussions of therapy, and the interplay is critical for the clinician to understand before starting the discussion.
2. Elicit patient, surrogate, and family understanding: an often neglected and critical step, starting with broad questions focused on determining if the coming news will come as a surprise or if they are aware of the possibility of a poor prognosis. In the modern era, the overwhelming majority of patients and families seek outside information, beyond the treating clinician, when facing a grave prognosis, and it is very common that they will have at least some concept of what the future may hold.[44] Understanding, framing, and either supporting or refuting the perspective the patient and family have is critical for a therapeutic alliance and future advanced

care planning. Discordance between preexisting understanding and the physician-delivered information can underlie situations in which the prognostic information is rejected by the patient and family.

3. Deliver the prognostic information: after determining how the family would like the information delivered, an honest assessment of prognosis always includes a range of scenarios, ranging from best to worse case and including the most likely scenario.[45] The psychological burden of this uncertainty, which is difficult for experienced clinicians, can be exceptionally difficult for patients and families. The difficulty grappling with the unknown should be acknowledged and the family guided compassionately and thoughtfully. When time may be short, guiding patients and families to focus on personal goals can help to inoculate them against the distressing feelings associated with the knowledge of limited time. The framing of the prognostic information can strongly influence the decisions a patient or their families may or may not make. A mindful clinician will frame prognostic estimates in both positive and negative light (within 6 months, 70% of patients with this problem will be dead and 30% will remain alive), as well as stressing that they are providing an estimate based on experience with similar patients in the past.
4. Respond to the emotions: grim prognoses often trigger strong and negative reactions. Physicians need to be sensitive to this distress and remain physically and emotional available for support. The NURSE mnemonic of emotional response (Name-Understand-Respect-Support-Explore) model can be a helpful framework in this setting. There is an overwhelming desire that is driven by deeply held altruistic values, to try to minimize the hurt associated with a grim prognosis. It is critically important not to offer false hope to patients or their families. The underlying truth of the clinical situation cannot be changed, and providing false hope prevents patients and their families from preparing for impending death.
5. Plan for the next steps: the delivery of bad news and a grim prognosis is not the end of a therapeutic clinical relationship. It is incredibly important to plan for follow-up, either in the outpatient or inpatient setting, to answer questions, clarify the prognosis, or provide additional support as the patient and family grapple with the prognosis.

ADVANCED CARE PLANNING: DOCUMENTS

The advanced care planning process can result in a formal document, which can take several forms and carry varying degrees of legal weight. Unfortunately, only about 1 in 3 patients will have completed an advanced directive or living will before presenting with a serious medical condition.[46] It is important to remember that formal documents are typically thought of as implying that an advanced care planning discussion has taken place, but a document necessarily implies neither a full advanced care planning discussion has taken place nor does the discussion always yield a formal advance care plan document. These documents are not the primary goal of the discussion because the intent of an advanced care planning meeting is to ensure that a patient's treatment team understands their values, priorities, and goals, and supports the patient in choosing or deciding to pursue medical interventions that are in pursuit of the same.[33]

It is also important to keep in mind that formal documentation of advanced care planning discussions are typically acted on only when patients have lost the ability to make decisions for themselves, and thus can be revoked by a patient with decision-making capacity or their surrogate at any time. It is important to recall that, whereas this is generally true, there are documents that ask patients if they want their surrogate to take effect before the moment of incapacity or only after they are deemed to lack capacity, and review of the wording of any document is strongly advised. That being said, a successful advanced care planning meeting assures that not only the physicians, patient, and family present talk about future care, but that those wishes can be recorded and memorialized in a way that they will follow a patient across their journey through the health care system and be easily obtainable in an urgent situation.[22] With increasing access to the electronic medical record, advanced care planning documents should be uploaded in a format that maximizes accessibility for all.

One of the biggest concerns about the formal documentation that accompanies advanced care planning is assuring that they are honored when they are needed most. In a survey of physicians using a series of hypothetical scenarios and a conflict between the advanced care planning documentation, the prognosis, and family/friend input—there was adherence to patient's documented wishes less than half the time.[47] These data suggest that physicians appear to consider information in addition to the documentation when helping to guide care for patients who cannot speak for themselves. Although the ethical implications of this finding are likely outside the scope of this article, it is important to recall that these advanced care planning documents are the patient reaching forward in time to make their wishes known and should be given the appropriate weighting. This section is meant as an introduction for medical professionals and not as an authoritative legal resource.

1. Durable Power of Attorney for Healthcare, also known as a Healthcare Proxy or Health Care Power of Attorney: these documents record a patient's choice of a designated proxy and are signed legal documents that authorize one person to make the medical decisions on another's behalf.[48] In addition to this, these documents can provide guidance to the medical teams and surrogate decision maker(s) when a clinical situation does not exactly match previous discussions. Within the United States, individual states have specific forms, and it is advisable to use a state-specific form to reduce the chances of a challenge to a patient's selected surrogate. In an ideal world, at the time a Healthcare Durable Power of Attorney is enacted, the patient would have a discussion with their surrogate regarding their preferences for health care in the event of an incapacitating illness, severe injury, or prolonged disability, although this is not mandatory.
2. Living Will: this is a document expressing patient preferences for life-sustaining treatments and cardiopulmonary resuscitation (CPR) as well as for future medical care in general. Typically written to take effect in the setting of a terminal or profound illness/injury with limited chance for a recovery, they are often designed to limit heroic, invasive, and low-benefit interventions at the end of life. The ideally constructed living will details not only a patient's wishes for CPR and other life-sustaining medical treatment, but also their preferences in a wide range of medical situations. These documents can be limited in applicability, as they may not detail a course of action for every scenario and there are typically state laws guiding their implementation and design. Importantly, the preferences described in a living will cannot necessarily be extrapolated to inform related but not prespecified decisions. Surrogates may, however, draw on the living will as a guide to a patient's preferences.[49]
3. Physician/Practitioner/Provider Orders of Life Sustaining Treatment (POLST) or Medical Orders for Life Sustaining Treatment (MOLST) form: in distinction to Living Wills and Health Care Power of Attorney designations, POLST/MOLST forms are a coordinated effort across the spectrum of care to create a form that can be rapidly identified, interpreted, and used by paramedics, emergency

department staff, residential facilities, surgeons, and critical care physicians. Established and supported in the United States on the state level, POLST/MOLST forms do have a degree of variation across states. Although limited in scope, POLST/MOLST forms are medical orders, signed by practitioners, and portable in the 40 states where programs have been established.[50] The POLST/MOLST form is designed to ensure that patients' preferences to use or limit life-sustaining medical treatments are equally honored, regardless of their physical location.[51] This means that these orders can be applied in all health care facilities and by all emergency services in the region where they are recognized.[52] Building a consistent system and supporting wide training of a broad swathe of medical providers is imperative.[53] The implementation of this system in Oregon resulted in nearly two-thirds of Oregonians who died in 2013, dying at home, whereas only 40% of persons in the rest of the United States did so. The rate of intensive care unit use in the last 30 days of life in Oregon was 18%, compared with 23% in Washington and 29% in the rest of the United States.[53] POLST/MOLST programs fill an important gap where other advanced directive documents fail, namely limiting unwanted resuscitative measures in the urgent/emergent setting when patients are unable to speak reliably for themselves.[51,54] The POLST/MOLST Web site (www.POLST.org) has sample downloadable forms, educational materials, descriptions of the core elements of a POLST/MOLST paradigm program, and information on how to build the coalition of health care professionals necessary to start such a program. POLST/MOLST forms are generally applicable for patients who have a reasonably serious illness or frailty, and their treating practitioner would not be surprised if they died in the coming year. Although a firm declaration of prognosis is not required for a POLST/MOLST form, these are documents designed to apply to patients with a relatively limited life expectancy and thus may not be universally applicable.

4. Others: it should be noted that other instruments exist; however, they are either uncommon or limited in their application. They are included here to provide a picture of the diversity of advanced care planning tools available.
   - Five Wishes: a program of the Aging with Dignity project, "Five Wishes" is a legal advanced directive that is, designed specifically for the lay public to help them decide what is important to them. It specifically speaks to medical, personal, emotional, and spiritual wishes at the end of life, and helps the patient structure discussions with their family and physicians.
   - Values History: a document that seeks to ascertain which facets of life are most important to a given individual to help define their preferences around the time of death. Although important to explore with a patient, it is not clear whether the document is useful to physicians at the bedside.
   - Combined Directives: an increasingly common combination of a living will, Durable Power of Attorney, and values history. A single document that meets many advanced care planning needs, clinicians are encouraged to see if combined directives meet local statutory requirements.
   - Instructional Directives: proposed in an attempt to avoid the limitations of the living will, these ask patients to decide in advance which of multiple options they would prefer in a variety of hypothetical scenarios. Although very detailed, it is also a large and complicated document that may overwhelm a patient's ability to complete it, and does not address declining function in the later years of life. There is also no discussion of the goal of the interventions and no potential to distinguish between short-term and long-term use of an intervention for a potentially reversible versus chronically progressive condition.

PITFALLS IN ADVANCED CARE PLANNING

1. Not starting or starting the discussion too late: one of the biggest challenges to a thoughtful and empathetic advanced care planning process is getting started. Too often, the unfounded fears about removing hope or harm to the physician-patient relationship keep clinicians from beginning. The best advanced care planning discussions are longitudinal and require several visits or discussions over a period of time. Failing to undertake an advanced care planning process in a seriously ill patient is planning for them to have a time-pressured conversation at the time of decompensation. In a Cochrane review of decision aids, most studies demonstrated that shared decision making added no additional time from the usual care model.[55] Most importantly, the skills to navigate these discussions can be learned and practiced.[56]
2. Expecting a "home run": once the conversation has been started, the astute clinician understands that advanced care planning often extends over the course of multiple conversations. It is frequently not possible to address all issues in the same encounter, particularly when the initial impetus for the conversation is the delivery of serious news. Often the delivery of this news and the emotional response take up the entirety of the emotional and intellectual energy of participants. Clinicians need to be mindful of patients being overwhelmed with serious news and not having the intellectual facility to process more information and engage in serious decision making. Goals, decision making, and surrogacy discussions therefore need to be deferred. In these situations, matching information delivery, processing, and content to the mindset and emotional state of the patient and their family/surrogates is key.
3. Biasing the conversation based on their own beliefs: this often is manifested when clinicians use "goals of care" as a euphemism for a discussions about comfort-focused measures. Clinicians often have firmly held beliefs about what is reasonable, appropriate, and compassionate in the setting of a seriously ill patient, but it is imperative that their personal beliefs do not bias the discussion and exploration of a patient's values. This can be particularly difficult when families or patients ask a variation of "what would you do?" Keeping in mind that a significant fraction of patients would depart from their initial preference to follow a recommendation by a physician, answering this question requires skill and tact.[57] Drawing from the psychiatry literature, it may be best to avoid answering the question directly but to explore the reasons they asked it and emphasize the need to align medical decisions to the values of the PATIENT and not the physician.[58] In this same vein, clinicians must acknowledge their own feelings during serious clinical decline, or when a patient is dying, as these events prompt self-blame when the reality is that the underlying disease is progressive and incurable.[10,59]
4. Fear of removing hope: in the setting of a seriously ill patient, the hope for cure or return to a pre-illness/pre-injury state of health may be slim to none. Even in this setting, surgeons will sometimes err on the side of offering operative intervention, despite the knowledge that operative intervention would be nonbeneficial, for fear of removing hope.[10] Accurately reflecting the current situation and anticipated future course is particularly challenging in the end stages of a chronically deteriorating illness, such as cancer, which is commonly conceptualized as a "battle" and transitioning away from cure-based therapies is equated with "surrendering." This often is framed in the setting of "he/she is a fighter" and acknowledging that staying focused on achieving the patient's goals in

the reality of the situation is critical.[59] This fear is likely overexaggerated as providing high-quality palliative care promotes stronger clinician-patient relationships, reduces fragmentation of care, and can easily be integrated with other therapeutic interventions.[3,5] Prognostic disclosures, if done well, actually contribute to improved patient satisfaction, reduced incidence of anxiety and depression, a more realistic expectation of the future, and potentially a stronger therapeutic alliance.[40–43]

5. Outside pressure: the relationship between a given patient and their treatment team should be inviolate. The reality of modern medical care is that clinicians often feel pressure from administrators, insurance companies, referring physicians, their own conceptualization of profession obligations, and lawyers. In particular, trauma and vascular surgeons involved in the care of critically ill and complex patients commonly report external pressure to operate in situation in which an operation is not expected to be beneficial; neither changing the ultimate outcome nor providing palliation. This pressure comes not only from patients and their families but also from referring physicians and their own conceptualization of professional responsibility.[10,60] Exploring a patient's values and goals early in the clinical course is likely the best bulwark against these pressures, as it frames the entire conversation about interventions and care within the patient's overall goals. In particularly dire situations, inclusion of a palliative care consultation service or a trusted partner can help to defend against outside decision-making pressures.

SUMMARY

The biggest mistake that clinicians make when considering a patient's goals of care is failing to start the advanced care planning process. Deciding to begin planning for the future is as simple as asking patients what matters most to them, what they are afraid of, and who they would want to speak for them if they would not be able to. Within an elective setting, in a nonseriously ill patient, this often is enough to open a goals of care discussion. As patients progress through increasing severity of illness and are faced with abrupt deteriorations, time-pressured discussions about high-risk/low-reward interventions can be based on that initial understanding of values, hopes, and fears. All physicians who care for patients who are, or may become, seriously ill are strongly encouraged to take advantage of periods of clinical calm to start the advanced care planning process (**Box 1**).

Box 1
Resource guide

POLST/MOLST Web sites

- https://www.health.ny.gov/professionals/patients/patient_rights/molst/
- https://www.health.ny.gov/forms/doh-5003.pdf
- https://oregonpolst.org/

Five Wishes Web site

- https://fivewishes.org/shop/order/product/five-wishes

There are myriad guides available in the professional and popular literature that provide guidelines to conduct goals of care discussions. In addition to the approach presented in this article, the approach of the Vital Talk consortium, a nonprofit focused on disseminating research into patient communication, is particularly instructive.

- https://www.vitaltalk.org/topics/reset-goals-of-care/

REFERENCES

1. Organization WH. WHO Definition of Palliative Care. Available at: http://www.who.int/cancer/palliative/definition/en/. Accessed November 20, 2018.
2. Care NCfHaP. Clinical practice guidelines for quality palliative care. 4th edition. Richmond (VA): National Consensus Project for Quality Palliative Care; 2018.
3. Quill TE, Abernethy AP. Generalist plus specialist palliative care–creating a more sustainable model. N Engl J Med 2013;368(13):1173–5.
4. Weissman DE, Meier DE. Identifying patients in need of a palliative care assessment in the hospital setting: a consensus report from the Center to Advance Palliative Care. J Palliat Med 2011;14(1):17–23.
5. Scibetta C, Kerr K, McGuire J, et al. The costs of waiting: implications of the timing of palliative care consultation among a cohort of decedents at a comprehensive cancer center. J Palliat Med 2016;19(1):69–75.
6. Shah KK, Tsuchiya A, Wailoo AJ. Valuing health at the end of life: a review of stated preference studies in the social sciences literature. Soc Sci Med 2018; 204:39–50.
7. Olsen JA. Priority preferences: "end of life" does not matter, but total life does. Value Health 2013;16(6):1063–6.
8. Kwok AC, Semel ME, Lipsitz SR, et al. The intensity and variation of surgical care at the end of life: a retrospective cohort study. Lancet 2011;378(9800):1408–13.
9. Politi MC, Studts JL, Hayslip JW. Shared decision making in oncology practice: what do oncologists need to know? Oncologist 2012;17(1):91–100.
10. Morris RS, Ruck JM, Conca-Cheng AM, et al. Shared decision-making in acute surgical illness: the surgeon's perspective. J Am Coll Surg 2018;226(5):784–95.
11. Detering KM, Hancock AD, Reade MC, et al. The impact of advance care planning on end of life care in elderly patients: randomised controlled trial. BMJ 2010; 340:c1345.
12. Hammes BJ, Rooney BL. Death and end-of-life planning in one midwestern community. Arch Intern Med 1998;158(4):383–90.
13. Molloy DW, Guyatt GH, Russo R, et al. Systematic implementation of an advance directive program in nursing homes: a randomized controlled trial. JAMA 2000; 283(11):1437–44.
14. Teno JM, Gruneir A, Schwartz Z, et al. Association between advance directives and quality of end-of-life care: a national study. J Am Geriatr Soc 2007;55(2): 189–94.
15. Wright AA, Zhang B, Ray A, et al. Associations between end-of-life discussions, patient mental health, medical care near death, and caregiver bereavement adjustment. JAMA 2008;300(14):1665–73.
16. Brinkman-Stoppelenburg A, Rietjens JA, van der Heide A. The effects of advance care planning on end-of-life care: a systematic review. Palliat Med 2014;28(8): 1000–25.
17. Auriemma CL, Nguyen CA, Bronheim R, et al. Stability of end-of-life preferences: a systematic review of the evidence. JAMA Intern Med 2014;174(7):1085–92.
18. Kim YS, Escobar GJ, Halpern SD, et al. The natural history of changes in preferences for life-sustaining treatments and implications for inpatient mortality in younger and older hospitalized adults. J Am Geriatr Soc 2016;64(5):981–9.
19. Messinger-Rapport BJ, Baum EE, Smith ML. Advance care planning: beyond the living will. Cleve Clin J Med 2009;76(5):276–85.
20. Bischoff K, O'Riordan DL, Marks AK, et al. Care planning for inpatients referred for palliative care consultation. JAMA Intern Med 2018;178(1):48–54.

21. Tulsky JA. Beyond advance directives: importance of communication skills at the end of life. JAMA 2005;294(3):359–65.
22. Hickman SE, Hammes BJ, Moss AH, et al. Hope for the future: achieving the original intent of advance directives. Hastings Cent Rep 2005. Spec No:S26-S30.
23. Marson DC, Hawkins L, McInturff B, et al. Cognitive models that predict physician judgments of capacity to consent in mild Alzheimer's disease. J Am Geriatr Soc 1997;45(4):458–64.
24. Voss H, Vogel A, Wagemans AMA, et al. Advance care planning in palliative care for people with intellectual disabilities: a systematic review. J Pain Symptom Manage 2017;54(6):938–60.e1.
25. Yun YH, Kwon YC, Lee MK, et al. Experiences and attitudes of patients with terminal cancer and their family caregivers toward the disclosure of terminal illness. J Clin Oncol 2010;28(11):1950–7.
26. Hornung CA, Eleazer GP, Strothers HS 3rd, et al. Ethnicity and decision-makers in a group of frail older people. J Am Geriatr Soc 1998;46(3):280–6.
27. Blank K, Robison J, Doherty E, et al. Life-sustaining treatment and assisted death choices in depressed older patients. J Am Geriatr Soc 2001;49(2):153–61.
28. Seckler AB, Meier DE, Mulvihill M, et al. Substituted judgment: how accurate are proxy predictions? Ann Intern Med 1991;115(2):92–8.
29. Uhlmann RF, Pearlman RA. Perceived quality of life and preferences for life-sustaining treatment in older adults. Arch Intern Med 1991;151(3):495–7.
30. Emanuel EJ, Emanuel LL. Proxy decision making for incompetent patients. An ethical and empirical analysis. JAMA 1992;267(15):2067–71.
31. Shalowitz DI, Garrett-Mayer E, Wendler D. The accuracy of surrogate decision makers: a systematic review. Arch Intern Med 2006;166(5):493–7.
32. Lynn J. Conflicts of interest in medical decision-making. J Am Geriatr Soc 1988; 36(10):945–50.
33. Sudore RL, Fried TR. Redefining the "planning" in advance care planning: preparing for end-of-life decision making. Ann Intern Med 2010;153(4):256–61.
34. Moore CD, Reynolds AM. Clinical update: communication issues and advance care planning. Semin Oncol Nurs 2013;29(4):e1–12.
35. Ahalt C, Walter LC, Yourman L, et al. "Knowing is better": preferences of diverse older adults for discussing prognosis. J Gen Intern Med 2012;27(5):568–75.
36. Moulton B, King JS. Aligning ethics with medical decision-making: the quest for informed patient choice. J Law Med Ethics 2010;38(1):85–97.
37. King JS, Moulton BW. Rethinking informed consent: the case for shared medical decision-making. Am J Law Med 2006;32(4):429–501.
38. Weeks JC, Catalano PJ, Cronin A, et al. Patients' expectations about effects of chemotherapy for advanced cancer. N Engl J Med 2012;367(17):1616–25.
39. Soylu C, Babacan T, Sever AR, et al. Patients' understanding of treatment goals and disease course and their relationship with optimism, hope, and quality of life: a preliminary study among advanced breast cancer outpatients before receiving palliative treatment. Support Care Cancer 2016;24(8):3481–8.
40. Chochinov HM, Tataryn DJ, Wilson KG, et al. Prognostic awareness and the terminally ill. Psychosomatics 2000;41(6):500–4.
41. Enzinger AC, Zhang B, Schrag D, et al. Outcomes of prognostic disclosure: associations with prognostic understanding, distress, and relationship with physician among patients with advanced cancer. J Clin Oncol 2015;33(32):3809–16.
42. Fenton JJ, Duberstein PR, Kravitz RL, et al. Impact of prognostic discussions on the patient-physician relationship: prospective cohort study. J Clin Oncol 2018; 36(3):225–30.

43. Pruyn JF, Rijckman RM, van Brunschot CJ, et al. Cancer patients' personality characteristics, physician-patient communication and adoption of the Moerman diet. Soc Sci Med 1985;20(8):841–7.
44. Boyd EA, Lo B, Evans LR, et al. "It's not just what the doctor tells me:" factors that influence surrogate decision-makers' perceptions of prognosis. Crit Care Med 2010;38(5):1270–5.
45. Taylor LJ, Nabozny MJ, Steffens NM, et al. A framework to improve surgeon communication in high-stakes surgical decisions: best case/worst case. JAMA Surg 2017;152(6):531–8.
46. Yadav KN, Gabler NB, Cooney E, et al. Approximately one in three US adults completes any type of advance directive for end-of-life care. Health Aff (Millwood) 2017;36(7):1244–51.
47. Hardin SB, Yusufaly YA. Difficult end-of-life treatment decisions: do other factors trump advance directives? Arch Intern Med 2004;164(14):1531–3.
48. Sabatino CP. The evolution of health care advance planning law and policy. Milbank Q 2010;88(2):211–39.
49. Silveira MJ, Kim SY, Langa KM. Advance directives and outcomes of surrogate decision making before death. N Engl J Med 2010;362(13):1211–8.
50. Braun UK. Experiences with POLST: opportunities for improving advance care planning: editorial and comment on: "use of physician orders for life-sustaining treatment among California nursing home residents." J Gen Intern Med 2016; 31(10):1111–2.
51. Fromme EK, Zive D, Schmidt TA, et al. Association between physician orders for life-sustaining treatment for scope of treatment and in-hospital death in Oregon. J Am Geriatr Soc 2014;62(7):1246–51.
52. Hickman SE, Nelson CA, Moss AH, et al. The consistency between treatments provided to nursing facility residents and orders on the physician orders for life-sustaining treatment form. J Am Geriatr Soc 2011;59(11):2091–9.
53. Tolle SW, Teno JM. Lessons from Oregon in embracing complexity in end-of-life care. N Engl J Med 2017;376(11):1078–82.
54. Hickman SE, Nelson CA, Perrin NA, et al. A comparison of methods to communicate treatment preferences in nursing facilities: traditional practices versus the physician orders for life-sustaining treatment program. J Am Geriatr Soc 2010;58(7):1241–8.
55. Stacey D, Legare F, Lewis K, et al. Decision aids for people facing health treatment or screening decisions. Cochrane Database Syst Rev 2017;(4):CD001431.
56. Rodriguez HP, Anastario MP, Frankel RM, et al. Can teaching agenda-setting skills to physicians improve clinical interaction quality? A controlled intervention. BMC Med Educ 2008;8:3.
57. Mendel R, Traut-Mattausch E, Frey D, et al. Do physicians' recommendations pull patients away from their preferred treatment options? Health Expect 2012;15(1): 23–31.
58. Mendel R, Hamann J, Traut-Mattausch E, et al. 'What would you do if you were me, doctor?': randomised trial of psychiatrists' personal v. professional perspectives on treatment recommendations. Br J Psychiatry 2010;197(6):441–7.
59. Duska LR. Acknowledging the limitations of treatment: surrendering to reality. Oncologist 2015;20(8):854–5.
60. Pecanac KE, Schwarze ML. Conflict in the intensive care unit: nursing advocacy and surgical agency. Nurs Ethics 2018;25(1):69–79.

Discussing Prognosis and Shared Decision-Making

Joshua Sommovilla, MD[a,*], Kimberly E. Kopecky, MD, MSCI[b], Toby Campbell, MD[c,d]

KEYWORDS

- Shared decision-making • Prognostication • Prognostic awareness • Decision aid
- Best case/worst case

KEY POINTS

- Effective conversations in high-stakes situations share similarities with surgical procedures: they are well planned, follow an organized sequence of steps, and use specific tools and techniques to improve outcomes.
- Responding to patient emotion after breaking bad news is an essential requirement before proceeding to discussion of treatment options.
- Shared decision-making is a communication framework that encourages bidirectional sharing of information and promotes relationship-centered care.
- "Best case/worst case" is a decision-making tool that uses scenario planning to paint a picture of life after a particular treatment choice.

INTRODUCTION

In high-stakes surgical situations, decision-making occurs against the backdrop of patients who face life-altering changes in their health. Whether be due to a recurrent cancer, severe trauma, or high-risk acute or chronic surgical illness, patients and their families are in crisis. Confronted with a situation that belies a simple fix, surgeons struggle to balance the hope of improving a problem with the fear of doing harm and prolonging suffering. Nevertheless, surgeons bear the responsibility of guiding patients through high-risk decision-making in these situations that are both medically and emotionally complex.

High-stakes surgical decisions comprise a portion of a bigger conversation, one that usually begins with reviewing a test result or delivering other news that portends

Disclosure Statement: The authors have nothing to disclose.

[a] Division of Hospice and Palliative Medicine, University of Wisconsin-Madison, Madison, WI, USA; [b] Department of Surgery, Stanford University, 300 Pasteur Drive, H3591, Stanford, CA 94305, USA; [c] Department of Medicine, Division of Hematology, Oncology, and Palliative Care, University of Wisconsin-Madison, 1111 Highland Ave, Madison, WI 53705, USA; [d] School of Nursing, University of Wisconsin -Madison, Madison, WI, USA

* Corresponding author. Ochsner Clinic Foundation, Colon and Rectal Surgery Department, New Orleans, LA 70121, USA

E-mail address: jsommovilla@gmail.com

Surg Clin N Am 99 (2019) 849–858

https://doi.org/10.1016/j.suc.2019.06.011

0039-6109/19/

something serious. The conversations include multiple discrete components: breaking bad news, responding to patients' reactions and emotions, discussing the prognostic implications, reviewing treatment options, eliciting goals and values, making a treatment recommendation, arriving at a decision, and then obtaining informed consent. Surgeons often rely on their training, experience, available standards of care, and evidence-based practice to navigate this tricky terrain with patients. In palliative care training, the investigators learned that it is helpful to organize conversations in distinct phases and apply specific tools to improve communication (**Fig. 1**). The goal of this article is to review some approaches that surgeons can consider for optimizing communication with patients and families in high-stakes situations.

DISCUSSING SERIOUS NEWS

Many of the difficult conversations surgeons have with patients occur in the context of a piece of data, test result, or "news" that portends a serious, life-altering change. This news may occur in a variety of clinical settings, such as a new cancer diagnosis, surveillance imaging results, a serious traumatic injury, or an acute or progressive chronic surgical problem in a highly comorbid patient. Sometimes, patients are in acute pain and distress. Although the surgeons have become accustom to these medically and surgically complex problems on a daily basis in surgical practice, this is a pivotal juncture in their patient's life. These discussions require the same care and attention to detail as an operation, with the steps of the conversation planned and thought-out to the fullest extent possible. As with a complex operation, these high-stakes conversations may take unexpected turns that require slight adjustments to specific content or intentional sequencing of each step in the conversation, but the overall structure generally remains the same. Consider the following case:

Mr Johnson is a 70-year-old teacher who presents to the emergency department (ED) with emesis and abdominal pain. He has a history of stage III rectal cancer diagnosed a year ago. He underwent neoadjuvant chemotherapy and radiation, followed by low anterior resection by one of your partners. He has chronic obstructive pulmonary disease, renal insufficiency (baseline Cr 3.5), and rheumatoid arthritis for which he takes daily prednisone. His last surgery was complicated by pneumonia, a 7-day intensive care unit stay, a month in a nursing home, and persistent hypoxemia requiring supplemental oxygen during activity. You are evaluating him in the ED for abdominal pain and emesis. His computed tomographic scan shows a high-grade small bowel obstruction secondary to peritoneal carcinomatosis with evidence of liver metastasis.

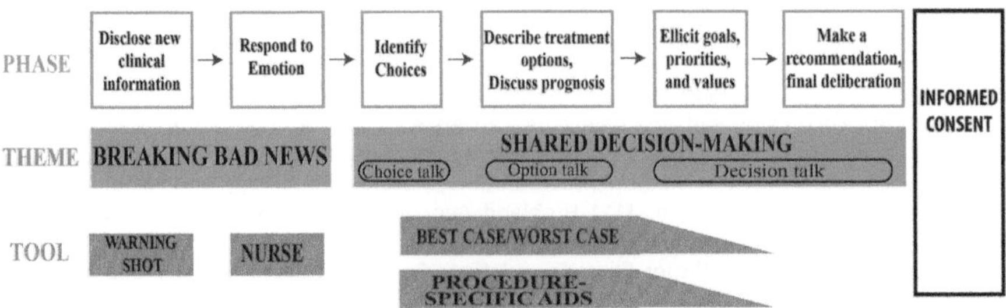

Fig. 1. Organizational guide to breaking bad news, discussing prognosis, and shared decision-making with patients. As conversations progress through phases with distinct themes, specific tools can help surgeons navigate these discussions with patients facing decisions in the context of serious life-limiting illness.

As **Fig. 1** illustrates, surgeons need to cross several hurdles before discussing treatment options and making shared decisions with patients such as Mr Johnson:

- Presenting bad news with a concise "warning shot"
- Responding to the patient's emotional response while avoiding "cognitive traps."
- Asking permission and creating space to discuss the implications of the results

Surgeons should expect a strong emotional response when disclosing bad news. This emotion is sometimes disguised as a cognitive question—the cognitive trap—and physicians can easily fall into the trap by responding to the literal question with medical information and ignoring the emotion (as illustrated in **Table 1**). Responding to the emotion, however, is an essential step for the patient in order to process the life-altering medical news and regain the ability to think clearly about medical decisions. Returning to the earlier case, **Table 1** illustrates a surgeon relaying bad news and responding to emotion.

The NURSE mnemonic is an useful tool that categorizes empathic statements that can be used in emotionally fraught conversations (**Table 2**).

Using these phrases and communication tools such as NURSE allows the surgeon and patient to climb down from an emotionally heightened state and return to a place where practical discussion is more feasible. Patients often initiate multiple emotional statements early in these conversations and may require repeated empathic responses before they are prepared to discuss more.[1] Once the emotion has been addressed, it is often helpful to use a question or ask permission to transition across phases of the discussion.

TAB

In this instance, the question "would you like to talk about what that means?" serves as a transition to discussing the significance of a malignant bowel obstruction. This simple question can be quite effective at creating space for a prognostic conversation with patients and may lessen the likelihood of skipping immediately from the discussion of bad news to "next steps."[2]

PROGNOSTIC TOOLS AND DISCUSSING PROGNOSIS

With the conversation now headed toward discussing treatment options and possible outcomes, we need to be prepared to discuss prognosis. In these circumstances it is important patients understand that life will not be the same, regardless of the chosen treatment. For our patient with metastatic rectal cancer, it is important to convey that the condition is incurable. This may seem intuitive for the surgeon, but prognostic understanding is not inherently obvious to many patients. Therefore, it is important to withhold assumptions and elaborate on pertinent information when patients have given permission to engage in these discussions. A recent review of patients with colorectal cancers showed that nearly 80% of patients with metastatic disease believed that a cure was likely.[3] Prognostic expectations affect patients' treatment decisions, so it is essential to communicate prognostic information clearly and in a way that has real-life contextual meaning for the patient.

The first step in this process is gathering the appropriate information to frame this part of the discussion. Multiple prognostic tools exist to estimate postoperative outcomes for surgical patients and to estimate mortality risk in various terminal medical illnesses. Most of these prognostic tools are available online. The American College of Surgeons NSQIP risk calculator (https://riskcalculator.facs.org/RiskCalculator/) is commonly used and easily accessible for many general surgery procedures. For

Table 1
Surgeon-patient conversation

Surgeon	Patient	Intent
Mr Johnson, would now be an okay time to discuss the results of your CT scan?	…sure.	Asks permission to discuss results and potential bad news
It's not good news. (pause) The scan shows that your cancer has returned. (pause) It's causing a blockage in the intestines which is why you have pain and nausea. [silence]	What? Are you sure? Dr Jones assured me that I was cancer free. I don't understand. *Could you possibly be looking at someone else's CAT scan?*	• Note the concise and measured delivery, done with a thoughtfully measured pace, making sure the patient is ready for the next piece of information. • The warning shot "it's not good news" helps organize the patient's thinking for the news, so they do not misinterpret the test results as good or stable news. • Leaves silence for expression of emotion • Notice the *cognitive trap* in patient response and watch how the doctor does not directly answer that question but rather interprets it as an expression of shock and responds to that emotion instead.
I can see this is shocking. (pause) I wish I had different news.	I was finally starting to feel better. We were making plans to go visit my kids. [turns to wife, starts to tear up]	• Avoids cognitive trap (didn't say, "yes, I reviewed the images with the radiologist myself.") • Names the emotions seen • Notice the surgeon is not immediately transitioning to a treatment plan but leaving space for the patient to process.
You did everything we asked. You did everything right. This isn't fair…	Yeah. It's not. I really wasn't expecting this.	• The surgeon is continuing to provide space to the patient to process this news by using empathic statements, in this case a praise statement and a statement of understanding.
This is really unfair…	Yeah, it sucks… [silence]… but, what do I do now?	Surgeon is assessing the patient's readiness to move into a treatment discussion.

(*continued on next page*)

Table 1
(*continued*)

Surgeon	Patient	Intent
Well, I mentioned before how the imaging shows that your cancer is back and causing an intestinal blockage... Would you like to talk about what that means?	Yes, I would.	• Repeats the news; *asks permission* to move to the next phase of conversation • The "what this means?" question is a convention that creates space to discuss meaning of test results, prognosis, and treatment options while giving patients control over the flow of information
Well, it means the cancer has returned. The horrible part about that is it means it is no longer curable. It also means, because of the bowel obstruction, this cancer is now threatening your life. [silence]		

trauma patients, the Injury Severity Score and Geriatric Trauma Outcome Score both model trauma severity and mortality risk. In patients with cancer, validated prognostic nomograms are available through some cancer centers, including Memorial Sloan Kettering and MD Anderson.

When using these tools and risk calculators, it is important to recognize that they provide information in a physician-directed manner.[4] They speak in the language of percentages and specific complications, which often lack context and meaning if relayed as such to the patient. Cancer survival nomograms in particular are easily misinterpreted by patients.[5] When relaying prognostic information, it is important to focus on outcomes of relevance to the patient: not just survival, but how their life and daily functions might change in the future. When prognostic information is conveyed in the context of a patient's quality of life, the discussion of prognosis and treatment options

Table 2
NURSE phrases for responding to emotion

Skill	Intent	Example
*N*aming	Acknowledge the emotion that you are noticing	"This must be so devastating to hear"
*U*nderstanding	Legitimize the emotion	"Anybody would be devastated to hear this news, it's so unfair"
*R*especting	Praise statements	"You've been so brave through all of your cancer treatments"
*S*upporting	Ally with patient	"This is not what we were hoping for, I will be here with you through this"
*E*xploring	Seek elaboration	"What are you most afraid of?"

Data from Fischer G, Tulsky J, Arnold R: Communicating a poor prognosis, in Portenoy R, Bruera E (eds): Topics in Palliative Care . New York, NY, Oxford University Press, 2000.

often blend together, which promotes decisions that align with a patient's goals and values.

DISCUSSING TREATMENT OPTIONS: THE LIMITATIONS OF INFORMED CONSENT IN PRACTICE

Providing informed consent is an essential cornerstone of ethical surgical practice, but even when done well the informed consent process is not itself adequate for high-stakes surgical decision-making. Grounded in the ethical principle of patient autonomy,[6] informed consent focuses on describing the risks, benefits, and alternatives to a particular treatment. In practice, however, obtaining informed consent is unfortunately often relegated to the most junior person on the surgical team to obtain a signature.[7] Informed consent, when done in this way, often fails to elicit patient goals and preferences, makes no attempt to align treatment options with stated goals, and neglects to offer an informed recommendation. Studies of informed consent for elective and emergency surgery show that patients frequently feel discouraged from asking questions about the proposed treatment options and intimidated by complex forms.[8] In one study, 22% of patients could not recall which type of physician asked them to sign the informed consent paperwork and 18% reported that they were not given enough time to think about the proposed procedure or the consent form document before they were asked to sign it. Even more disturbing, almost 1 in 4 patients undergoing elective surgery and 2 in 5 patients undergoing emergency surgery agreed that they had no choice but to sign the informed consent document.[8] Presuming that legal documentation occurs immediately after an appropriate discussion of risks, benefits, and alternatives, these statistics are sobering. Furthermore, when junior level trainees were asked to list the risks, benefits, and alternatives associated with relatively common surgical interventions, as is done in practice, they were only able to answer questions correctly approximately 50% of the time.[9] When done well by qualified practitioners, informed consent may provide adequate information to patients about a particular treatment option[6] but it is not designed as a tool to support decision-making.

SHARED DECISION-MAKING

Shared decision-making centers around a physician and patient building a relationship during a deliberative process. In doing so, a patient is supported in expressing values, preferences, and "what matters most" to them, while being provided with the information necessary to make an informed decision. As such, it is neither patient- nor physician-centered, but relationship-centered.[10] The communication framework has been conceptually described by Elwyn as existing in 3 phases:[11]

Choice talk: Make sure that the patient is aware that there is a choice to be made. Justify that there is a reason this is a *choice*, there is uncertainty about what may happen, and that the right choice may be different for different people.

Option talk: Describe the treatment options and their likely outcomes. Rather than going over a list of potential complications, patients should understand how different options might affect their day-to-day life moving forward.

Decision talk: Elicit patient values and preferences. Discuss these in the context of the treatment options and likely outcomes outlined in (2), providing support in decision-making.

These 3 phases are helpful in arriving at a shared decision that incorporates the surgeon's medical knowledge with the patient's values.

BEST CASE/WORST CASE: A WIDELY APPLICABLE SHARED DECISION-MAKING TOOL

There are several validated tools and guides available to assist with shared decision-making conversations. Some of these tools are generalizable and can be adapted to different situations in which difficult decisions are made. In the authors' experience, one very helpful such tool is "Best Case/Worst Case" (BC/WC). This is a scenario-planning tool based on Elwyn's conceptual model that was designed for "in the moment" decision-making.[12]

An example of the BC/WC, applied to the previous case, is shown in **Fig. 2**. Although this is shown typed here, the authors have found that this scenario planning is best done as a "live" pen and paper diagram completed either just before or while together with the patient. Another example can be found in a training video at https://www.youtube.com/watch?v=FnS3K44sbu0.

Information is arranged spatially; each treatment option is first listed side-by-side. For each option, a range of anticipated outcomes is represented by a vertical line with a star at the top (best case) and a box at the bottom (worst case). The length of the line can be adapted to reflect the range of the expected outcome for each option. Finally, circle is drawn along the line to reflect the "most likely" scenario anticipated for each treatment option.

For each treatment option, the surgeon describes and writes down the most important practical outcomes for each scenario. While creating the visual tool with the patient, the surgeon is simultaneously creating a verbal narrative of the outcomes described in the tool. This narrative should be rich in information based on the surgeon's experience but should also emphasize the patient experience of the anticipated outcomes.

The BC/WC tool is effective at promoting the "choice" and "option" phases of Elwyn's model mentioned earlier. After creating the tool and the associated narrative with the patient, the surgeon still needs to elicit the patient's values and provide decision support. This can be done with simple open-ended questions, such as "what do you think about these options?" and "what's most important to you now?" After learning more about the patient's values, hopes, and fears, the surgeon can move on to making a recommendation about how to proceed.

In this case, one can imagine the influence on their recommendation if Mr Johnson were to respond to his BC/WC discussion with "well, after spending a month in the nursing home last time, I just don't think I want to go through that again." In this framework, informed consent is still part of the preoperative conversation, but it occurs only after the part of the conversation in which a decision is reached.

PROCEDURE-SPECIFIC DECISION AIDS

One of the benefits to using BC/WC is that it can be adapted to any patient, regardless of disease process or surgical options. For surgeons who treat a narrower range of conditions, more specific decision aids exist or can be developed to improve communication with patients about particular treatment options. Such aids should guide patients facing a medical decision by making choices explicit, providing easy-to-understand information, and aligning patients' goals and values with their treatment options.

Condition-specific decision aids have shown effectiveness in performing these functions[13] and they can be adapted in format and setting. Patients with breast cancer confront complex therapeutic decisions as such; this cohort of patients has been studied in the use of surgical decision aids.[14] In a randomized controlled trial, the use of a "Decision Board" by surgeons during clinic visits improved patient knowledge

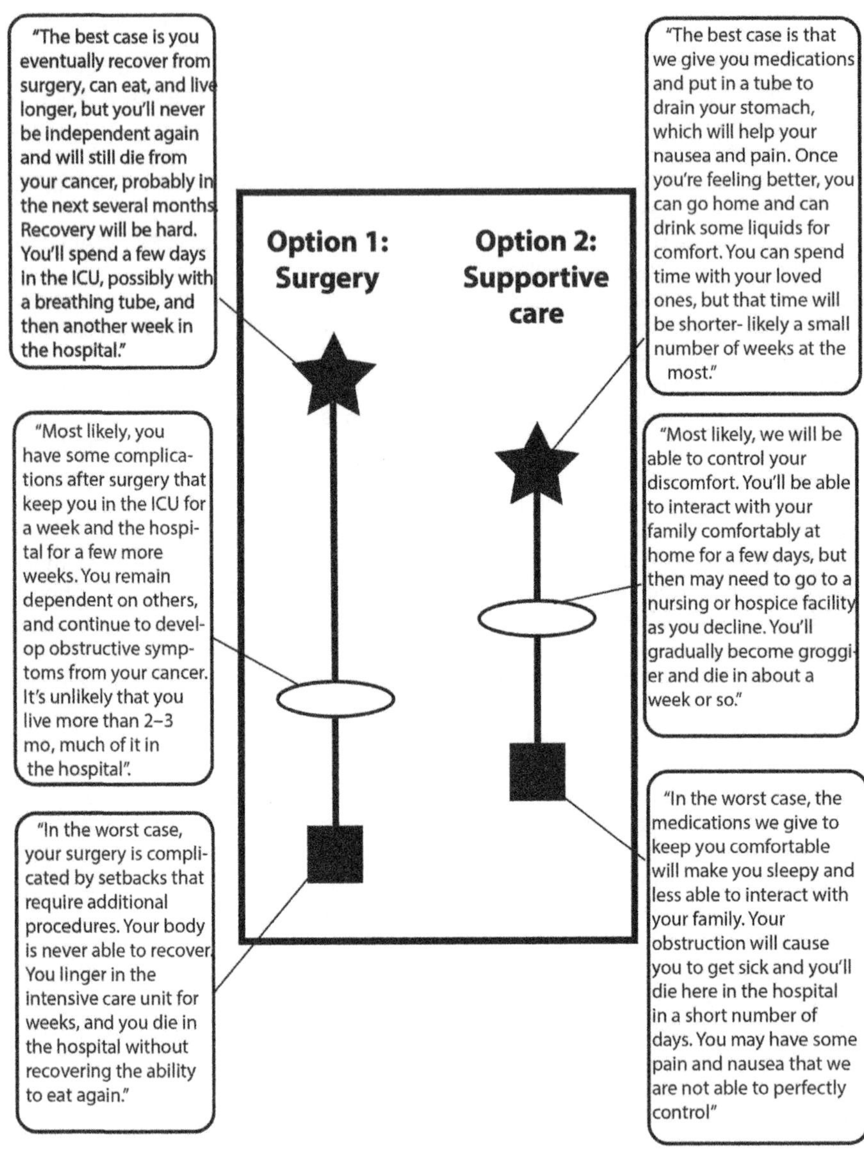

Fig. 2. BC/WC shared decision-making tool. BC/WC visual aid created during discussion with patient. For each treatment option, the star represents the best-case and the square represents the worst-case scenario, with a line connecting the two. A circle is drawn to show the most likely scenario. Notice the line length is longer when the range of anticipated outcomes is wider. In this figure, the texts represent what the surgeon would be saying. In reality, the text on the visual tool would usually be abbreviated bullet points (eg, "Die in hospital").

and satisfaction with decisions while decreasing decisional conflict.[15] The board consisted of visual and written information comparing mastectomy with breast-conserving multimodal therapy under 4 headings: treatment choice, side effects, results of treatment choice for the breast, and results of treatment choice for survival.

Table 3
Supplementary resources

Resource	Where to Find
Best Case/Worst Case	https://www.hipxchange.org/BCWC
NURSE Statements	https://www.vitaltalk.org/guides/responding-to-emotion-respecting/
American College of Surgeons NSQIP Risk Calculator	https://riskcalculator.facs.org/RiskCalculator/
Model of Shared Decision-Making	https://jamanetwork.com/journals/jamasurgery/fullarticle/2701816 (see manuscript Figure)

Other aids aim to promote shared decision-making even earlier in the evaluation process. A web-based decision aid given before their first clinic visit effectively improved patient knowledge and decreased the sense of urgency to make a decision.[16]

SUMMARY

Surgeons take on a great responsibility when guiding patients through major decisions that affect life-limiting illnesses. Sound decision-making in these scenarios requires patients to understand their prognosis and treatment options and surgeons to understand their patients' values and preferences. Shared decision-making provides a communication model that promotes collaboration around this information. By using conversation tools such as "BC/WC" and other disease-specific decision aids, surgeons can promote more effective relationship-centered decision-making with their patients (**Table 3**).

REFERENCES

1. Pollak KI, Arnold RM, Jeffreys AS, et al. Oncologist communication about emotion during visits with patients with advanced cancer. J Clin Oncol 2007;25(36):5748–52.
2. Cortez D, Maynard DW, Campbell TC. Creating space to discuss end-of-life issues in cancer care. Patient Educ Couns 2018. https://doi.org/10.1016/j.pec.2018.07.002.
3. Weeks JC, Cook EF, O'Day SJ, et al. Relationship between cancer patients' predictions of prognosis and their treatment preferences. JAMA 1998;279(21):1709–14.
4. Kopecky KE, Urbach D, Schwarze ML. Risk calculators and decision aids are not enough for shared decision making. JAMA Surg 2018. https://doi.org/10.1001/jamasurg.2018.2446.
5. Balachandran VP, Gonen M, Smith JJ, et al. Nomograms in oncology: more than meets the eye. Lancet Oncol 2015;16(4):e173–80.
6. Jones JW, McCullough LB, Richman BW. A comprehensive primer of surgical informed consent. Surg Clin North Am 2007;87(4):903–18, viii.
7. Wood F, Martin SM, Carson-Stevens A, et al. Doctors' perspectives of informed consent for non-emergency surgical procedures: a qualitative interview study. Health Expect 2016;19(3):751–61.
8. Akkad A, Jackson C, Kenyon S, et al. Informed consent for elective and emergency surgery: questionnaire study. BJOG 2004;111(10):1133–8.

9. Angelos P, DaRosa DA, Bentram D, et al. Residents seeking informed consent: are they adequately knowledgeable? Curr Surg 2002;59(1):115–8.
10. Wensing M, Elwyn G, Edwards A, et al. Deconstructing patient centred communication and uncovering shared decision making: an observational study. BMC Med Inform Decis Mak 2002;2:2.
11. Elwyn G, Durand MA, Song J, et al. A three-talk model for shared decision making: multistage consultation process. BMJ 2017;359:j4891.
12. Taylor LJ, Nabozny MJ, Steffens NM, et al. A framework to improve surgeon communication in high-stakes surgical decisions: best case/worst case. JAMA Surg 2017;152(6):531–8.
13. Stacey D, Légaré F, Lewis K, et al. Decision aids for people facing health treatment or screening decisions. Cochrane Database Syst Rev 2017;(4):CD001431.
14. Waljee JF, Rogers MAM, Alderman AK. Decision aids and breast cancer: do they influence choice for surgery and knowledge of treatment options? J Clin Oncol 2007;25(9):1067–73.
15. Whelan T, Levine M, Willan A, et al. Effect of a decision aid on knowledge and treatment decision making for breast cancer surgery: a randomized trial. JAMA 2004;292(4):435–41.
16. Tucholka JL, Yang D-Y, Bruce JG, et al. A randomized controlled trial evaluating the impact of web-based information on breast cancer patients' knowledge of surgical treatment options. J Am Coll Surg 2018;226(2):126–33.

Perioperative Advance Directives: Do Not Resuscitate in the Operating Room

Michael E. Shapiro, MD[a,*], Eric A. Singer, MD, MA, MS[b]

KEYWORDS

• Perioperative care • Goals of care • DNR • Palliative operations

KEY POINTS

- Important to establish a patient's goals of care before an invasive, operative procedure.
- The Do Not Resuscitate (DNR) discussion is not an aim in itself, but should be the last phase of a goals of care discussion.
- DNR should not be automatically suspended before an operation, but there should be a discussion and a decision by the patient about intraoperative resuscitation preoperatively.
- Palliative operations can be justified in patients with a standing DNR.

INTRODUCTION

Increasingly, surgeons, anesthesiologists, and nurses are confronted with the request to operate on patients with preexisting "Do Not Resuscitate" (DNR) orders (see Framing Case, later in this article). There is much uncertainty and confusion regarding the proper approach to managing advance directives for these patients. Many believe that DNR orders must be suspended before an operation, and there is concern that clinicians put themselves at risk when operating on a patient with an extant DNR order. There are both clinical and ethical reasons, in specific patients, to either suspend, or not suspend the DNR order in the perioperative period, and, most importantly, such

Disclosure Statement: The authors have nothing to disclose. E.A. Singer receives research support from Astellas/Medivation.
Funding: This work is supported by a grant from the National Cancer Institute (P30CA072720).
[a] Department of Surgery, Rutgers New Jersey Medical School, 185 South Orange Avenue, MSB G-526, Newark, NJ 07103, USA; [b] Section of Urologic Oncology, Division of Urology, Department of Surgery, Rutgers Robert Wood Johnson Medical School, Rutgers Cancer Institute of New Jersey, 195 Little Albany Street Room 4563, New Brunswick, NJ 08903, USA
* Corresponding author.
E-mail address: Michael.shapiro@rutgers.edu
; @shapirotx (M.E.S.)

Surg Clin N Am 99 (2019) 859–865
https://doi.org/10.1016/j.suc.2019.06.006
0039-6109/19/

decisions should be the subject of shared decision-making between surgeon and patient, or surrogate decision-makers. In this article, we describe the factors that contribute to these decisions, and current policy.

Attempts to resuscitate or re-animate the dead have been made since antiquity, with occasional success beginning in the eighteenth century. Modern approaches to reversing cardiac asystole or ventricular fibrillation date to the early 1950s, with external electrical pacing[1] and alternating current defibrillation,[2] followed a few years later by DC countershock.[3] Careful reading of these publications reveals that although defibrillation successfully reversed the electrical anomaly, at least transiently, few patients (only 1 of 4 in the initial article by Zoll[1]) survived to hospital discharge. Further, because there were inadequate techniques for effective ventilation and oxygenation, defibrillation was successful only when initiated soon after onset of the arrhythmia. For this reason, it was hypothesized that cardiac arrest in the operating room (OR), where there is continuous observation and monitoring of the patient, would be most amenable to defibrillation and a successful outcome.

OUTCOMES OF RESUSCITATION

Current data on in-hospital cardiopulmonary resuscitation (CPR) are not much improved since the early work of Zoll[2] and Lown and colleagues.[3] Although approximately 40% of patients who undergo CPR in the hospital will have return of spontaneous circulation (ROSC),[4] only 10% will survive to hospital discharge.[5] Of those, only 25% will survive in excess of 5 years, and a significant percentage will be confined to chronic care facilities or have neurologic disabilities. Younger, previously healthy patients, those with witnessed arrest, and initial rhythm of ventricular fibrillation tend to do better.[6,7] Nonetheless, the current public perception of CPR, fueled by TV medical dramas, is that it is frequently (or even usually) successful, allowing most patients to both survive and return to a normal neurologic status.

As noted, electrical defibrillation was initially proposed for a restricted group of rhythms and settings, such as cardiac arrest in the OR. Through the 1960s, however, with the development of more standardized techniques, CPR became routine therapy for any patient who died in hospital. To avoid confusion and distress as to which patients should or should not undergo CPR, the American Medical Association recommended in 1974 that decisions not to resuscitate be formally entered in patients' progress notes and communicated to all attending staff.[6] In 1976, the first proposed hospital policy regarding "orders not to resuscitate" was published.[8] This policy pointed out the "growing concern that it may be inappropriate to apply technologic capabilities to the fullest extent in all cases and without limitation." Rabkin and colleagues[8] also pointed out that "it is the general policy of hospitals to act affirmatively to preserve the life of all patients, including persons who suffer from irreversible terminal illness," and thus mandated attempts at resuscitation in all patients without a DNR order. This created the perverse situation in which resuscitation became the sole medical intervention requiring a written order, and usually patient consent, *not* to perform.[9]

INDICATIONS FOR DO NOT RESUSCITATE ORDERS

When might it be appropriate for a patient, or the patient's surrogate or physician to consider an order not to resuscitate? Respect for patient autonomy recognizes the patient's right to refuse unwanted interventions, and to provide guidance consistent with the patient's goals of care. Cardiac arrest is the final common pathway of the dying process. A DNR order should be merely one, and not the most important, decision that patients and families make in defining their preferences for end-of-life care.[10] When an attempt at resuscitation merely prolongs the process of dying, rather than contributing to meaningful (in the opinion of the patient) life, it cannot be seen as consistent with the ethical principle of beneficence. The vast majority of patients who die in hospital do so with an existing DNR order, and review of these cases failed to find any ethical objections in those patients.[11,12] Briefly, there are 3 situations in which a DNR decision is appropriate[13]:

1. When a patient makes an informed decision to decline CPR
2. In those situations in which CPR is known to be ineffective
3. When the physician and patient (or surrogate, if the patient lacks capacity) recognize the burdens of CPR would outweigh the benefits.

For patients or families to make such decisions, it is crucial for them to have a realistic view of their disease process, the likely outcome of CPR, the chance for ROSC and survival to hospital discharge and the potential morbidity of attempts at CPR, including anoxic brain injury and physical trauma. Indeed, when patients are better informed about CPR procedures and outcomes, fewer are inclined to elect CPR.[14]

An ongoing controversy regarding DNR is the dilemma created when physicians and other clinicians believe CPR to be nonbeneficial, but the patient, or family, insists on resuscitation. Many states permit physicians to institute unilateral DNR orders, with appropriate notification to the patient or surrogate, but some require the order to be rescinded if the patient or family objects.[15] It has also been suggested that an attempt at resuscitation may provide “symbolic comfort” to the family, even when certain to fail, or likely to cause physical discomfort to the patient.[10]

When evaluating the place of perioperative DNR orders, it is important to consider whether cardiac arrest and resuscitation in the OR, interventional radiology suite, or cardiac catheterization laboratory, is different from cardiac arrest elsewhere in the hospital. Both CPR and defibrillation were initially developed for use in the OR, and then spread to other venues in and outside the hospital. Cardiac arrest in the OR may be related to the patient’s underlying disease process, that is, the reason for the DNR order in the first place, or it may be related to an anesthetic or surgical complication. Resuscitative efforts in the OR generally have better outcomes than elsewhere in the hospital (after all, the patient is being continuously monitored, with an anesthetist standing by), and when the arrest is attributable to the anesthetic, the recovery rate can be as high as 92%.[16] In addition, many of the usual resuscitative maneuvers (intubation, ventilation, inotropic support) are a routine part of anesthetic care. The only additional features of CPR are chest compression and defibrillation. Whether a patient wishes an attempt at resuscitation it is not a 1-time decision; it should be reassessed when there is a change in a patient’s status, a new diagnosis, or in their required level of care, which certainly includes the OR.[17] Because the likelihood of success with resuscitation in the OR is higher than elsewhere, the calculation of risk and benefit is different, and the patient may come to a different decision regarding the value of DNR in the perioperative period. DNR does not imply that a patient wishes to die; rather, the patient may believe that the burdens of attempted resuscitation, or of surviving after resuscitation with a greatly diminished quality of life, does not comport with their preference for their end of life. A rapidly reversed cardiac arrest in the OR may portend a better postarrest state than when CPR is initiated on an unmonitored patient after an unknown duration of hypoxia.

A frequent question is why one would propose an operation for a patient with a DNR order. It is important to emphasize that DNR means only that; do not resuscitate. It does not in any way mean “do not treat,” and there are many palliative procedures associated with different levels of procedural risk and requiring various degrees of anesthesia that may contribute to pain relief, quality of life, or longevity, despite an underlying illness leading to the DNR. Such procedures may include tracheostomy, gastrostomy, stenting of ureters to relieve obstruction, fixation of pathologic fractures, or relief of malignant intestinal obstruction. As with any other operation, DNR or not, careful consideration and discussion of risks and potential benefit is critical to avoid unnecessary suffering in patients with a limited life span.

REQUIRED RECONSIDERATION

From an ethical viewpoint, it is inappropriate to require universal suspension of a DNR order before a patient can have an operation, or anesthetic, as it violates the patient's right to self-determination. Further, creating a situation in which a patient must rescind the DNR to undergo a desired procedure is coercive. The first official policy addressing DNR in the OR was promulgated by the American Society of Anesthesiologists (ASA) in 1993,[18] and amended several times since.[19] Similar policy statements were subsequently issued by the American College of Surgeons (ACS)[20,21] and the Association of Operating Room Nurses (AORN).[22] These policies agree that mandated suspension of a DNR order is not appropriate, but that a discussion with the surgeon, anesthesiologist, and patient/surrogate should take place to provide an explanation to the patient about the issues particular to the administration of anesthesia and the proposed procedure, and to ascertain the patient's wishes regarding the DNR order. The patient may then choose to suspend the DNR order, keep the DNR in place, or modify the DNR in some way (eg, if caused by an easily remediable problem, please attempt resuscitation; otherwise, please refrain from such attempts). It also should be determined the duration of the change in status, if any, such as when the patient leaves the post-anesthesia care unit, or has recovered from the anesthetic and/or operative procedure. This discussion must then be documented in the medical record, so that all members of the treatment team understand the parameters of care for the particular patient. There may be members of the OR team who have moral or ethical objections to participating in the care of the patient with a DNR in place; arrangements need to be in place to permit such individuals to withdraw from the case, providing an alternative team member in a timely fashion.[19,21,22]

Despite uniform agreement among the responsible societies 25 years ago, the adoption of these policies for "required reconsideration" has been slow. Between 1991 and 1997, the number of anesthesiology residency programs responding to a survey, and subsequent follow-up, noted the percentage that had DNR policies, and mandated suspension, dropped from 81% to 26%.[23] A significant number of those still with mandated suspension had not revised their policies following the ASA recommendations. Today, still, it is not uncommon for surgeons to be told by OR or anesthesia staff that they need to suspend the patient's DNR before they can come to the OR, even in hospitals that have clear policies to the contrary.

PROCEDURE-DIRECTED AND GOAL-DIRECTED INTERVENTIONS

The discussion and documentation of the decisions about resuscitation and end-of-life care may be documented in several ways. Unfortunately, all too often, the order not to attempt resuscitation is written simply as "DNR." This, obviously, provides little guidance to caregivers as to the patient's preferences and values. There are, in general, two more prescriptive approaches to these discussions, termed "procedure-directed" and "goal-directed" advance directives. Each has its own advantages and drawbacks. The procedure-directed approach specifies, in a check-box, or menu-type form specifically which procedures (eg, intubation, medications, chest compressions, defibrillation) the patient or surrogate believes are, or are not, appropriate. Such a form is particularly useful in the setting in which the staff who are faced with a patient in extremis do not know the patient intimately, where there are frequent shift changes, and where the on-call staff are not the patient's primary physician. The form is clear, straightforward, and easily interpreted by whoever is managing the patient (or, in a worst-case scenario, responding to the code). This approach is without situational nuance, however, and does not explain what sort of result is important to the patient; only what techniques might be used to get there.[23]

The alternative approach, termed "goal-directed," is to discuss, and document, the patient's detailed goals of care, allowing the patient's physicians to determine the best ways to achieve those goals.[23] This method of determining appropriate resuscitative measures requires the care team to have a detailed understanding of the patient's wishes and values, and is thus not useful in the setting of rapid team handoffs. It requires more time to do properly than the procedure-directed checklist, but often provides a deeper insight into the patient/surrogate values and preferred outcomes. In the OR, however, where both the attending surgeon and attending anesthesiologist have had the opportunity to have a real discussion of goals of care with the patient or the patient's surrogate, a goal-directed approach will provide more flexibility, and more accurately provide the care the patient would prefer. For example, a patient might state that he or she most fears survival with a severe cognitive deficit. The operative team would then recognize that the patient would accept resuscitative efforts requiring only a brief period to restore circulation, but not extensive interventions that would sustain life, but at the cost of almost certain anoxic brain injury. This would be more respectful of the patient than a statement or checklist noting "no defibrillation."

SUMMARY

The decision not to attempt resuscitation can be seen as merely one of a constellation of interventions at the end of life that should be considered to respect a patient's beliefs and right to autonomy. Some of those interventions include palliative surgical procedures requiring anesthesia, thus creating the dilemma of how to deal with the simultaneous administration of an anesthetic in a patient with a DNR order. The mandated universal suspension of DNR orders in the perioperative period is not respectful of the patient's autonomy, and often not appropriate to the clinical situation. On the other hand, cardiac arrest in the OR may result from different reversible or iatrogenic events, including anesthesia itself or intraoperative complications, and resuscitation in that setting may have superior outcomes. All of the professional organizations involved in providing treatment to patients in the OR (ASA, ACS, and AORN) have repeatedly promulgated guidelines calling for the establishment of hospital policies requiring reconsideration of DNR orders before operation, and documentation of the discussion in the medical record. Although procedure-directed DNR protocols are simpler to enact, and less ambiguous in the setting of multiple caregivers and frequent handoffs, the goal-directed approach gives surgeons and anesthesiologists more flexibility in providing the care that patients prefer, and is best suited to the operative setting. More extensive education is required of OR professionals and staff to resolve confusion about the appropriate care of the perioperative patient with a DNR order, and to avoid the misconception that such orders must be suspended in the perioperative period.

FRAMING CASE

Mrs. J is a 56-year-old woman who was diagnosed with locally advanced signet ring adenocarcinoma of the cecum in 2002. She underwent a right colectomy with partial cystectomy and adjuvant chemotherapy. In 2009, she underwent radical cystectomy with ileal conduit for localized bladder recurrence with additional adjuvant chemoradiation.

In 2018, she was admitted for a partial small bowel obstruction (SBO) due to tumor recurrence (biopsy proven). It resolved with nasogastric tube decompression. She was discharged to a rehabilitation facility. While there, she completed a MOLST form (Medical Order for Life Sustaining Therapy, sometimes also called a "POLST"; an advance directive indicating that she did not want intubation or resuscitation).

She has been receiving third-line chemotherapy as an outpatient but was just readmitted with a complete SBO. Her surgical oncologist thinks she can perform a laparoscopic lysis of adhesions and ileostomy. Given your expertise in palliative care, you are called to help the surgical/anesthesia/nursing team decide how best to address her advance directives.

1. What options do the patient and surgical/anesthesia/nursing team have?
   Options include keeping the advance directive in place during surgery, canceling the advance directive, or suspending the advance directive for a specified period of time. Required reconsideration is the recommended review process for this scenario. Procedure-directed or goal-directed advance directives can be kept in place.
2. If consensus cannot be reached, who gets to make the final decision?
   The patient or surrogate (if the patient lacks decision-making capacity) has the final word regarding perioperative advance directives. However, the surgeon/anesthesiologist/nurse cannot be forced to violate their conscience or provide care that is substandard or unsafe (such as performing an exploratory laparotomy with local anesthesia only). Providers whose conscience will not allow them to participate in the operation/procedure are obligated to recuse themselves and find an appropriate substitute.
3. What resources are available at your institution to help resolve this type of situation?
   Palliative care or ethics consultation can be a valuable resource. Palliative care specialists (including surgical palliative care providers) also can help explore a variety of surgical and nonsurgical treatment pathways.
4. What recommendations have professional societies (ACS, ASA, AORN) provided?
   The ACS, ASA, and AORN have all explicitly stated that it is inappropriate to automatically suspend a patient's advance directive (DNR). Required reconsideration is the standard of care.

REFERENCES

1. Zoll PM. Resuscitation of the heart in ventricular standstill by external electric stimulation. N Engl J Med 1952;247:768–71.
2. Zoll PM, Linenthal AJ, Gibson W, et al. Termination of ventricular fibrillation in man by externally applied electric countershock. N Engl J Med 1956;254:727–32.
3. Lown B, Neuman J, Amarasingham R, et al. Comparison of alternating current with direct current electroshock across the closed chest. Am J Cardiol 1962; 10:223–33.

4. Ebell MH, Becker LA, Barry HC, et al. Survival after in-hospital cardiopulmonary resuscitation. A meta-analysis. J Gen Intern Med 1998;13:805–16.
5. Peberdy MA, Ornato JP, Larkin GLL, et al. Survival from in-hospital cardiac arrest during nights and weekends. JAMA 2008;299:785–92.
6. Standards for cardiopulmonary resuscitation (CPR) and emergency cardiac care (ECC). V. Medicolegal considerations and recommendations. JAMA 1974; 227(Suppl):864–6.
7. Andersen LW, Holmberg MJ, Berg KM, et al. In hospital cardiac arrest: a review. JAMA 2019;321:1200–10.
8. Rabkin MT, Gillerman G, Rice NR. Orders not to resuscitate. N Engl J Med 1976; 295:364–6.
9. Loertscher L, Reed DA, Bannon MP, et al. Cardiopulmonary resuscitation and do-not-resuscitate orders: a guide for clinicians. Am J Med 2010;123:4–9.
10. Burns JP, Truog RD. The DNR order after 40 years. N Engl J Med 2016;375: 504–6.
11. Aune S, Herlitz J, Bang A. Characteristics of patients who die in hospital with no attempt at resuscitation. Resuscitation 2005;65:291–9.
12. Fritz Z, Heywood R, Moffat S, et al. Characteristics and outcome of patients with DNACPR orders in an acute hospital: an observational study. Resuscitation 2014; 85:104–8.
13. Mockford C, Fritz Z, George R, et al. Do not attempt cardiopulmonary resuscitation (DNACPR) orders: a systematic review of the barriers and facilitators of decision-making and implementation. Resuscitation 2015;88:99–113.
14. Schonwetter RS, Walker RM, Kramer DR, et al. Resuscitation decision making in the elderly: the value of outcome data. J Gen Intern Med 1993;8:295–300.
15. New Jersey Register, 10:8-1.1-3 (5/15/95).
16. Olsson GL, Hallen B. Cardiac arrest during anaesthesia: a computer-aided study in 250,543 anaesthetics. Acta Anaesthesiol Scand 1988;32:653–64.
17. Demme RA, Singer EA, Greenlaw J, et al. Ethical issues in palliative care. Anesthesiol Clin 2006;24:129–44.
18. American Society of Anesthesiologists, Ethical Guidelines for the anesthesia care of patients with do-not-resuscitate (DNR) orders or other directives that limit treatment: approved by the House of Delegates, October 10, 1993. Available at: http://www.asahq.org/standards-and-guidelines. Accessed July 11, 2019.
19. American Society of Anesthesiologists, Ethical Guidelines for the anesthesia care of patients with do-not-resuscitate (DNR) orders or other directives that limit treatment: approved by the ASA House of Delegates, reaffirmed October 17, 2018. Available at: https://www.asahq.org/standards-and-guidelines/. Accessed March 14, 2019.
20. American College of Surgeons. Statement of the American College of Surgeons on advance directives by patients: "do not resuscitate" in the operating room. Bull Am Coll Surg 1994;79:29.
21. American College of Surgeons. Statement on advance directives by patients: "Do not Resuscitate" in the operating room. Bull Am Coll Surg 2014;99:42–3.
22. Association of Operating Room Nurses. Perioperative care of patients with do-not-resuscitate (DNR) orders. 1994. Available at: https://www.aorn.org/guidelines/clinical-resources/position-statements. Accessed March 14, 2019.
23. Truog RD, Waisel DB, Burns JP. DNR in the OR; a goal-directed approach. Anesthesiology 1999;90:289–95.

Optimizing Pain Control During the Opioid Epidemic

Calista M. Harbaugh, MD[a,*], Pasithorn A. Suwanabol, MD, MS[a,b]

KEYWORDS

• Opioids • Narcotics • Pain management • Opioid epidemic • Surgery

KEY POINTS

- Excessive or unmonitored opioid prescribing may increase risk of opioid misuse, addiction, overdose, and diversion into the community.
- A stepwise approach to multimodal pain management should be used, beginning with nonopioid medications for opioid-naïve patients, and adjuvant therapies to address concomitant symptoms, such as anxiety.
- Patients with chronic opioid use likely require dose escalation for acute pain but should be followed closely for adequate pain management and dose de-escalation when feasible.
- Patients receiving an opioid prescription should be assessed for risk of opioid misuse or overdose, and naloxone coprescribing should be considered for high-risk patients.

INTRODUCTION

More than 100 million Americans experience chronic daily pain.[1] Moreover, it is estimated that more than 65.9 million outpatient surgical procedures are performed in the United States each year, resulting in acute pain.[2] Treatment of acute and chronic pain has long been centered on pharmacologic use of analgesics, including opioid analgesics. Opioid overdose deaths have risen drastically over the past 2 decades, however, and the risks of opioid use disorder from prescription opioids are increasingly recognized.[3] As a result, the paradigms from which pain has been assessed and managed are shifting. The purpose of this article is to (1) explore the relevance of the US opioid crisis to surgical prescribing; (2) introduce a stepwise therapy approach to perioperative and nonoperative pain management for surgical patients; (3) discuss nonopioid and adjuvant therapies for opioid-sparing approaches; and (4) review specific considerations for safe opioid stewardship.

Disclosures: The authors have no relevant financial relationships or conflicts of interest to disclose.

[a] Department of Surgery, University of Michigan, Ann Arbor, MI, USA; [b] General Surgery, 112 VAMC, 2215 Fuller Rd Ann Arbor, MI 48109-2399, USA

* Corresponding author. 1620 East Medical Center Drive, 2110 Taubman Center, Ann Arbor, MI 48109-5346.

E-mail address: calistah@med.umich.edu

Surg Clin N Am 99 (2019) 867–883

https://doi.org/10.1016/j.suc.2019.06.002

surgical.theclinics.com

THE US OPIOID CRISIS

Opioid Addiction in the United States

Opioid addiction in the United States has risen since the Civil War era when hypodermic morphine was liberally administered for severe wounds, gangrene, dysentery, malaria, and diarrhea.[4] To address the growing problem of morphine addiction, heroin was developed by Bayer Pharmaceuticals in 1889 as a nonaddictive cough suppressant substitute to morphine. A heroin addiction emerged into the 1960s and 1970s, largely among young minority men in metropolitan areas.[5] Unlike the heroin epidemic of the 1960s and 1970s, in which opioid use was initiated with intravenous heroin, the current wave of opioid addiction is initiated most commonly with prescription opioids.[6,7] Since the 1990s, opioid prescribing in the United States quadrupled, peaking at 81.2 prescriptions per 100 persons.[8]

Pain as the Fifth Vital Sign

Several events contributed to the rise in opioid prescribing. In 1995, "pain as the fifth vital sign" was introduced in the Presidential Address to the American Pain Society, emphasizing the undertreatment of pain.[9] In 2000, Congress declared that the next decade would be the "Decade for Pain Control and Research" and the Joint Commission linked standards for assessing and treating pain to hospital accreditation the following year.[10,11] From 1997 to 2015, the Food and Drug Administration approved more than 263 new opioid-containing medications, including 33 brand name products, such as OxyContin (Purdue Pharma, Stamford, CT).[12,13] These were heavily marketed using inappropriate citations of evidence that the risk of addiction from long-term opioid use was "less than 1%."[12,14,15]

Rise in Opioid-Related Overdose Deaths

Opioid-related overdose deaths closely have mirrored trends in opioid prescribing. Prescription opioid and heroin overdose deaths plateaued at 4.4 deaths per 100,000 persons and 4.9 deaths per 100,000 in 2017, respectively, with 60,000 opioid-related deaths in the United States that year. Deaths from synthetic and semi-synthetic opioids, however, such as fentanyl, continue to steeply rise, with a 70% increase from 2016 to 2017 to 9.0 deaths per 100,000 persons.[3] Opioid use disorder is now the seventh leading cause of disability-adjusted life years (ie, the sum of years of life lost and years lived with disability), and opioid-related overdose deaths have had the largest contribution to loss of life expectancy in the United States.[16,17] Rates of opioid exposure and overdose have increased in young children by more than 200% over the past 2 decades, at least partly due to increased accessibility of opioids in the home, and 160% in adolescents and young adults related to intentional misuse or self-harm.[18,19]

Legislative Response to the Opioid Epidemic

As the risks of opioid misuse and overdose have been increasingly recognized, states have rapidly enacted several policies to curb prescribing and identify high-risk patterns of opioid prescribing and/or use.[20] The most common policies include (1) prescription drug monitoring programs (PDMPs) and (2) opioid-prescribing limits. PDMPs are statewide databases in which all dispensed controlled substances are recorded. PDMPs help prescribers to identify when a patient is receiving prescriptions from multiple providers and help the state identify clinicians who are prescribing inappropriately. PDMPs have been associated with reductions in opioid dispensation and the risk of misuse.[21] Most states now have a PDMP, but policies vary as to requirements for providers to enroll and/or review the data prior to opioid prescribing. Furthermore, opioid prescribing limits vary widely by state. Given that many prescribing limits went into effect in 2017 to 2018, the effects have yet to be studied.

STEPWISE APPROACH TO PAIN MANAGEMENT

Despite the current environment, acute pain is common among surgical patients and must be managed optimally to mitigate the risk of chronic pain syndromes and persistent postoperative pain, which affects 450,000 individuals yearly.[22,23] In 1986, the World Health Organization developed a framework for providers managing chronic cancer-related pain (**Fig. 1**). This 3-step approach encompasses slow and incremental increased use of analgesics, beginning with nonopioids (step 1) and progressing through mild opioids (step 2) to strong opioids (step 3) based on patient-reported pain scores. In the management of neuropathic or nociceptive pain, adjuvants are recommended for patients with concomitant anxiety or depression.[24]

Although this approach was intended to promote comprehensive pain control for patients with terminal cancer, expanded use for patients with chronic noncancer pain has likely contributed to inappropriate overuse of opioids.[25] This stepwise approach to pain management, however, using nonopioid medications first, with use of adjuvant therapies guided by patient assessment, provides a useful framework to optimize pain relief while minimizing the side effects of opioids and risks of opioid misuse.[26] Providing patients with realistic descriptions of anticipated postoperative pain, along with management expectation setting through patient education and specifically written instructions prior to a procedure, may yield the best outcome.[27]

Pain is subjective, and assessment should address total pain and functional outcomes through a multidisciplinary and multimodal approach. Total pain is a palliative

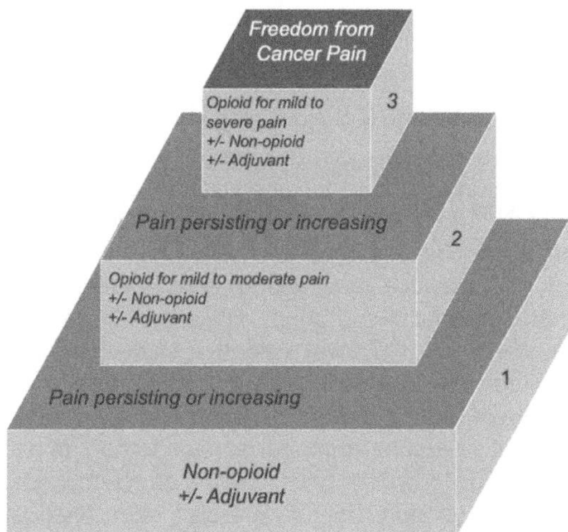

Fig. 1. WHO pain relief ladder. The World Health Organization developed a 3-step ladder to address pain relief in patients with cancer-related pain. Application of this model to non–cancer-related pain has likely contributed to the current overuse of opioids; however, the framework of a stepwise approach to therapy may be useful for the treatment of acute pain. (*Adapted from* World Health Organization. WHO's cancer pain ladder for adults. https://www.who.int/cancer/palliative/painladder/en/. Published 2019. Accessed January 24, 2019.)

care concept that embraces the aspects of a patient's well-being beyond the physical triggers and manifestations of pain, encompassing physical, psychological, social, emotional, and spiritual components.[28] Multidisciplinary care addresses all components through involvement of multiple disciplines, including pain or palliative care specialists, behavioral health providers or psychologists, physical and occupational therapy, and massage therapists. Multimodal therapy uses medications from multiple drug classes that act on pain receptors through diverse mechanisms of action.[26] Consideration of these principles is particularly important in the care of patients with serious life-limiting illness or injury and older adults. Comorbid conditions that include metabolic impairments and cognitive function understandably pose barriers for providers to safely prescribe many medications, however. For instance, older adult patients are historically undertreated for pain and, therefore, stand to benefit from both multidisciplinary and multimodal approaches to functional pain control.

NONOPIOID ANALGESICS

Acetaminophen

Acetaminophen is thought to inhibit prostaglandin formation in the central nervous system. Acetaminophen may be useful alone or in combination with nonsteroidal anti-inflammatory drugs (NSAIDs) for mild to moderate pain. Even for patients who are already on strong opioids, such as in the setting of advanced cancer, acetaminophen may provide additional benefit for pain and overall well-being.[29,30] There is a risk of hepatotoxicity with doses greater than 3 g per day but, with appropriate dosing, acetaminophen may be used long term. Unlike opioids where the dosing is limited by physiologic effects, nonopioid analgesic dosing is limited by end-organ toxicities. Although no benefit of parenteral acetaminophen administration has been shown over enteral dosing, parenteral acetaminophen has shown benefit over placebo after upper gastrointestinal (GI) tract surgery and plays a role in enhanced recovery after surgery (ERAS) protocols when oral dosing is not tolerated.[31–33]

Nonsteroidal Anti-inflammatory Drugs

NSAIDs inhibit type 2 cyclooxygenase (COX-2) enzymes that form inflammatory mediators, such as prostaglandins, in both the periphery and central nervous system. NSAIDs may be useful alone for mild to moderate pain or by providing synergistic opioid-sparing benefit.[30,34] In addition to blockade of COX-2, nonspecific NSAIDs (eg, aspirin, ibuprofen, and naproxen) block type 1 cyclooxygenase enzymes that enable the formation of protective prostaglandins of platelets, the GI tract, and the renal system, leading to platelet dysfunction; nausea, heartburn, and/or GI bleeding; and renal toxicity, respectively.[35] Newer selective COX-2 inhibitors (eg, celecoxib and rofecoxib) demonstrate reduced toxicities than their older counterparts.[36]

Ketorolac is a parenteral alternative NSAID for patients who are unable to take an oral formulation, frequently used in the perioperative setting as a single dose or in a scheduled manner for up to 5 consecutive days. Due to concern for postoperative bleeding from platelet dysfunction, use of ketorolac has previously been limited. A meta-analysis of randomized controlled trials found no significant increase in postoperative bleeding with ketorolac (2.5%) compared with controls such as placebo, acetaminophen, or metamizole (2.1%; $p = .72$).[37] Moreover, postoperative nausea and vomiting may be reduced with the use of ketorolac in the perioperative setting, likely due to sparing of opioids, although this effect is likely dependent on dose and route of administration.[37] Many ERAS protocols now recommend dosing of ketorolac before patients leave the operating room, if not contraindicated.[33]

Locoregional Interventions

Preemptive analgesia with local wound injection of bupivacaine prior to incision may reduce postoperative pain.[38] Intraperitoneal local anesthetic administration also may reduce postoperative pain and facilitate early recovery after major abdominal surgery due to transient blockade of vagal afferents.[39] It is unclear, however, whether the analgesic effect is local or systemic, because local anesthetic levels have been detected systemically within 2 minutes to 4 minutes of a bolus.[40]

Interventional strategies, such as regional infusions (eg, subcutaneous, epidural, intrathecal, or regional plexus) should be considered for surgical site-specific analgesia, in particular major thoracic and abdominal procedures.[41] Neuraxial analgesics may decrease postoperative ileus, pneumonia, venous thromboembolism, and myocardial infarction.[42–44] These findings likely are mediated by reduced systemic opioid use, which inhibits GI motility by activating endogenous opioid receptors in the central nervous system and GI tract.[45] Epidural analgesia with local anesthetics alone or in combination with epidural opioids may also block postsurgical sympathetic hyperactivity, which can contribute to postsurgical GI dysmotility.[45] It is postulated that major pulmonary and cardiovascular morbidity is mitigated with epidural analgesia by enhancing pain management and reducing stress caused by the pain, thus promoting increased physical activity and improved lung expansion.[46]

ADJUVANT THERAPIES

Adjuvant therapies are pharmaceuticals labeled for other indications that are frequently useful in the management of neuropathic or opioid-refractory pain, or treatment of concomitant symptoms, such as anxiety and depression (**Box 1**).[47] Neuropathic pain is caused by damage and subsequent hyperexcitability of nerve tissue, leading to distorted pain pathways frequently described as burning or shooting.

Corticosteroids

Corticosteroids may be used to treat pain, nausea and vomiting, fatigue, depression, anorexia, cachexia, and malaise in the palliative pain management setting due to anti-inflammatory effects, direct effects on pain pathways, and reduced peritumor

Box 1
Stepwise therapy for postoperative pain management

Step 1. Nonopioid analgesic and/or adjuvant therapy

Nonopioid analgesics

- Acetaminophen (oral, rectal, intravenous)
- NSAIDs (oral, intravenous)
- Preemptive intradermal or regional injection or infusion catheter
- Neuraxial analgesia (spinal, epidural, intrathecal)

Potential adjuvant therapies

- Corticosteroids
- Topical agents (NSAIDs, lidocaine, capsaicin)
- Anticonvulsants
- Ketamine
- Antidepressants
- α_2-Adrenergic agonists
- Osteoclast inhibitors
- Medical cannabinoids

Step 2. Short-acting opioid at the lowest effective dose, prescribed according to evidence-based procedure-specific guidelines (opioid-naïve patients) or using the appropriate dose escalation estimate (patients on chronic opioid therapy) edema.[30,48,49] Although there is no evidence to support one steroid over another, dexamethasone is frequently used due to its high glucocorticoid potency, low mineralocorticoid activity, and long half-life for once-daily or twice-daily dosing.[50] Short-term adverse effects include insomnia (mitigated by morning dosing), weight gain, fluid retention and edema, and mood changes. Long-term adverse effects of corticosteroids include immunosuppression, hypoadrenalism, and peptic ulcer disease resulting in GI bleed; these long-term adverse effects necessitate GI prophylaxis for long-term opioid use and ultimately prohibit long-term use specifically for pain management.

Topical Agents

Topical agents may provide local pain relief without the adverse effects of systemic analgesics; however, topical application is supported over oral formulation only if the therapeutic effect is peripheral (not central).[51] There are no data to support topical opioid use over oral formulations.[52,53] Diclofenac, a topical NSAID, has been found more effective than placebo in several acute soft tissue injury trials, without severe GI effects observed.[54,55] Ibuprofen gel has been found to have comparable efficacy to oral ibuprofen, and ibuprofen cream demonstrated a significant reduction in pain scores compared with placebo.[56,57] Although evidence is limited, 5% lidocaine patch may be superior to placebo and comparable to oral pregabalin in the treatment of neuropathic pain.[58] Similarly, capsaicin cream may be more effective in relieving neuropathic pain than placebo; however, a burning sensation may limit use.[59]

Anticonvulsants

Anticonvulsants, such as gabapentin, act by inhibiting certain voltage-dependent calcium channels in the central nervous system. Due to a high safety profile, gabapentin often is a first-line anticonvulsant considered for neuropathic pain. Sedation is the most common adverse effect. Alternative agents include clonazepam or pregabalin.[60,61] Oral gabapentin has been included in multimodal pain therapy in ERAS pathways, but there is concern for risk of misuse and increased risk of overdose with concomitant use of gabapentin and opioids.[62,63]

Ketamine

Ketamine, an *N*-methyl-D-aspartate receptor antagonist, has been studied extensively in the perioperative period. A recent Cochrane review of 130 studies encompassing 8341 patients and a multitude of surgical procedures found that perioperative ketamine may reduce postoperative opioid analgesic consumption, pain scores, and nausea and vomiting associated with opioid use.[64] Ketamine may be effective for management of opioid-induced hyperalgesia by modulating the sensitization process to opioids and attenuating a hyperalgesic response.[65]

Antidepressants

Some classes of antidepressants, primarily serotonin-norepinephrine reuptake inhibitors (SNRIs) and some tricyclic antidepressants (TCAs), may be useful for patients with concomitant anxiety or depression but should not be used in place of analgesics in the setting of perioperative and nonoperative pain management in surgical patients. Antidepressants may also provide analgesia for refractory neuropathic pain.[66–68] SNRIs, such as duloxetine and venlafaxine, provide analgesia but may be associated with sexual dysfunction and altered mentation.[68–70] At doses lower than antidepressant doses, TCAs, such as amitriptyline, nonspecifically inhibit reuptake of norepinephrine and serotonin-enhancing availability of monoamines in descending pain-modulating systems.[66,71] Because of their nonspecific mechanism of action, TCAs have several adverse effects, including cardiotoxicity, orthostatic hypotension, somnolence, altered mentation, and anticholinergic effects (dry mouth, urinary retention, and blurred vision), and are contraindicated with severe heart or prostate disease and narrow-angle glaucoma.

Other Adjuvant Therapies

Other potential adjuvants include α_2-adrenergic agonists, such as clonidine; osteoclast inhibitors for symptomatic bone pain; and anticholinergics, for pain related to a bowel obstruction. Medical cannabinoids may offer another potential opioid reduction strategy where legal (**Fig. 2**) but are primarily considered in the setting of chronic rather than acute or acute-on-chronic pain. The potential harms, however, include cognitive impairment and psychotic symptoms, even in the setting of chronic pain, and must be considered prior to recommendation.[72–74]

SPECIFIC CONSIDERATIONS FOR OPIOID PRESCRIBING

Opioid analgesics may be short term or long acting and carry varying levels of potency. Opioid quantity is communicated in oral morphine equivalents (OMEs) to calculate conversion between the different prescribed opioids (**Table 1**).[75]

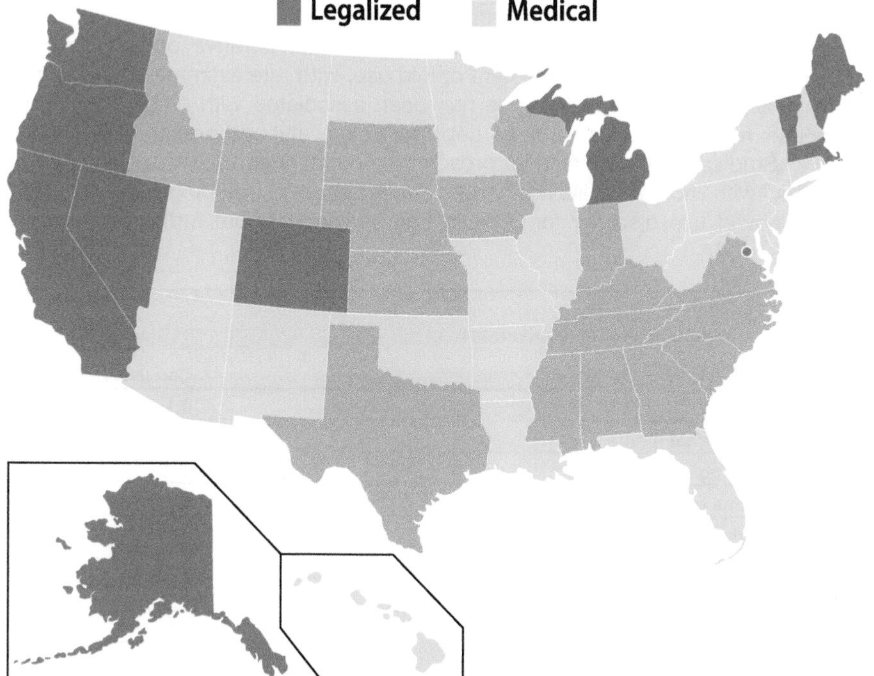

Fig. 2. States in which cannabinoids have been legalized for all or medical purposes only. Legalization of marijuana means that an individual cannot be penalized or convicted of a crime for the possession or use of cannabinoids for any purpose, given that the individual abides by state laws limiting consumption by age, location of use, and quantity. Medical legalization refers to the legalization for patients that qualify for specific medical reasons. Additional restrictions may apply, including on length of use. State designations are current as of February 2019. (*Data from* DISA Global Solutions. Map of Marijuana Legality by State. https://disa.com/map-of-marijuanal-legality-by-state. Published 2019. Accessed February 19, 2019.)

High-Risk Prescribing Practices

Providers are responsible for recognizing and avoiding high-risk prescribing patterns that may be associated with misuse and/or overdose. These include (1) high daily dose greater than 100 OMEs per day; (2) overlapping opioid, benzodiazepine, and sedative/hypnotic prescriptions by 7 or more days; (3) prescribing by multiple providers or filling at multiple pharmacies; (4) long-acting or extended-release formulations for acute pain conditions; and (5) opioid dose escalation by 50% or more.[76–79]

Opioid-Naïve Patients

Although opioids have been a cornerstone of surgical pain management, few data exist to guide how much opioid medication should be prescribed at the time of discharge. More doses of opioid pain medications often are prescribed than patients need,[80] leading to patients taking opioid analgesics for more days than actually needed. Physical dependence (chronic tolerance to the effects of a medication) may occur in as few as 7 days and withdrawal symptoms may be experienced if the medication is suddenly stopped. Evidence-based procedure-specific guidelines for opioid prescription quantity are becoming available and applicable to opioid-naïve patients.[81] Guidelines are meant to provide initial guidance but should be tailored according to postoperative inpatient opioid use and projected time to recovery based on extent of surgery and healing trajectory.[82]

Among opioid-naïve patients with exposure to postoperative opioids, there is concern for transition to new persistent opioid use, with rate estimates ranging from 5% to 10%.[83–86] New persistent use has been associated with preoperative substance use; mood disorders, such as depression; anxiety; and preoperative chronic pain.[83,85] Studies suggest that total prescription quantity and days' supply may be associated with increased likelihood of adverse effects, including new-long term use and opioid use disorder for chronic pain indications, but further evidence is

Table 1
Calculating morphine milligram equivalents

Opioid	Conversion Factor[a]
Codeine (mg/day)	0.15
Fentanyl transdermal (μg/h)	2.4
Hydrocodone (mg/day)	1
Hydromorphone (mg/day)	4
Methadone (mg/day)	
1–20	4
21–40	8
41–60	10
≥61–80	12
Morphine (mg/day)	1
Oxycodone (mg/day)	1.5
Oxymorphone (mg/day)	3

[a] These dose conversions are estimated and cannot account for all individual differences in genetics and pharmacokinetics.

Adapted from Centers for Disease Control and Prevention. Calculating Total Daily Dose of Opioids for Safer Dosage Available at https://www.cdc.gov/drugoverdose/pdf/calculating_total_daily_dose-a.pdf.

needed to understand the thresholds for increased risk among opioid-naïve patients treated for acute pain.[83,87,88]

Patients with Chronic Pain

In 2016, the Centers for Disease Control and Prevention released guidelines for opioid prescribing to patients with chronic noncancer pain. These guidelines should be considered when prescribing for patients with acute-on-chronic pain.[83] Similar to opioid-naïve patients, nonpharmacologic and nonopioid modalities are preferred, with multimodal approaches used when opioids are needed. Immediate-release formulations rather than long-acting/extended-release formulations should be initiated with the lowest effective dose.[89]

Before initiating opioid therapy for perioperative functional pain control in the setting of chronic pain, the treatment goal should be established and an opioid contract should be considered. Opioid contracts, also referred to as *narcotic agreements* or *pain contracts*, are not legally binding documents, and there are no established guidelines on how to administer and enforce them. Rather, opioid contracts or agreements should be considered to improve adherence, obtain informed consent, outline prescribing policies of the provider, and mitigate risk.[90] Urine drug testing may be performed at initiation to assess for preoperative opioid use. Intermittent urine drug testing may be indicated if there is concern that prescribed opioids are being diverted to someone other than the patient to whom they were prescribed.[89] With an established opioid contract, urine drug testing should be a known possibility so that there are no surprises and trust within the doctor-patient relationship is not violated.

Patients with Chronic Opioid Use

Surgeons should expect that patients with preoperative opioid use likely will require dose escalation in the short term to treat acute postoperative pain due to baseline tolerance. In addition, patients on chronic opioids may experience hyperalgesia secondary to long-term opioid use. For breakthrough dosing of enteral short-acting opioids, it is suggested that the dose should remain within 10% to 15% of the total daily dose.[91,92] Again, urine drug testing and an opioid contract should be considered. Clinicians should re-evaluate the benefits and harms of opioid therapy for any patient on opioid therapy at regular and frequent intervals. Conditions and needs change over time, indicating either de-escalation or escalation of dosing for best care.

After surgical recovery, the care transition to a primary care provider and/or pain specialist remains critically important to ensure opioid and adjunct dose escalation is calculated safely, adverse side effects are minimized, and analgesics are continued only as long as necessary.[93] Appropriate de-escalation is necessary to avoid withdrawal effects. Patients on long-acting opioids, such as morphine and oxycodone extended-release formulations, methadone, or buprenorphine, for chronic pain require consultation by palliative medicine or a pain specialist for assistance with dosing. Patients on medication-assisted treatment require consultation with the prescribing clinician for assistance with the inpatient and outpatient transitions in addition to a pain specialist around the time of surgery if on a partial opioid antagonist.

Patients at the End of Life

Pain is a common and distressing symptom for patients and their loved ones; yet, clinicians often lack the knowledge to adequately assess and manage physical pain as well as total pain. For patients with serious life-limiting illness who are transitioning to comfort-focused care, opioids may be appropriate regardless of prior attempted therapies.[89] It is important to recognize the best setting for receiving that care, and referral to hospice is recommended.

SAFE OPIOID STEWARDSHIP

With the ability to prescribe opioids comes the responsibility for safe opioid stewardship, which encompasses not only appropriate prescribing but also assessment for risk of substance misuse and overdose and coprescribing of naloxone for patients at elevated risk of overdose.

Substance Use Risk Assessments

The goal of risk assessment is to identify those at moderate to high risk of future misuse, abuse, and/or diversion (intentional transfer of a controlled substance). Indication of elevated risk should trigger increased preventive efforts and lower threshold for intervention in the setting of aberrant behaviors that do not comply with the agreed-on treatment plan.[94,95] Risk assessment instruments encompass 3 types: (1) misuse prior to initiating long-term therapy; (2) misuse in patients currently using opioids; and (3) nonopioid general substance abuse. **Table 2** provides an outline of commonly used risk assessment tools.

Screener and opioid assessment measure for patients with pain–revised

The Screener and Opioid Assessment Measure for Patients with Pain–Revised (SOAPP-R) is used to assess the risk of opioid abuse in patients with chronic pain. Adult patients with pain not associated with malignancy use a self-reported rating scale, which has been demonstrated to have strong predictive validity, reliability, and internal consistency.[96]

Opioid risk tool

The Opioid Risk Tool (ORT) is another self-reported checklist used for a similar patient population to assess risk of aberrant behaviors when introduced to opioid therapy.[97]

Current opioid misuse measure

The Current Opioid Misuse Measure (COMM) is used in adults with chronic nonmalignant pain already on long-term opioid therapy to monitor aberrant medication-related behaviors. This is a self-reported scale with strong internal consistency and reliability.[98]

Table 2
Examples of instruments assessing opioid and nonopioid risk

Instrument	Category	Number of Items	Administered by	Indicator of Risk by Score
SOAPP-R[96]	Patients considered for long-term opioid therapy	24	Patient	Positive screen: ≥18
ORT[97]	Patients considered for long-term opioid therapy	5	Patient	Low risk: ≤3 Moderate risk: 4–7 High risk: ≥8
COMM[98]	Patients on long-term opioid therapy	17	Patient	Positive screen: ≥9
CAGE-AID[99]	Nonopioid general substance use	4	Clinician	Positive screen: ≥1

Cut down, annoyed, guilty, eye-opener, adapted to include drugs tool
The Cut Down, Annoyed, Guilty, Eye-Opener, Adapted to Include Drugs (CAGE-AID) tool is a commonly administered instrument to screen for illicit or nonprescribed drugs and alcohol. Presence of nonopioid substance use disorders is also a risk for transition to new chronic opioid use in opioid-naïve patients initiated on opioids. Screening for drug and alcohol use can be performed with several instruments.[99]

Naloxone Coprescribing for Patients at High Risk of Overdose

Increased access to naloxone is associated with a 9% to 11% reduction in opioid-related deaths and more than 26,000 overdose reversals since 1996.[100,101] Coprescribing of naloxone is supported by patients, the government, and international health organizations.[89,102–104] Consideration of coprescribing naloxone should be made in the following scenarios: high opioid dosing greater than or equal to 100 OMEs per day; concomitant benzodiazepine prescription; history of substance use disorder; underlying mental health conditions; comorbid medical conditions, such as respiratory disease and sleep apnea that increase susceptibility to respiratory distress; or in individuals who may be able to assist another at risk of opioid overdose.[105] Both patients and providers find coprescribing to be acceptable, and this practice does not have a negative impact on liability risk for providers.[106,107]

SUMMARY

Pain management is a critical aspect of symptom management in surgical care. Although paradigms with which pain management is approached are evolving within the context of the current opioid crisis, the underlying principles of functional pain control remain the same. Acute, chronic, and acute-on-chronic pain management should be managed using multimodal therapy and multidisciplinary care. Approaching treatment plans with compassion and patient engagement may help with early expectation setting and encourage a goal-directed focus. When opioid prescribing is indicated, clinicians should avoid high-risk prescribing practices that are associated with increased risk of opioid misuse, use disorder, and overdose; perform appropriate risk screening; and consider naloxone coprescribing. The opioid crisis has heightened awareness of the risks for opioid misuse, abuse, addiction, and overdose with medical use of prescription opioids alone and in combination with other prescribed pharmaceuticals and recreational drugs and alcohol. Clinicians' duty is to alleviate suffering responsibly and with a multidisciplinary approach so that the most comprehensive patient care is provided, risk of harm minimized, and provider liability decreased.

REFERENCES

1. Relieving pain in America: a blueprint for transforming prevention, care, education, and research. Mil Med 2016;181(5):397–9.
2. National Center for Health Statistics. Health, United States, 2016: with chartbook on long-term trends in health. Hyattsville (MD): National Center for Health Statistics (US); 2017.
3. Scholl L, Seth P, Kariisa M, et al. Drug and opioid-involved overdose deaths - United States, 2013-2017. MMWR Morb Mortal Wkly Rep 2018;67(5152): 1419–27.
4. Courtwright DT. Opiate addiction as a consequence of the civil war. Civ War Hist 1978;24(2):101–11.
5. Greene MH. An epidemiologic assessment of heroin use. Am J Public Health 1974;64(Suppl 12):1–10.

6. Cicero TJ, Ellis MS, Surratt HL, et al. The changing face of heroin use in the United States: a retrospective analysis of the past 50 years. JAMA Psychiatry 2014;71(7):821–6.
7. Muhuri P, Gfoerer J, Davies C. Associations of nonmedical pain reliever use and initiation of heroin use in the United States. Rockville (MD): Center for Behavioral Health Statistics and Quality, SAMHSA. CBHSQ Data Review; 2013.
8. Guy GP Jr, Zhang K, Bohm MK, et al. Vital Signs: Changes in Opioid Prescribing in the United States, 2006-2015. MMWR Morb Mortal Wkly Rep 2017;66(26): 697–704.
9. Morone NE, Weiner DK. Pain as the fifth vital sign: exposing the vital need for pain education. Clin Ther 2013;35(11):1728–32.
10. A bill to designate the calendar decade beginning on January 1, 2001, as the "Decade of Pain Control and Research". In. S.3163. 2D ed2001.
11. The Joint Commission. Joint commission statement on pain management. Oakbrook Terrace (IL): The Joint Commission; 2016.
12. Van Zee A. The promotion and marketing of oxycontin: commercial triumph, public health tragedy. Am J Public Health 2009;99(2):221–7.
13. Chai G, Xu J, Osterhout J, et al. New opioid analgesic approvals and outpatient utilization of opioid analgesics in the United States, 1997 through 2015. Anesthesiology 2018;128(5):953–66.
14. Porter J, Jick H. Addiction rare in patients treated with narcotics. N Engl J Med 1980;302(2):123.
15. Leung PTM, Macdonald EM, Stanbrook MB, et al. A 1980 letter on the risk of opioid addiction. N Engl J Med 2017;376(22):2194–5.
16. Mokdad AH, Ballestros K, Echko M, et al. The state of US health, 1990-2016: burden of diseases, injuries, and risk factors among US states. JAMA 2018; 319(14):1444–72.
17. Dowell D, Arias E, Kochanek K, et al. Contribution of opioid-involved poisoning to the change in life expectancy in the United States, 2000-2015. JAMA 2017; 318(11):1065–7.
18. Gaither JR, Leventhal JM, Ryan SA, et al. National trends in hospitalizations for opioid poisonings among children and adolescents, 1997 to 2012. JAMA Pediatr 2016;170(12):1195–201.
19. Allen JD, Casavant MJ, Spiller HA, et al. Prescription opioid exposures among children and adolescents in the United States: 2000-2015. Pediatrics 2017; 139(4) [pii:e20163382].
20. Parker AM, Strunk D, Fiellin DA. State responses to the opioid crisis. J Law Med Ethics 2018;46(2):367–81.
21. Bao Y, Wen K, Johnson P, et al. Assessing the impact of state policies for prescription drug monitoring programs on high-risk opioid prescriptions. Health Aff (Millwood) 2018;37(10):1596–604.
22. Kehlet H, Jensen TS, Woolf CJ. Persistent postsurgical pain: risk factors and prevention. Lancet 2006;367(9522):1618–25.
23. Peters ML, Sommer M, de Rijke JM, et al. Somatic and psychologic predictors of long-term unfavorable outcome after surgical intervention. Ann Surg 2007; 245(3):487–94.
24. World Health Organization. WHO's cancer pain ladder for adults 2019. Available at: https://www.who.int/cancer/palliative/painladder/en/. Accessed January 24, 2019.
25. Ballantyne JC, Kalso E, Stannard C. WHO analgesic ladder: a good concept gone astray. BMJ 2016;352:i20.

26. U.S. Department of Health and Human Services. Draft Report on Pain Management Best Practices: Updates, Gaps, Inconsistencies, and Recommendations. Washington, DC: Department of Health and Human Services; 2018.
27. Moreno MA, Furtner F, Rivara FP. How parents can help children cope with procedures and pain. Arch Pediatr Adolesc Med 2011;165(9):872.
28. Mehta A, Chan LS. Understanding the concept of "total pain": a prerequisite for pain control. J Hosp Palliat Nurs 2008;10(1):26–32.
29. Stockler M, Vardy J, Pillai A, et al. Acetaminophen (paracetamol) improves pain and well-being in people with advanced cancer already receiving a strong opioid regimen: a randomized, double-blind, placebo-controlled cross-over trial. J Clin Oncol 2004;22(16):3389–94.
30. Candido KD, Perozo OJ, Knezevic NN. Pharmacology of acetaminophen, nonsteroidal antiinflammatory drugs, and steroid medications: implications for anesthesia or unique associated risks. Anesthesiol Clin 2017;35(2):e145–62.
31. Jibril F, Sharaby S, Mohamed A, et al. Intravenous versus oral acetaminophen for pain: systematic review of current evidence to support clinical decision-making. Can J Hosp Pharm 2015;68(3):238–47.
32. Lee Y, Yu J, Doumouras AG, et al. Intravenous Acetaminophen Versus Placebo in Post-bariatric Surgery Multimodal Pain Management: a Meta-analysis of Randomized Controlled Trials. Obes Surg 2019;29(4):1420–8.
33. Helander EM, Webb MP, Bias M, et al. A comparison of multimodal analgesic approaches in institutional enhanced recovery after surgery protocols for colorectal surgery: pharmacological agents. J Laparoendosc Adv Surg Tech A 2017;27(9):903–8.
34. Eisenberg E, Berkey CS, Carr DB, et al. Efficacy and safety of nonsteroidal anti-inflammatory drugs for cancer pain: a meta-analysis. J Clin Oncol 1994;12(12):2756–65.
35. Davies NM, Reynolds JK, Undeberg MR, et al. Minimizing risks of NSAIDs: cardiovascular, gastrointestinal and renal. Expert Rev Neurother 2006;6(11):1643–55.
36. Lanza FL, Chan FK, Quigley EM, Practice Parameters Committee of the American College of Gastroenterology. Guidelines for prevention of NSAID-related ulcer complications. Am J Gastroenterol 2009;104(3):728–38.
37. Gobble RM, Hoang HL, Kachniarz B, et al. Ketorolac does not increase perioperative bleeding: a meta-analysis of randomized controlled trials. Plast Reconstr Surg 2014;133(3):741–55.
38. Ong CK, Lirk P, Seymour RA, et al. The efficacy of preemptive analgesia for acute postoperative pain management: a meta-analysis. Anesth Analg 2005;100(3):757–73, table of contents.
39. Kahokehr A. Intraperitoneal local anesthetic for postoperative pain. Saudi J Anaesth 2013;7(1):5.
40. Kahokehr A, Sammour T, Vather R, et al. Systemic levels of local anaesthetic after intra-peritoneal application–a systematic review. Anaesth Intensive Care 2010;38(4):623–38.
41. Chou R, Gordon DB, de Leon-Casasola OA, et al. Management of postoperative pain: a clinical practice guideline from the American Pain Society, the American Society of Regional Anesthesia and Pain Medicine, and the American Society of Anesthesiologists' Committee on Regional Anesthesia, Executive Committee, and Administrative Council. J Pain 2016;17(2):131–57.

42. Ballantyne JC, Carr DB, deFerranti S, et al. The comparative effects of postoperative analgesic therapies on pulmonary outcome: cumulative meta-analyses of randomized, controlled trials. Anesth Analg 1998;86(3):598–612.
43. Pöpping DM, Elia N, Van Aken HK, et al. Impact of epidural analgesia on mortality and morbidity after surgery: systematic review and meta-analysis of randomized controlled trials. Ann Surg 2014;259(6):1056–67.
44. Mohamad MF, Mohammad MA, Hetta DF, et al. Thoracic epidural analgesia reduces myocardial injury in ischemic patients undergoing major abdominal cancer surgery. J Pain Res 2017;10:887–95.
45. Kurz A, Sessler DI. Opioid-induced bowel dysfunction: pathophysiology and potential new therapies. Drugs 2003;63(7):649–71.
46. Pöpping DM, Elia N, Marret E, et al. Protective effects of epidural analgesia on pulmonary complications after abdominal and thoracic surgery: A meta-analysis. Arch Surg 2008;143(10):990–9.
47. Mercadante S, Portenoy RK. Opioid poorly-responsive cancer pain. Part 3. Clinical strategies to improve opioid responsiveness. J Pain Symptom Manage 2001;21(4):338–54.
48. Vanston J. Corticosteroids- the double-edged sword of palliative care. AAHPM Quarterly. Chicago: American Academy of Hospice and Palliative Care Medicine; 2016.
49. Mercadante SL, Berchovich M, Casuccio A, et al. A prospective randomized study of corticosteroids as adjuvant drugs to opioids in advanced cancer patients. Am J Hosp Palliat Care 2007;24(1):13–9.
50. Uritsky TJ, Atayee RS, Herndon CM, et al. Ten tips palliative care pharmacists want the palliative care team to know when caring for patients. J Palliat Med 2018;21(7):1017–23.
51. Derry S, Wiffen PJ, Kalso EA, et al. Topical analgesics for acute and chronic pain in adults - an overview of Cochrane Reviews. Cochrane Database Syst Rev 2017;(5):CD008609.
52. McCarberg B, D'Arcy Y. Options in topical therapies in the management of patients with acute pain. Postgrad Med 2013;125(sup1):19–24.
53. Jorge LL, Feres CC, Teles VE. Topical preparations for pain relief: efficacy and patient adherence. J Pain Res 2010;4:11–24.
54. Mueller EA, Kirch W, Reiter S. Extent and time course of pain intensity upon treatment with a topical diclofenac sodium patch versus placebo in acute traumatic injury based on a validated end point: post hoc analysis of a randomized placebo-controlled trial. Expert Opin Pharmacother 2010;11(4):493–8.
55. Predel HG, Koll R, Pabst H, et al. Diclofenac patch for topical treatment of acute impact injuries: a randomised, double blind, placebo controlled, multicentre study. Br J Sports Med 2004;38(3):318–23.
56. Whitefield M, O'Kane CJA, Anderson S. Comparative efficacy of a proprietary topical ibuprofen gel and oral ibuprofen in acute soft tissue injuries: a randomized, double-blind study. J Clin Pharm Ther 2002;27(6):409–17.
57. Campbell J, Dunn T. Evaluation of topical ibuprofen cream in the treatment of acute ankle sprains. J Accid Emerg Med 1994;11(3):178–82.
58. Rehm S, Binder A, Baron R. Post-herpetic neuralgia: 5% lidocaine medicated plaster, pregabalin, or a combination of both? A randomized, open, clinical effectiveness study. Curr Med Res Opin 2010;26(7):1607–19.
59. McCleane G. Topical application of doxepin hydrochloride, capsaicin and a combination of both produces analgesia in chronic human neuropathic pain:

a randomized, double-blind, placebo-controlled study. Br J Clin Pharmacol 2000;49(6):574–9.
60. Swerdlow M, Cundill JG. Anticonvulsant drugs used in the treatment of lancinating pain. A comparison. Anaesthesia 1981;36(12):1129–32.
61. O'Connor AB, Dworkin RH. Treatment of neuropathic pain: an overview of recent guidelines. Am J Med 2009;122(10, Supplement):S22–32.
62. Gomes T, Juurlink DN, Antoniou T, et al. Gabapentin, opioids, and the risk of opioid-related death: a population-based nested case–control study. PLoS Med 2017;14(10):e1002396.
63. Montastruc F, Loo SY, Renoux C. Trends in first gabapentin and pregabalin prescriptions in primary care in the United Kingdom, 1993-2017. JAMA 2018; 320(20):2149–51.
64. Brinck EC, Tiippana E, Heesen M, et al. Perioperative intravenous ketamine for acute postoperative pain in adults. Cochrane Database Syst Rev 2018;(12):CD012033.
65. Choi E, Lee H, Park HS, et al. Effect of intraoperative infusion of ketamine on remifentanil-induced hyperalgesia. Korean J Anesthesiol 2015;68(5):476–80.
66. Verdu B, Decosterd I, Buclin T, et al. Antidepressants for the treatment of chronic pain. Drugs 2008;68(18):2611–32.
67. Onghena P, Van Houdenhove B. Antidepressant-induced analgesia in chronic non-malignant pain: a meta-analysis of 39 placebo-controlled studies. Pain 1992;49(2):205–19.
68. Saarto T, Wiffen PJ. Antidepressants for neuropathic pain. Cochrane Database Syst Rev 2007;(4):CD005454.
69. Rowbotham MC, Goli V, Kunz NR, et al. Venlafaxine extended release in the treatment of painful diabetic neuropathy: a double-blind, placebo-controlled study. Pain 2004;110(3):697–706.
70. Wernicke JF, Pritchett YL, D'Souza DN, et al. A randomized controlled trial of duloxetine in diabetic peripheral neuropathic pain. Neurology 2006;67(8):1411–20.
71. Max MB, Lynch SA, Muir J, et al. Effects of desipramine, amitriptyline, and fluoxetine on pain in diabetic neuropathy. N Engl J Med 1992;326(19):1250–6.
72. Lucas P. Rationale for cannabis-based interventions in the opioid overdose crisis. Harm Reduct J 2017;14(1):58.
73. Nugent SM, Morasco BJ, O'Neil ME, et al. The effects of cannabis among adults with chronic pain and an overview of general harms: a systematic review. Ann Intern Med 2017;167(5):319–31.
74. Mücke M, Phillips T, Radbruch L, et al. Cannabis-based medicines for chronic neuropathic pain in adults. Cochrane Database Syst Rev 2018;(3):CD012182.
75. Calculating total daily dose of opioids for safer dosage. Centers for Disease Control, U.S. Department of Health and Human Services. Available at: https://www.cdc.gov/drugoverdose/pdf/calculating_total_daily_dose-a.pdf. Accessed January 17, 2019.
76. Yang Z, Wilsey B, Bohm M, et al. Defining risk of prescription opioid overdose: pharmacy shopping and overlapping prescriptions among long-term opioid users in medicaid. J Pain 2015;16(5):445–53.
77. Bohnert AS, Logan JE, Ganoczy D, et al. A detailed exploration into the association of prescribed opioid dosage and overdose deaths among patients with chronic pain. Med Care 2016;54(5):435–41.
78. Park TW, Saitz R, Ganoczy D, et al. Benzodiazepine prescribing patterns and deaths from drug overdose among US veterans receiving opioid analgesics: case-cohort study. BMJ 2015;350:h2698.

79. Liu Y, Logan JE, Paulozzi LJ, et al. Potential misuse and inappropriate prescription practices involving opioid analgesics. Am J Manag Care 2013;19(8):648–65.
80. Hill MV, McMahon ML, Stucke RS, et al. Wide variation and excessive dosage of opioid prescriptions for common general surgical procedures. Ann Surg 2017;265(4):709–14.
81. Opioid prescribing recommendations for surgery. 2019. Available at: https://opioidprescribing.info. Accessed February 1, 2019.
82. Hill MV, Stucke RS, Billmeier SE, et al. Guideline for discharge opioid prescriptions after inpatient general surgical procedures. J Am Coll Surg 2018;226(6):996–1003.
83. Brummett CM, Waljee JF, Goesling J, et al. New persistent opioid use after minor and major surgical procedures in us adults. JAMA Surg 2017;152(6):e170504.
84. Alam A, Gomes T, Zheng H, et al. Long-term analgesic use after low-risk surgery: a retrospective cohort study. Arch Intern Med 2012;172(5):425–30.
85. Sun EC, Darnall BD, Baker LC, et al. Incidence of and risk factors for chronic opioid use among opioid-naive patients in the postoperative period. JAMA Intern Med 2016;176(9):1286–93.
86. Clarke H, Soneji N, Ko DT, et al. Rates and risk factors for prolonged opioid use after major surgery: population based cohort study. BMJ 2014;348:g1251.
87. Shah A, Hayes CJ, Martin BC. Factors influencing long-term opioid use among opioid naïve patients: an examination of initial prescription characteristics and pain etiologies. J Pain 2017;18(11):1374–83.
88. Brat GA, Agniel D, Beam A, et al. Postsurgical prescriptions for opioid naive patients and association with overdose and misuse: retrospective cohort study. BMJ 2018;360:j5790.
89. Dowell D, Haegerich TM, Chou R. CDC guideline for prescribing opioids for chronic pain - United States, 2016. MMWR Recomm Rep 2016;65(1):1–49.
90. Arnold RM, Han PK, Seltzer D. Opioid contracts in chronic nonmalignant pain management: objectives and uncertainties. Am J Med 2006;119(4):292–6.
91. Portenoy RK, Lesage P. Management of cancer pain. Lancet 1999;353(9165):1695–700.
92. Davis MP, Dalal S, Goforth H, et al. Pain assessment and management. Chicago: American Academy of Hospice and Palliative Medicine; 2017.
93. Klueh MP, Hu HM, Howard RA, et al. Transitions of care for postoperative opioid prescribing in previously opioid-naïve patients in the USA: a retrospective review. J Gen Intern Med 2018;33(10):1685–91.
94. Anghelescu DL, Ehrentraut JH, Faughnan LG. Opioid misuse and abuse: risk assessment and management in patients with cancer pain. J Natl Compr Canc Netw 2013;11(8):1023–31.
95. Peglow SL, Binswanger IA. Preventing opioid overdose in the clinic and hospital: analgesia and opioid antagonists. Med Clin North Am 2018;102(4):621–34.
96. Butler SF, Budman SH, Fernandez KC, et al. Cross-validation of a screener to predict opioid misuse in chronic pain patients (SOAPP-R). J Addict Med 2009;3(2):66–73.
97. Webster LR, Webster RM. Predicting aberrant behaviors in opioid-treated patients: preliminary validation of the opioid risk tool. Pain Med 2005;6(6):432–42.
98. Butler SF, Budman SH, Fernandez KC, et al. Development and validation of the current opioid misuse measure. Pain 2007;130(1–2):144–56.

99. Brown RL, Rounds LA. Conjoint screening questionnaires for alcohol and other drug abuse: criterion validity in a primary care practice. Wis Med J 1995;94(3):135–40.
100. Rees DI, Sabia JJ, Argys LM, et al. With a little help from my friends: the effects of naloxone access and good samaritan laws on opioid-related deaths. National Bureau of Economic Research Working Paper Series. 2017; No. 23171.
101. Wheeler E, Jones TS, Gilbert MK, et al, Centers for Disease Control and Prevention (CDC). Opioid overdose prevention programs providing naloxone to laypersons - United States, 2014. MMWR Morb Mortal Wkly Rep 2015;64(23):631–5.
102. World Health Organization. Community management of opioid overdose 2014. Available at: http://apps.who.int/iris/bitstream/handle/10665/137462/9789241548816_eng.pdf. Accessed January 15, 2019.
103. Centers for Disease Control. CDC guideline for prescribing opioids for chronic pain. Available at: https://www.cdc.gov/drugoverdose/pdf/Guidelines_At-A-Glance-a.pdf. Accessed February 19, 2019.
104. U.S. Department of Health & Human Services. Naloxone: the opioid reversal drug that saves lives. Available at: https://www.hhs.gov/opioids/sites/default/files/2018-12/naloxone-coprescribing-guidance.pdf. Accessed February 19, 2019.
105. Coffin PO, Behar E, Rowe C, et al. Nonrandomized intervention study of naloxone coprescription for primary care patients receiving long-term opioid therapy for pain. Ann Intern Med 2016;165(4):245–52.
106. Behar E, Rowe C, Santos GM, et al. Acceptability of naloxone co-prescription among primary care providers treating patients on long-term opioid therapy for pain. J Gen Intern Med 2017;32(3):291–5.
107. Davis CS, Burris S, Beletsky L, et al. Co-prescribing naloxone does not increase liability risk. Subst Abus 2016;37(4):498–500.

Ostomy Management

A Model of Interdisciplinary Care

Emily B. Rivet, MD, MBA

KEYWORDS

• Ostomy • Stoma • Colostomy • Ileostomy • Palliative care • QoL

KEY POINTS

- Ostomies are indicated for a variety of intestinal conditions, and a basic understanding of their management is appropriate for clinicians of all disciplines.
- The impact of ostomies on quality of life is complex, with both positive and negative effects.
- Close collaboration with wound ostomy and continence (WOC) nursing professionals leads to optimal ostomy outcomes.

There are an estimated 1 million patients living with a stoma in North America, and approximately 120,000 stomas are created in the United States annually.[1] Stomas are indicated in several disease processes including malignancy, inflammatory bowel disease, neurologic problems, urologic disease, traumatic injury, and diverticulitis. Stomas are classified as either ileostomies or colostomies depending on whether they are created from the small or large intestine, respectively (**Figs. 1** and **2**). The term ileal conduit is reserved to describe a stoma formed for the passage of urine (**Fig. 3**). Ostomy anatomy is further characterized by how proximally they are formed and whether they are configured as an end, loop (**Figs. 4** and **5**), or end-loop. There are also more complex stoma configurations that are sometimes used in the context of technical challenges. Ostomy anatomy affects the viscosity and composition of the output, likelihood of parastomal herniation or prolapse, ease of appliance management, and quality of life (QoL). It is important to be cognizant that patients with stomas have varied perspectives on their experience and, for many, living with an ostomy significantly improves QoL. Palliative care specialists interacting with patients with ostomies should understand best practices in ostomy management, common complications, and when to refer to an enterostomal nursing specialist. Furthermore, it is important to be able to counsel patients considering ostomy formation for the treatment of serious illness, especially advanced malignancy.

Disclosure: The author has nothing to disclose.
Virginia Commonwealth University Health System, 1200 East Broad Street, PO Box 980519, Richmond, VA 23298-0519, USA
E-mail address: Emily.rivet@vcuhealth.org

Surg Clin N Am 99 (2019) 885–898
https://doi.org/10.1016/j.suc.2019.06.007

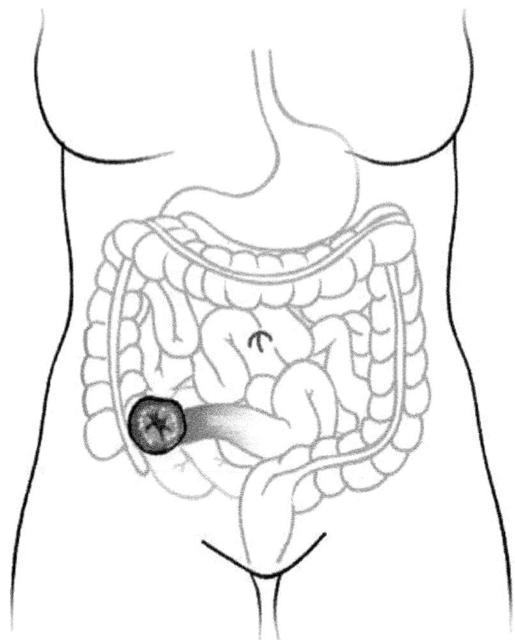

Fig. 1. Ileostomy. (Printed with permission from Lohitha Kethu.)

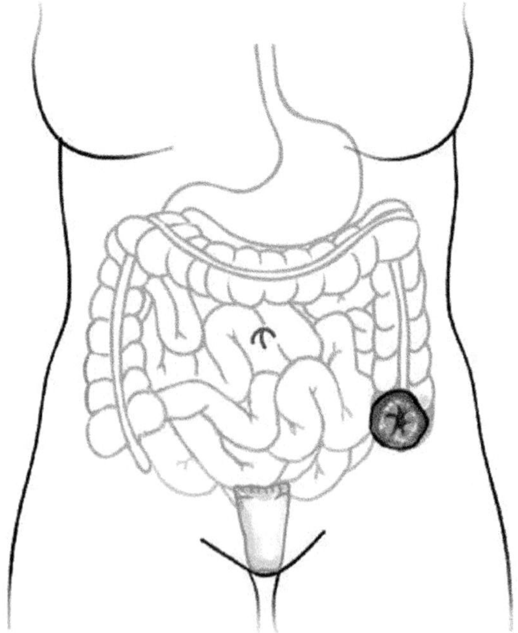

Fig. 2. Colostomy. (Printed with permission from Lohitha Kethu.)

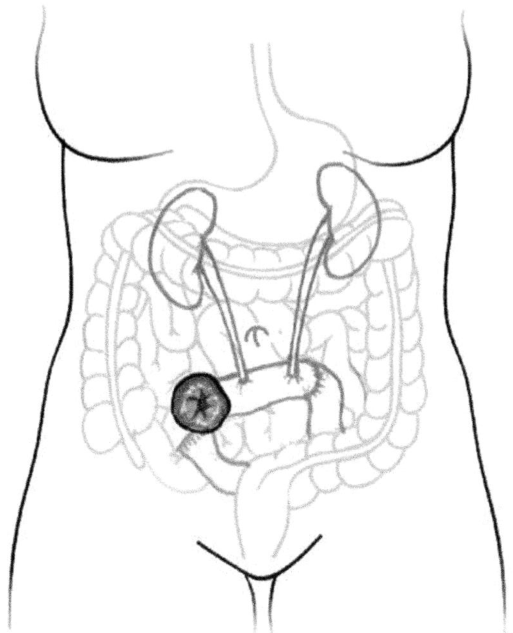

Fig. 3. Ileal conduit. (Printed with permission from Lohitha Kethu.)

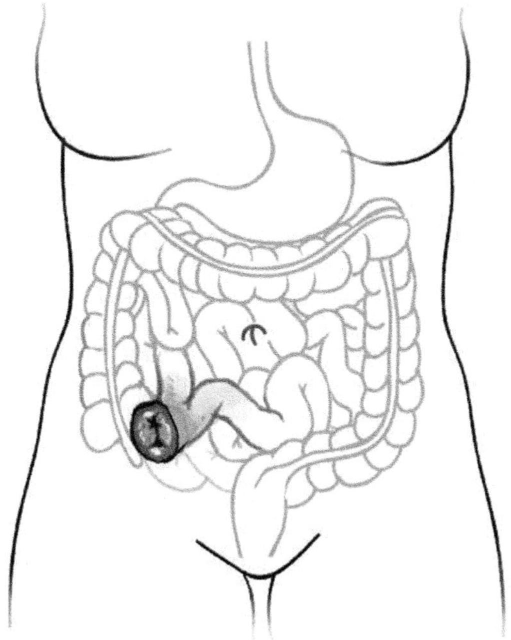

Fig. 4. Loop ileostomy. (Printed with permission from Lohitha Kethu.)

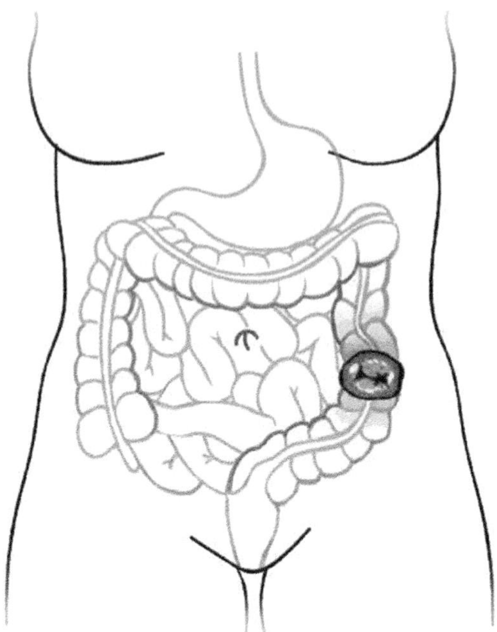

Fig. 5. Loop colostomy. (Printed with permission from Lohitha Kethu.)

Regardless of the indication or permanency of the stoma, early and continued involvement of wound ostomy and continence (WOC) nursing professionals is strongly advised. Ideally, a preoperative appointment should be used for stoma site marking in the supine (**Fig. 6**), seated (**Fig. 7**), and standing positions. In addition, preoperative appointments are important for patient and caregiver education on the medical and psychosocial sequelae of ostomy surgery. In emergent cases, education for patients and caregivers should begin early postoperatively; however, even in these circumstances, preoperative stoma site marking deserves attention. The stoma should be placed in the rectus abdominis on a 5-cm flat surface, and, in ambulatory patients, the preoperative mark should be evaluated in multiple positions. The stoma site marking should be made considering the expected type of ostomy (ileostomy vs colostomy and end vs loop), body habitus, abdominal contour (avoiding skin folds, the expected surgical incision, the umbilicus, previous surgical sites, and belt line), visual acuity, and dexterity.[2] In an analysis of over 1000 patients with end and loop ileostomies and colostomies, 364 experienced a major stoma-related complication including parastomal hernia, prolapse, retraction, fistula, stricture, bleeding, and ischemia. Of these 364 patients, 70% were not preoperatively marked, and in multivariate analysis preoperative marking was independently associated with reduced complication rates (odds ratio = 0.64; 95% CI, 0.48–0.84; P = .001).[3] Similarly, observational studies have consistently demonstrated that preoperative stoma site marking is associated with significantly fewer postoperative complications.[4–7] To reiterate the role of preoperative marking, the WOC Nurses Society, the American Society of Colon and Rectal Surgeons, and the American Urologiccal Society have published a joint position statement detailing the process and emphasizing the importance of stoma site marking.[2] This position statement, which can be accessed at https://www.ostomy.org/wp-content/uploads/2018/01/wocn_ascrs_stoma_site_marking_fecal_2014.pdf

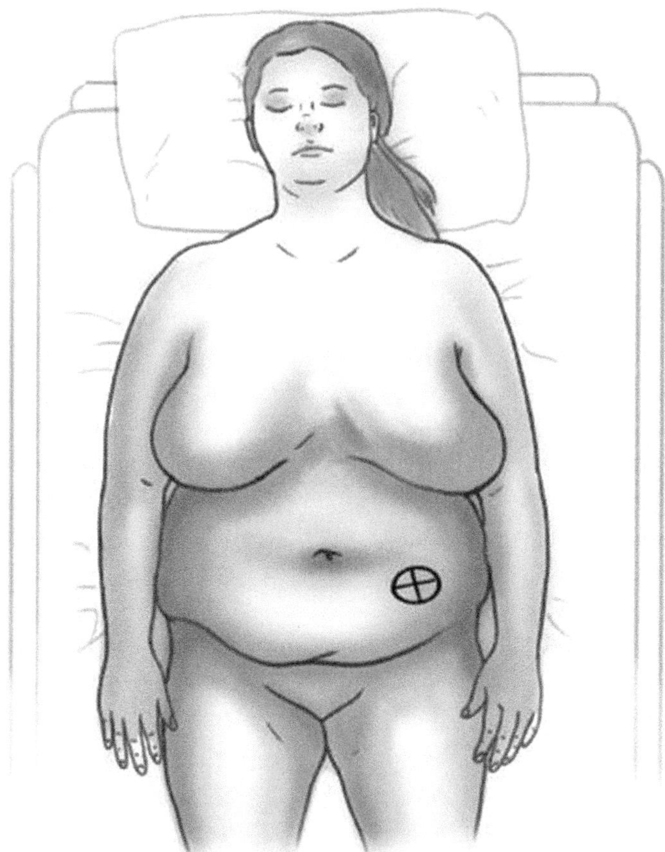

Fig. 6. Stoma marking supine. (Printed with permission from Lohitha Kethu.)

is an extremely valuable resource for best practice principles for stoma marking and should be referenced when circumstances create the need for stoma formation without an available WOC nurse to mark the site.

When considering ostomy output, generally the more proximal the stoma is formed the less viscous or formed the effluent. When the output is more liquid, there is an increased likelihood of nutritional and pharmacologic malabsorption and, therefore, the preferred location for the formation of ileostomies is often the distal ileum, just proximal to the cecum. However there are situations in which more proximal ileostomies or jejunostomies may be appropriate. In these cases, the need for antimotility agents, along with the risk of both nutritional and pharmacologic malabsorption, should be anticipated. Although there is no universal definition of excessive ostomy output, often when the volume exceeds 1200 mL/24 h, infectious causes should be ruled out, water and electrolyte balance assessed, and rehydration with intravenous fluid considered. The type of fluid should be tailored to the patient's electrolyte and volume status. In some patients, restricting hyper- or hypotonic fluids may reduce the volume of ostomy output; however, many require antimotility medications to prevent dehydration and acute kidney injury (**Table 1**). Patients with high-output stomas, particularly jejunostomies and ileostomies, are vulnerable to hyponatremia,

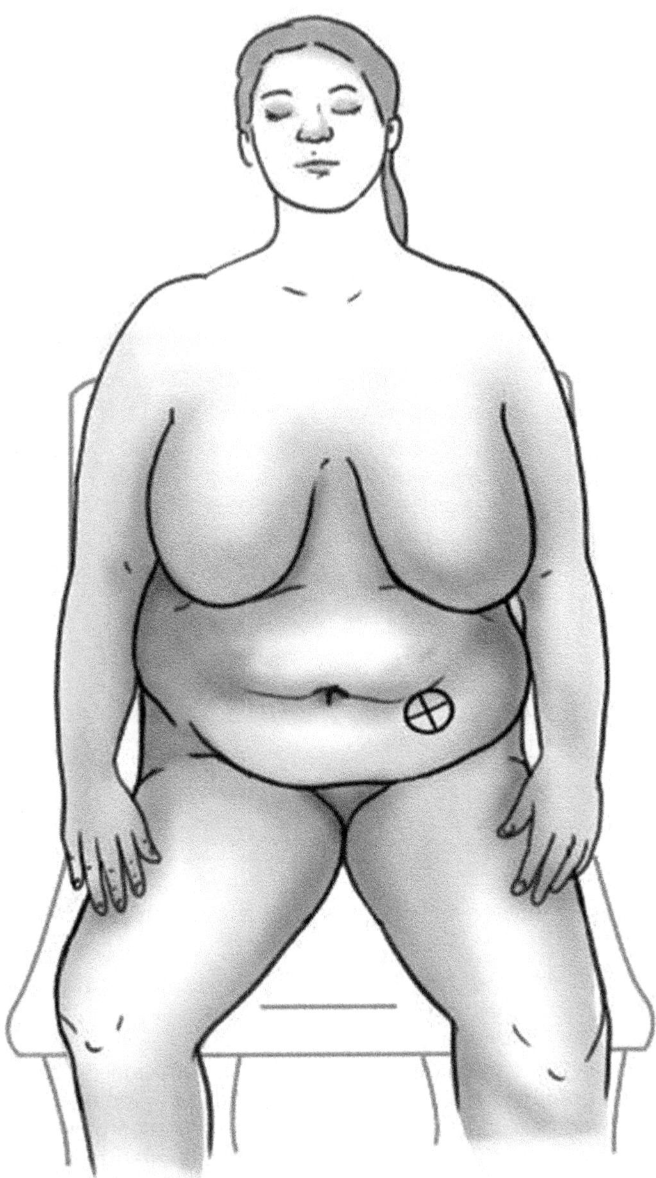

Fig. 7. Stoma marking sitting. (Printed with permission from Lohitha Kethu.)

hypomagnesemia, and vitamin (B12, A, D, E, and K) or micronutrient deficiencies. When assessing a patient's hydration status, urinary sodium or urine urea if the patient is taking diuretics, can be considered as a source of objective information.

Colostomies generally are fashioned from the distal colon and typically produce formed output similar to feces (see **Fig. 2**). Colostomies formed in the ascending or transverse colon are generally avoided unless intended to be temporary because the output is more difficult to manage, and transverse colostomies (**Fig. 8**) are more likely to develop prolapse and parastomal hernia. **Fig. 9** shows a colostomy with

Table 1
High-output ostomy management

	Stepwise Management of High-Output Ostomy (>1200 mL/24 h)	
	Intervention	**Options & Maximum Dosing**
First line	A. Rule out infectious causes B. Restrict (<1000 mL/d) fluids: • Hypotonic: water, tea, coffee, fruit juice, ETOH, dilute salt solutions • Hypertonic: coca cola, many sip feeds	—
Second line	Antimotility medications	Loperamide 4 mg QID
Thirrd line		Codeine 15–60 mg QID
Fourth line		Atropine/diphenoxylate (Lomotil) 2.5–5 mg TID
Fifth line		Tincture of opium (not with codeine)
Sixth line	Antisecretory drugs	Octreotide, omeprazole, cholestyramine

prolapse. Lastly, loop ostomies are configured so that the end of both the proximal and distal bowel are contiguous with the skin. This is typically done to facilitate future ostomy reversal or when there is concern for distal obstruction in an effort to avoid creation of a closed intra-abdominal bowel segment at risk for perforation. For surgeons, it is important to remember that even intestinal segments in discontinuity will

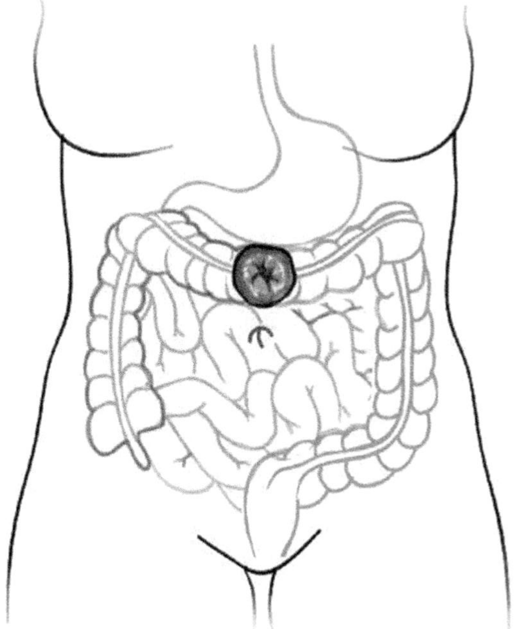

Fig. 8. Transverse colostomy. (Printed with permission from Lohitha Kethu.)

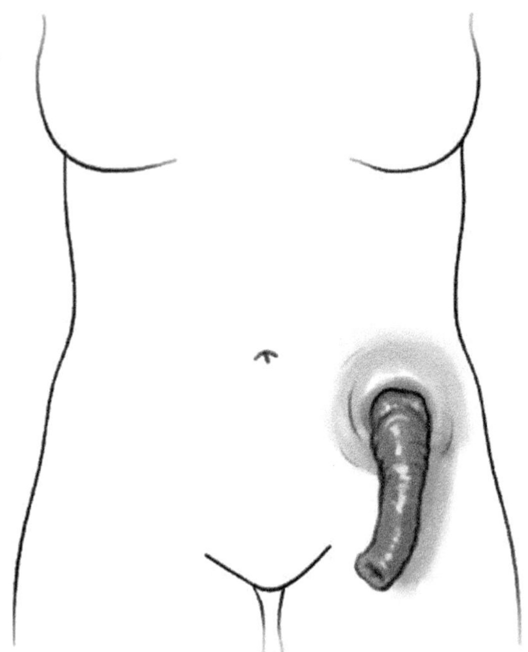

Fig. 9. Colostomy prolapse. (Printed with permission from Lohitha Kethu.)

produce fluid and mucus and thus will build up material that needs an outflow mechanism.

The rate of postoperative complications for patients receiving ostomies is high. Historically, up to 70% of patients receiving an ostomy were reported to experience a complication; however, even recent risk-adjusted data suggest that at certain centers complications occur in nearly 60% of patients.[8,9] Ostomy-specific complications can be classified as early (within 30 days of surgery) or late (greater than 30 days from surgery) and major (retraction, prolapse, stenosis, parastomal hernia, and necrosis) or minor (peristomal skin breakdown [PSB], mucocutaneous separation, and cutaneous infections). The complication rates vary widely owing to the follow-up duration and whether PSB is considered a complication. PSB is common and arguably should be considered a postoperative complication as it is influenced by the type of stoma,[6,10] the selected stoma site,[5] and the height of protrusion above the skin.[10,11] **Figs. 10** and **11** show a normal ileostomy and colostomy, whereas **Fig. 12** depicts a flush ileostomy. In addition, this common problem increases health care use.[12] For patients with appliance wear times under 48 hours or experiencing PSB, skin preparations or changing the type of appliance can be considered. In general, patients with soft, flaccid abdomens may benefit from a firm wafer, whereas patients with firm abdominal wall tissue would benefit from more flexible wafers. Convex rings are useful for patients with retracted or flush stomas because they can funnel the effluent and reduce the frequency of leaks. Other common peristomal skin issues that can be easily identified and treated empirically include allergic contact dermatitis and candidiasis. For contact dermatitis, an alternative appliance and/or adhesive is often required, and for candidiasis, topical antifungal powder (prescription Nystatin or 2% miconazole over the counter) is useful. If PSB persists, evaluation and treatment by a WOC nurse has been shown to improve skin condition and decrease appliance leaks and accessory product use.[13]

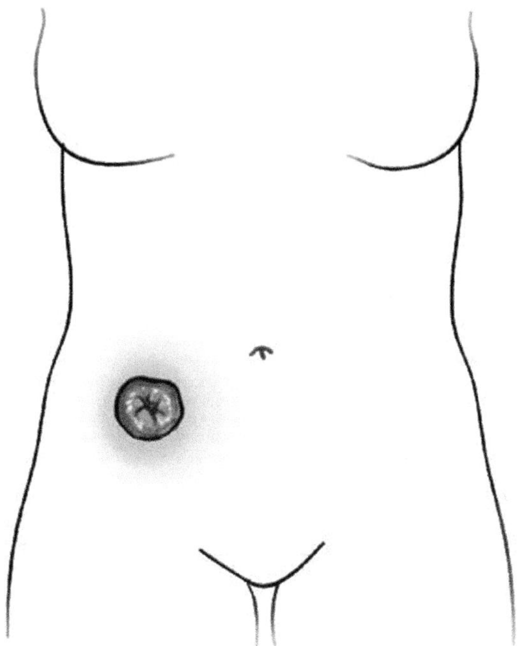

Fig. 10. Normal ileostomy height. (Printed with permission from Lohitha Kethu.)

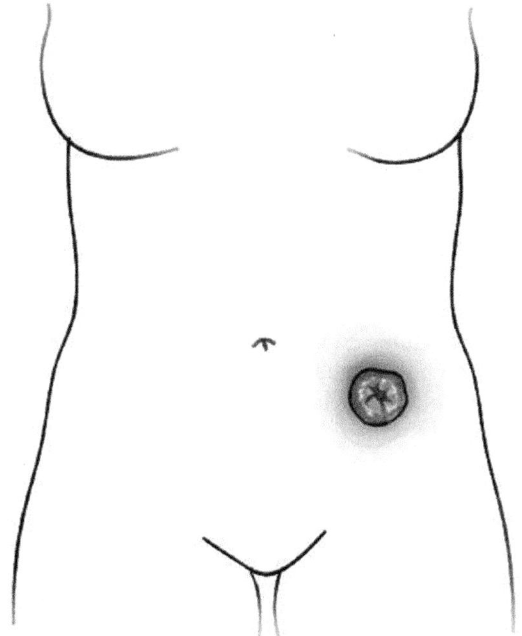

Fig. 11. Normal colostomy height. (Printed with permission from Lohitha Kethu.)

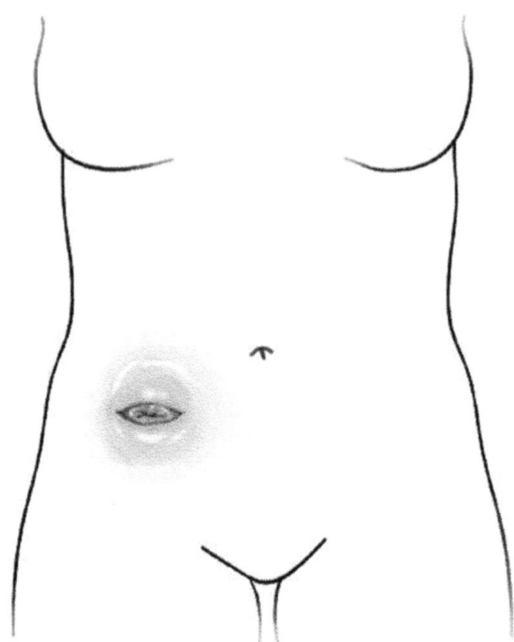

Fig. 12. Flush ileostomy. (Printed with permission from Lohitha Kethu.)

The formation of an ostomy induces significant changes in patient body image, function, and QoL. Postoperative QoL is a nuanced topic influenced by the involvement of a WOC nurse,[4] cause of disease, patient age,[14,15] complications,[15,16] and the time from surgery.[15,17,18] The overall negative impact of an ostomy on QoL is well described, and the literature suggests that avoiding a stoma is preferred.[19] However, in a meta-analysis comparing self-expanding metallic stents (SEMS) with palliative surgery for malignant bowel obstruction (MBO), patients who had surgery had significantly higher rates of relief of obstruction (93.1% vs 99.8%, P = .0009), and among the studies that reported failure rates (299 patients over 10 studies), 12.7% of patients who received SEMS required a subsequent stoma.[20] Regardless, a proportion of patients with colorectal cancer (CRC) have lesions close to the anal canal or are otherwise not amenable to stent placement, and a diverting ostomy is indicated. A retrospective study on patients with CRC undergoing palliative surgery reported a median survival of nearly 3.5 months and 18% of patients lived beyond 1 year. This suggests that this cohort can be expected to develop ostomy-related complications.[21] From a QoL perspective, there are few data on palliative surgery alone and that the data must be extrapolated from literature on therapeutic intervention or comparing stenting with ostomy creation.

Among patients with CRC, a population-based study of 2299 patients showed that older (≥76 years) patients with ostomies had reduced physical functioning, whereas younger patients with ostomies experienced significant impact on global health status and physical, role, and social functioning compared with similarly aged nonostomy patients and healthy controls.[14] Among the elderly, the magnitude of this effect was clinically insignificant, whereas younger patients with ostomies saw the greatest impact on QoL. Lastly, a study of over 700 long-term CRC survivors showed that health-related QoL and generic QoL both improved significantly over time, and psychological distress trended downward. In this analysis, patients with poorer optimism and low social support (single, no pet) had poorer adjustment over 5 years.[17] Although these data should be interpreted cautiously in a palliative situation, younger patients with CRC without social support who are ineligible for stenting should be expected to experience the greatest negative impact on QoL. Cost-effective interventions such as preoperative education, stoma site marking, and involvement of a WOC nurse can reduce complications and improve QoL. When stenting or surgery are therapeutic options, the risks and benefits of both palliative procedures should be carefully considered and discussed with the patient.[20]

Although patients with CRC represent most cases that palliative care specialists will interact with, other causes of disease should be considered and may require longer-term support. The fact that QoL data from CRC cannot be extrapolated to other indications becomes clear when assessing patients with spinal cord injury (SCI). In a meta-analysis and several case series of patients with SCI who received ostomies for several reasons, QoL significantly improved after surgery.[22–27] In 1 study, after a mean of 5.5 years after surgery, most patients were satisfied with their stoma (88s % with right-sided colostomies, 100% with left-sided colostomies, and 83% with ileostomies) and most would have preferred surgery sooner (63% right-sided and 77% left-sided ileostomy 63%).[25]

Palliative care specialists often encounter 2 kinds of patients with ostomies. The first group of patients are those with an existing ostomy created for a condition unrelated to the issue that led to referral to palliative care. In this population, the goal is to maintain the ostomy care regimen and make adjustments as needed with alterations in oral intake and PSB. The second group are patients in whom ostomy formation is being considered for palliation. In general, palliative principles of empathetic and patient-centered communication, thoughtful discussions of prognosis, and a multidisciplinary approach, particularly with involvement of an enterostomal therapy nurse, is recommended (**Box 1**). Depending on resources and the clinical context, primary and specialty palliative care consultation may be both beneficial and appropriate.

Box 1
Discussing ostomy as a therapeutic option

Protocol for discussions regarding ostomies

1. *Set* the scene. It is a serious discussion and should be given appropriate time and space. Find out who the patient does (and does NOT) want to be present for the discussion
2. Assess the patient's *perception.* Many patients with conditions that can result in the need for an ostomy have already heard things about ostomies, had friends or family members with ostomies, or independently researched this option. Find out what they know and think before you tell them your opinion. For example, "Have you ever thought about an ileostomy as an option?"
3. Obtain the patient's *invitation.* Ask, "Would it be OK to talk about an ileostomy as a treatment option?"
4. Provide *knowledge.* Give this information in small chunks and use nontechnical words appropriate for the health literacy of the patient. "A colostomy involves bringing the end of the large intestine to the skin, so the poop can come out into a special bag."
5. Address emotions with *empathy.* Consideration of an ostomy can prompt a large spectrum of reactions including relief, anger, and grief at the loss of perceived normalcy. Be prepared to support all of these emotions.
6. Strategy and *summary.* Assess the patient's understanding of the discussion, answer questions, and formulate next steps.

Data from Baile WF1, Buckman R, Lenzi R, et al. SPIKES—A six-step protocol for delivering bad news: application to the patient with cancer. Oncologist. 2000;5(4):302-11.

Table 2
Points to consider for palliative ostomy formation for malignant bowel obstruction

Patient factors	Family, caregiver support/ability to manage ostomy Prognosis (recovery time vs expect life span)
Disease factors	Anatomy of obstructing process (proximal vs distal, focal vs diffuse) Anticipated efficacy of treatment alternatives (stent, gastric decompression, medical management)

The most common condition for consideration of palliative ostomy formation is MBO. For MBO, there are several possible interventions including decompressive gastric tube placement, ostomy formation, medical management, SEMS placement, surgical bypass, and surgical resection without ostomy formation, among others, which vary by clinical context. The benefits of ostomy formation should be considered in the context of patient prognosis and anticipated complexity of the surgical technique. Surgical intervention should be avoided when the recovery will take up much of a patient's life expectancy. For example, patients with MBO due to stage IV ovarian or pancreatic cancer, have a median survival after their first admission of less than 3 months.[28] Similarly, a systematic review showed that mortality was high (6%–32%) after palliative surgery for peritoneal carcinomatosis, and that hospitalization alone took up a significant portion of the patient's remaining life.[29] Patient and disease factors are both important considerations when discussing palliative surgery in the context of MBO, **Table 2**. When a multidisciplinary approach to patient care is adopted to include the disciplines of surgery and palliative care, coupled with the preferences of the patient, one is able to achieve outcomes that are acceptable to all involved.

ACKNOWLEDGMENTS

The author thanks Anthony Loria, BS, Annette Dean, BSN, RN, and Karunasai Mahadevan, BS.

REFERENCES

1. McGee MF. JAMA PATIENT PAGE. Stomas. JAMA 2016;315(18):2032.
2. Salvadalena G, Hendren S, McKenna L, et al. WOCN Society and ASCRS position statement on preoperative stoma site marking for patients undergoing colostomy or ileostomy surgery. J Wound Ostomy Continence Nurs 2015;42(3):249–52.
3. Arolfo S, Borgiotto C, Bosio G, et al. Preoperative stoma site marking: a simple practice to reduce stoma-related complications. Tech Coloproctol 2018;22(9):683–7.
4. Person B, Ifargan R, Lachter J, et al. The impact of preoperative stoma site marking on the incidence of complications, quality of life, and patient's independence. Dis Colon Rectum 2012;55(7):783–7.
5. Bass EM, Del Pino A, Tan A, et al. Does preoperative stoma marking and education by the enterostomal therapist affect outcome? Dis Colon Rectum 1997;40(4):440–2.
6. Pittman J, Rawl SM, Schmidt CM, et al. Demographic and clinical factors related to ostomy complications and quality of life in veterans with an ostomy. J Wound Ostomy Continence Nurs 2008;35(5):493–503.

7. Baykara ZG, Demir SG, Karadag A, et al. A multicenter, retrospective study to evaluate the effect of preoperative stoma site marking on stomal and peristomal complications. Ostomy Wound Manage 2014;60(5):16–26.
8. Robertson I, Leung E, Hughes D, et al. Prospective analysis of stoma-related complications. Colorectal Dis 2005;7(3):279–85.
9. Sheetz KH, Waits SA, Krell RW, et al. Complication rates of ostomy surgery are high and vary significantly between hospitals. Dis Colon Rectum 2014;57(5): 632–7.
10. Parmar KL, Zammit M, Smith A, et al, Greater Manchester and Cheshire Colorectal Cancer Network. A prospective audit of early stoma complications in colorectal cancer treatment throughout the Greater Manchester and Cheshire colorectal cancer network. Colorectal Dis 2011;13(8):935–8.
11. Persson E, Berndtsson I, Carlsson E, et al. Stoma-related complications and stoma size - a 2-year follow up. Colorectal Dis 2010;12(10):971–6.
12. Meisner S, Lehur P-A, Moran B, et al. Peristomal skin complications are common, expensive, and difficult to manage: a population based cost modeling study. PLoS One 2012;7(5):e37813.
13. Erwin-Toth P, Thompson SJ, Davis JS. Factors impacting the quality of life of people with an ostomy in North America: results from the Dialogue Study. J Wound Ostomy Continence Nurs 2012;39(4):417–22 [quiz: 423–4].
14. Verweij NM, Bonhof CS, Schiphorst AHW, et al. Quality of life in elderly patients with an ostomy - a study from the population-based PROFILES registry. Colorectal Dis 2018;20(4):O92–102.
15. Arndt V, Merx H, Stegmaier C, et al. Restrictions in quality of life in colorectal cancer patients over three years after diagnosis: a population based study. Eur J Cancer 2006;42(12):1848–57.
16. Vonk-Klaassen SM, de Vocht HM, den Ouden MEM, et al. Ostomy-related problems and their impact on quality of life of colorectal cancer ostomates: a systematic review. Qual Life Res 2016;25(1):125–33.
17. Chambers SK, Meng X, Youl P, et al. A five-year prospective study of quality of life after colorectal cancer. Qual Life Res 2012;21(9):1551–64.
18. Bekkers MJ, van Knippenberg FC, van Dulmen AM, et al. Survival and psychosocial adjustment to stoma surgery and nonstoma bowel resection: a 4-year follow-up. J Psychosom Res 1997;42(3):235–44.
19. Young CJ, De-Loyde KJ, Young JM, et al. Improving quality of life for people with incurable large-bowel obstruction: randomized control trial of colonic stent insertion. Dis Colon Rectum 2015;58(9):838–49.
20. Zhao X-D, Cai B-B, Cao R-S, et al. Palliative treatment for incurable malignant colorectal obstructions: a meta-analysis. World J Gastroenterol 2013;19(33): 5565–74.
21. Pickard C, Thomas R, Robertson I, et al. Ostomy creation for palliative care of patients with nonresectable colorectal cancer and bowel obstruction. J Wound Ostomy Continence Nurs 2018;45(3):239–41.
22. Hocevar B, Gray M. Intestinal diversion (colostomy or ileostomy) in patients with severe bowel dysfunction following spinal cord injury. J Wound Ostomy Continence Nurs 2008;35(2):159–66.
23. Bølling Hansen R, Staun M, Kalhauge A, et al. Bowel function and quality of life after colostomy in individuals with spinal cord injury. J Spinal Cord Med 2016; 39(3):281–9.
24. Branagan G, Tromans A, Finnis D. Effect of stoma formation on bowel care and quality of life in patients with spinal cord injury. Spinal Cord 2003;41(12):680–3.

25. Safadi BY, Rosito O, Nino-Murcia M, et al. Which stoma works better for colonic dysmotility in the spinal cord injured patient? Am J Surg 2003;186(5):437–42.
26. Munck J, Simoens C, Thill V, et al. Intestinal stoma in patients with spinal cord injury: a retrospective study of 23 patients. Hepatogastroenterology 2008; 55(88):2125–9.
27. Rosito O, Nino-Murcia M, Wolfe VA, et al. The effects of colostomy on the quality of life in patients with spinal cord injury: a retrospective analysis. J Spinal Cord Med 2002;25(3):174–83.
28. Lilley EJ, Scott JW, Goldberg JE, et al. Survival, healthcare utilization, and end-of-life care among older adults with malignancy-associated bowel obstruction: comparative study of surgery, venting gastrostomy, or medical management. Ann Surg 2018;267(4):692–9.
29. Paul Olson TJ, Pinkerton C, Brasel KJ, et al. Palliative surgery for malignant bowel obstruction from carcinomatosis: a systematic review. JAMA Surg 2014;149(4): 383–92.

Palliative Wound Care

Less Is More

Emily H. Beers, MD

KEYWORDS

• Palliative • Wound care • Malignant wound • Radiation wound • Pressure ulcer

KEY POINTS

- Palliative wound care is a complex discipline that encompasses both the physical and psychological suffering of patients with wounds and advanced illness.
- This type of care differs from standard wound care in many ways, with the primary goal being relief of symptoms as opposed to wound healing.
- Historic wound treatments are enjoying revived interest in the palliative care setting, which has spurred further research into their mechanisms and efficacy.
- There is a paucity of well-controlled trial data about the various products used in palliative wound care.
- The physical symptoms of palliative wounds engender complex emotional responses in patients and caregivers that can cause social isolation, diminished physical intimacy, and delay in treatment if not addressed empathically by providers.

INTRODUCTION

Wound care is the oldest discipline in medicine and serves as a metaphor for all that medical science has strived to accomplish since earliest man—knitting back together what has been rent asunder. Clay tablets from 2200 BC describe the acts of washing, plastering, and bandaging wounds, and Egyptian papyri discuss the application of lint, honey, and grease, which we now know in turn likely facilitated drainage of exudate, served as an antibacterial, and provided a moist wound healing environment.[1,2] Throughout the many ages of human civilization we have tried to understand wounds and how to cure them, and although today's modern world has thousands of specialized dressings we find that ancient remedies such as honey and silver remain part of a canon whose powers we are only now beginning to more deeply understand. "Palliation" means to alleviate suffering, and when that suffering comes from a physical wound the patient has a connection to the oldest, deepest roots of the healing arts.

Disclosure Statement: Nothing to disclose.

Division of Geriatric, Hospital, Palliative and General Internal Medicine, Keck Hospital and Norris Cancer Center, University of Southern California, 2020 Zonal Avenue, IRD 306, Los Angeles, CA 90033, USA

E-mail address: Emily.Beers@med.usc.edu

Surg Clin N Am 99 (2019) 899–919

https://doi.org/10.1016/j.suc.2019.06.008

surgical.theclinics.com

0039-6109/19/

An additional but integral part of the palliative model is treatment of not just the physical wound but the psychological, emotional, and even spiritual/existential distress engendered by these injuries.[3,4] What in another case could be just an erosion of the skin in this context can be thought as breakdown of boundary between the self and the outer world, and that relentless reminder of the disease creates a profound sense of isolation when "living within a body that cannot be trusted."[5,6] Palliative wound care is thus a unique territory of medical science, one that prioritizes comfort above all things at a fragile time in a patient's life so far beyond the miracles of modern medicine that it at times shares more features with ancient Egyptian life than our current world. Proper palliative treatment of wounds thus involves knowledge of the types of issues advanced illness creates, and how treatment is often more than an intent to cure.

Malignant Wounds

Malignant wounds are those directly related to tumor infiltration of superficial structures such as skin and lymphatics, and they afflict approximately 10% to 15% of patients with cancer in the course of their illness.[7,8] Given their association with poorly controlled local or distant disease, they are often considered "nonhealable," and although the body of evidence is scant it seems true that healing of these wounds is surpassingly rare.[9] Given that malignant fungating wounds are the most aggressive and difficult to manage, the treatment selections herein can be more broadly applied to other wounds in the palliative care setting. Cancers most likely to lead to malignant wounds are breast, head and neck, primary skin, gastrointestinal (GI), and lung.[3] These wounds cause significant symptoms in those affected including pain, mass effect, exudate, odor, pruritus, and bleeding.[10] Pain is the most frequently encountered symptom (noted in up to 30% of patients), but malodor often eclipses it in terms of negative impact on a patient's quality of life. Malodor causes a visceral response in patients, caregivers, and staff and can lead to feelings of inadequacy in all who encounter them and increase isolation for patients who fear the inescapable social stigma.[11] These wounds externalize the disease process to the point of forced confrontation with the illness, and at the same time create a profound barrier to physical touch and intimacy that could otherwise be so therapeutic. Studies about the lived experience of both patients and nurses suggest that malignant wounds represent some of the hardest cases these clinicians encounter.[12] Treatment of malignant wounds thus must address the severe, multidimensional physical symptomatology but also acknowledge the psychic distress.

Systemic opioids remain the mainstay of treatment of wound pain, but the side-effect burden of these medicines is high and the social cost of widespread opioid use has proved devastating. One opioid-sparing tool used in the palliative and hospice setting is topical opioids, which have minimal systemic absorption unless used on large wounds (>60 cm^2 in the representative study), where bioavailability from that wound was estimated at 20%.[13,14] A meta-analysis of 27 publications about topical opioids in palliative treatment of cutaneous wounds showed significant reduction in pain in 23 of the studies, minimal systemic absorption, and incidentally found a higher likelihood of positive treatment effect when treating malignant and pressure wounds as opposed to vascular ulcers.[15]

Treatments to reduce wound odor have also been extensively studied given the debilitating consequences patients face when dealing with this challenge. Although bacteriologic assessment of malignant wounds shows several common aerobic species, anaerobes are thought to be the major causative feature of malodorous wounds.[16,17] To date the most commonly investigated antibacterial treatment is topical metronidazole. Limited existing data suggest that systemic oral administration is not effective, likely due to poor penetrance of systemic antibiotics into the necrotic tissues of a malignant wound.[18] Topical metronidazole however remains an off-label but common treatment of wound odor, and despite heterogeneous data numerous studies have shown significant improvement with a negligible side-effect profile.[19–22] This is most commonly administered as a 0.75% metronidazole gel (MetroGel 75), although empirical data from hospice workers have shown that crushed metronidazole 500 mg tablets sprinkled into the wound bed are effective and more economical, as cost containment is usually of paramount importance in a hospice business model.[23] The most common treatment pattern is once daily application under a non-adherent dressing such as Vaseline gauze or absorbent foam for a 14-day total course.

Although bacterial bioburden is thought to be the main culprit in wound odor, many other nonantibiotic topical therapies have been increasingly investigated given fears of antibiotic resistance. Although large randomized trials are essentially absent, there are various other products on the market reflecting growing interest in nonantibiotic treatment including such agents as charcoal, silver, and honey. Although knowledge of silver's antimicrobial properties extends back to Hippocrates, the more recent technology creating nanoparticles that are easily incorporated into other substrates has massively increased silver's popularity as an antibacterial agent, in everything from wound dressings to underwear and pillowcases. Silver nanoparticles are thought to be toxic via binding to bacterial cell walls and increasing both membrane permeability and production of harmful reactive oxygen species, which leads to cell death.[24] There is some evidence from small trials suggesting that silver-containing dressings can reduce wound odor in malignant fungating wounds, and a larger volume of mixed-quality evidence also supporting their use in chronic wounds of other causes.[25–28] The barrier to broader use in the palliative/hospice setting is cost, and although more expensive silver-containing dressings may actually reduce cost in venous ulcer populations with a chance of expected healing, unfortunately palliative and malignant wounds do not have the same long-term expectations and create a challenge in bearing the increased expense.[29]

Activated charcoal is a fine powder created from superheating a carbonaceous fuel to create a microporous structure that can have surface-area-to-volume ratio of up to 3000 m^2 per gram.[30] The submicroscopic channels within the particles create a large area for adsorption of the volatile chemicals released by malignant wounds such as cadaverine, putrescine, and sulfur.[14] Charcoal is usually applied as an active agent within a dressing substrate (ACTISORB, CarboFLEX, etc) matched to the level of exudate and type of drainage of the wound. Unfortunately the few studies that have been conducted are mostly descriptive, so use of charcoal products is dictated by which product is on the formulary.[31,32]

Honey has also been increasingly studied as a wound-healing agent, with a millennia-long history of use in wound care dating back to the ancient Egyptians who used honey, animal grease, and lint as one of the first recorded adherent dressings.[33] After the development of antibiotics and subsequent antibiotic resistance, more traditional remedies such as honey had resurgence of interest in the literature. The pioneering work on this research was led by a New Zealand scientist, Peter Molan, who first published about the antibacterial properties of monofloral Mānuka honey harvested from *Leptospermum scoparium* trees after finding it to be the most antibacterial of a large sample of varietals.[34] Although initial research was coincident to his location in New Zealand, Mānuka honey has since been found the most antibacterial of all honey species, and the bulk of commercially available honey and specialty dressings (MEDIHONEY) are made of pure Mānuka honey.[35] Honey's low pH causes increased release of bactericidal reactive oxygen species and deactivates harmful proteases that can impair wound healing, and its high osmolarity has a hygroscopic effect that dehydrates bacteria and increases lymph transit through the wound base.[36] The antibacterial properties of honey continue to be understood and are currently thought to be related to various active compounds including dicarbonyl methylglyoxal, hydrogen peroxide, and other complex peptides that alter bacterial cell morphology and both disrupt and prevent biofilm formation.[37] The pooled analysis of honey as a general wound-healing agent shows mixed results, but more specific studies relating to wound malodor tend toward positive results.[38,39]

When more aggressive intervention is being considered, negative-pressure wound therapy (NPWT) is a newer model of wound care that first came to market in 1997 and whose use has exploded in the past decades. In just 6 years following their initial reimbursement by Medicare, in 2001 payments for NPWT devices increased by 583%.[40] NPWT has been shown in numerous studies to be an effective therapy that can improve healing times and wound outcomes, although the heterogeneity of trial types limits meta-analysis.[41–43] It has also been shown to improve quality of life in patients with disabling wounds, despite a slight reported decrease in the first week of therapy possibly secondary to anxiety associated with the more complicated device.[44] In general, NPWT has remained contraindicated by manufacturers for malignant wounds because of concerns for growth or spread of malignancy, but there is a paucity of evidence to support such concern.[45] Despite this historic prohibition there are a small number of case studies examining the possible role of NPWT in a palliative context, and they all showed positive results after palliative resection of malignant lesions with NPWT closure.[46–49] Palliation with NPWT in these cases caused reduction in exudate, odor, and pain, given fewer dressing changes and should be considered as an option for patients healthy enough to undergo palliative resection but not well enough to tolerate major reconstruction. Traditional NPWT devices were durable medical equipment intended for use over multiple patients, but newer pump technology is single use and has shown dramatic cost savings—an important consideration when making decisions about the treatment for palliative and hospice care.[50,51] Unfortunately hospice is not able to bill for NPWT unless it is unrelated to the patient's terminal condition, and thus the selected patients who may benefit from this therapy must have those costs absorbed and averaged over all other care that hospice provides.

Bleeding is another distressing symptom faced by patients with malignant wounds, and although much less common than pain, odor, or exudate, there is a more urgent feeling of threat to life with bleeding and patients almost universally reporting fear that they will "bleed to death."[6] As with any fragile wound, core management includes atraumatic dressing changes and use of nonadherent materials such as vaseline gauze (Xeroform, Adaptic) or nonstick gauze (Telfa). Although standard hemostatic agents common in the operating room setting can be used on malignant wounds, the cost of things such as thrombin or fibrin spray unfortunately excludes them from the toolkit of most palliative and hospice providers. Alginate dressings are a common category of hemostatic dressing; derived from seaweed extracts, they release large amounts of calcium when the fibers contact wound fluid, which enhances the normal clotting process.[52] Because of this, alginate dressings should only be used for wounds with moderate to heavy exudate, and although proved to be effective hemostatic agents it is unclear that alginate alone can control more than gentle bleeding.[53,54] An older, inexpensive agent with newly discovered uses in palliative wound care is Mohs paste. There is an increasing number of case series reporting topical application of Mohs paste (controlled-release zinc chloride) to palliate bleeding malignant wounds with excellent results.[55–61] Another older agent with potential benefit in the palliative realm is oxymetazoline nasal spray (Afrin). Although it has been used for decades in the management of epistaxis, it is an over-the-counter option with the potential to minimize wound surface bleeding via its alpha adrenergic effects and with no reported systemic side effects.[62–67]

Pressure Ulcers

Given their fragility and large number of risk factors, palliative patient populations have the highest incidence of all types of wounds—amongst those pressure ulcers dominate, comprising up to 60%.[1] The skin is the largest organ in the body and constitutes 10% to 15% of body weight. Normal age-related changes to skin include loss of sweat glands, thinning via shrinkage and loss of collagen and elastic fibers, and decreased vascularity, all of which lead to an overall decline in barrier function with increased susceptibility to injury.[68] The term "skin failure" is used throughout the literature to mean everything from TENS/Stevens-Johnsons systemic reactions to pressure ulceration from hypoperfusion in the acutely ill, but the broader concept of skin as an organ susceptible to failure like the heart or kidneys is a useful idea when caring for palliative care and hospice patients given their higher likelihood of all forms of skin injury.[69,70]

Another important concept when dealing with palliative and hospice patients with pressure ulcers is the concept of the "unavoidable pressure injury." The term SCALE (Skin Changes At Life's End) was introduced by an expert panel in 2008 to describe the group of wound phenomena that result from the complex failure of homeostatic mechanisms at end of life.[71] This panel formalized the notion that given the irreversible issues faced in the palliative population, not all pressure wounds can be avoided—although simple on its face, this was an important and unique assessment in a time where quality metrics and payment are tied to such issues. An unavoidable pressure ulcer was later defined as"*one that may occur even though providers have evaluated the individual's clinical condition and PU risk factors have been evaluated and defined and interventions have been implemented that are consistent with individual needs, goals, and recognized standards of practice*" and "*one that occurs even though providers have monitored and evaluated the impact of preventive interventions and revised these approaches as appropriate.*"[72] The most classic example of unavoidable pressure injury at the end of life is the Kennedy terminal ulcer (KTU). The phenomenon was originally described by Jean-Martin Charcot in the nineteenth century as "decubitus ominosis" after observing a category of pressure ulcers that seemed to herald death.[73] His neuropathic theory for these ulcers has since been discredited, and the phenomenon was largely forgotten until the 1980s when Karen Lou Kennedy (a nurse practitioner in Fort Wayne, Indiana) reviewed her skin/wound data from a long-term care facility and found that 55.7% of patients who died with a pressure ulcer had onset of that ulcer 6 weeks or fewer before death.[74] Further investigation found that there are 2 main presentations of the KTU (**Fig. 1**, **Table 1**)[75]:

As opposed to "classic" KTU, the "3:30 syndrome" version was so dubbed for the rapidity of change—the original anecdote noted the patient's skin was normal when examined in the morning and by 3:30 PM shift change the ulcer had emerged.[76]

A few prospective studies of patients with palliative ulcers exist, and those have shown that only early ulcers have a chance of healing. The likelihood of healing a Stage I or a Stage II pressure ulcer was reported as 9% to 25%, and no Stage III or Stage IV ulcers healed.[77,78] Although that is a small healed percentage, knowing that some ulcers can heal is helpful guidance. The factors associated with increased likelihood of ulcer healing in these studies were age less than 70 years, Palliative Performance Scale score greater than 30, and interestingly in one article, use of artificial

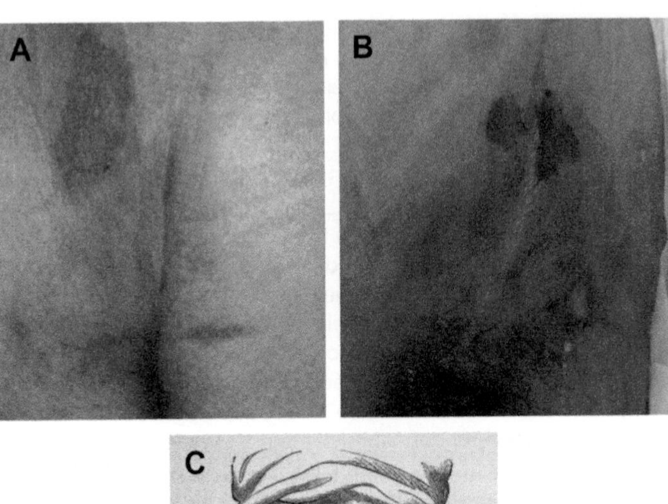

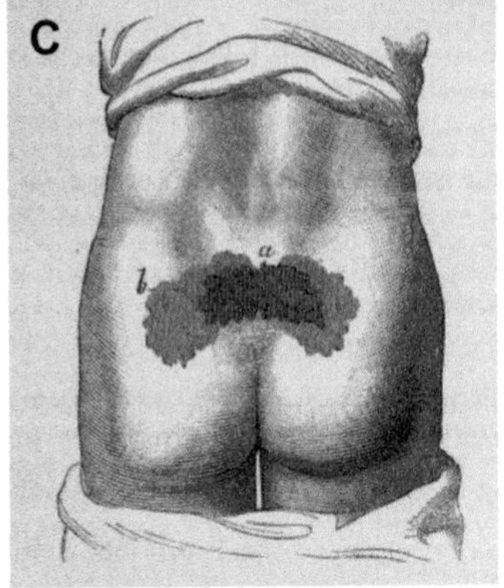

Fig. 1. Features of Kennedy terminal ulcers. (*A*) Image of a "3:30 syndrome" KTU. (*B*) Image of a classic KTU. (*C*) Original description in Charcot's 1877 Lectures on Diseases of the Nervous System (a - mortified portion, b - erythematous zone).

nutrition.[53,79] The use of tube feeding at end of life has been controversial and remains a challenging topic for palliative care providers, patients, and families: in fact withholding or stopping tube feeding is frequently misconstrued as euthanasia.[80] Most studies examining artificial nutrition for treatment or prevention of pressure ulcers in palliative populations are related to dementia, and pooled meta-analysis of many patient types does not suggest that tube feeding at end of life is useful for this

Table 1
Features of Kennedy terminal ulcers

	"Classic" KTU	"3:30 Syndrome" KTU
Shape	Irregular pear, butterfly, or horseshoe shape	Irregular, small, black, macular
Location	Bilateral sacrum or coccyx	Unilateral buttock
Onset	Sudden onset	Sudden onset
Color and progression	Red or purple, +/– skin erosion, progresses to yellow and/or black	Purple/black, rapidly enlarging, no skin erosion
Timeline	2 wk to several mo before death	8–24 h before death

indication.[81–83] However, subgroup analysis shows that certain carefully selected populations may benefit from tube feeds even in a palliative scenario, such as those with anatomic preclusion of oral intake from head and neck cancer or upper GI cancer and those with a good performance status.[84]

Dressing choice for management of pressure ulcers in palliative and hospice shares principles with those outlined in malignant wounds. The basic steps in pressure ulcer management include: cleansing/debridement, management of exudate, slough, or infection, protection of the periwound skin, and dead space management. Many products used in palliative and hospice care are chosen to serve dual purposes, with an agent selected to both cleanse and debride or treat infection and absorb exudate. Many newer, more expensive products are outside the scope of this review given lack of access in the palliative setting, but some of the core agents used in management of pressures ulcers are outlined later.

WOUND CLEANSING AND DEBRIDEMENT

Cleansing of a wound is one of the oldest treatments in medicine, part of the irrevocably intuitive understanding that most sentient creatures have: the concept of "licking one's wounds" reflects the animal practice of wound care and concomitant retreat to heal. We know that bacteria can promulgate and develop into recalcitrant biofilms within hours, so prompt and regular wound cleansing can reduce wound bioburden.[85,86] Pressure ulcers in the palliative setting are often chronic and encumbered with slough and eschar, which are prime grounds for bacterial replication and maintenance. Ideal wound-cleansing agents are antiseptic with broad spectrum activity, have ability to penetrate eschar and biofilm, have low potential for development of resistance, and minimal toxicity to normal tissues. Often in the palliative care setting where dressing changes must be weighed in terms of burden versus benefit, the cleansing and debriding agents overlap. One major category of cleansing compounds with the longest history and continued palliative use is the halide family, with active ingredients such as chlorine or iodine.

In the preantibiotic era, traumatic war wound infections were a major threat to life and the source of much research. Chemist Henry Drysdale Dakin did many experiments leading to the discovery that sodium hypochlorite (a.k.a. NaOCl, household bleach) had excellent antiseptic properties. This led to development of Dakin's solution, a buffered 0.5% bleach that has been used to treat infected or at-risk wounds since 1916.[87] The bactericidal efficacy of Dakin's solution is driven by its concentration of reactive chlorine species in the form of HOCl, OCl^-, and Cl_2, which causes increased membrane permeability from direct lipid damage and irreversible protein cross-linking from disulfide bonds leading to cellular dysfunction and death.[88] Unfortunately, Dakin's solution has been shown to be directly cytotoxic to the very cells recruited to heal these wounds such as keratinocytes, fibroblasts, and macrophages, even in concentrations as low as 0.0025%.[89,90] Dakin's solution is still widely used in palliative and hospice settings for its cost-efficiency, and it has been shown to have bactericidal efficacy against a broad range of microorganisms including *Pseudomonas aeruginosa*, *Escherichia coli*, *Proteus mirabilis*, *Serratia marcescens*, *Enterobacter cloacae*, group D enterococci, *Bacteroides fragilis*, *Streptococcus mitis*, *Staphylococcus epidermidis* (both methicillin- and non–methicillin-resistant), and fungi including *Candida albicans*.[91] However, there are 2 pitfalls of Dakin's solution: (1) the half-life of reactive chlorine species in Dakin's solution is short, with greater than 90% of its activity degraded after 15 minutes, and (2) the pH of the solution is ~10, which can be irritating to skin.[65] Dakin's original research was aware of half-life limitation, and thus his suggestion for use included a continuous irrigation system designed by his Nobel-laureate surgeon colleague Dr Alexis Carrel (**Fig. 2**).[92] Although Dakin's solution is still used in modern academic centers in the standard once or twice daily application of gauze, the most modern update of his original research includes negative-pressure wound dressings with periodic instillation and dwell of the solution (NPWT-id), which have been shown to promote granulation tissue formation and improve healing times compared with standard NPWT[93,94]. As for the pH issue, the newer approach to chlorine-based solutions is production of hypochlorous acid (HOCl, marketed as Vashe, Puracyn Plus, Dermacyn, etc), which has a skin-compatible pH of 5.5 and shows similar bactericidal efficacy and minimal tissue toxicity.[95,96] Both Dakin's solution and hypochlorous acid solutions are mild debriding agents as well and can be used in wounds with slough, and the multiple effects work to reduce wound odor.

Iodine is the other halide that has been used for over a century as an antimicrobial therapy. It comes in various formulations such as povidone iodine, cadexomer iodine, and iodine-impregnated dressings. Iodine is similar to chlorine in that it is a strong oxidizer, causing cross-linking and disruption of membrane proteins and enzymes leading to cell dysfunction and death.[97] Almost no studies exist examining iodine specifically in the context of palliative pressure ulcers or wounds, so support for its use must be extrapolated from studies involving other chronic wounds such as venous and diabetic ulcers.[98] Numerous studies have shown conflicting evidence about iodine's effects on wound healing in vivo versus in vitro, although current opinion suggests the mixed results may be related to detergents in some formulations that are to blame. Multiple reviews and trials show that iodine is effective at reducing bacterial load and disrupting biofilm and is a cost-effective treatment that can reduce healing

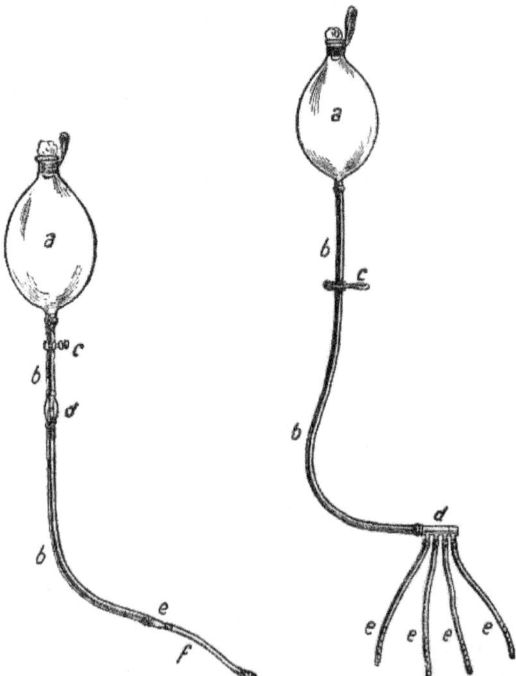

Fig. 2. Carrel-Dakin wound irrigation device. (a) reservoir; (b) irrigation tube; (c) screw pinchcock; (d) drop-counter; (e) distributing tube; (f) Conducting tube with terminal orifice.

times in chronic wounds.[99–103] Iodine is not typically used as a debriding agent despite some shared properties with chlorine, but cadexomer iodine has a microscopic structure that allows it to absorb 6 times its weight in fluid and thus it is used as a drying antiseptic for wounds that have heavy exudate.[104] It's combination of absorptive and antibacterial properties make it another good choice to reduce wound odor.

Yet another long-used agent with revived modern interest is acetic acid. It has been known to have antibacterial properties since the early twentieth century, with specific action against *Pseudomonas* discovered in relation to burn wounds.[105] Given the increasing preponderance of antibiotic-resistant *Pseudomonas* species and their frequent contribution to wound symptoms such as odor, acetic acid should be reconsidered as a dual-purpose topical agent to both debride and manage infection.[106] A recent prospective randomized trial showed 1% acetic acid applied twice daily on gauze was effective at eradicating multidrug-resistant *Pseudomonas* from wounds 3 times as fast as control.[107] Given its broad antiseptic effect without potential for rapid resistance, there has been a recent increase in research on the effects of acetic acid on wounds with biofilms, which all demonstrate its efficacy at eradicating wound infection.[108–112]

The last wound-modifying agent worth noting that is used mostly in the palliative realm is phenytoin. Phenytoin was initially discovered and utilized as an antiepileptic medication in 1938, with initial publications already indicting gingival hyperplasia as a side effect.[113] This unexpected accelerated tissue growth response lead clinicians to investigate how and if this secondary effect could be harnessed to improve wound healing in other areas. Early studies used the oral form of the drug for periodontal patients, who showed reduction in pain, reduced inflammation, and improved healing time.[114] Trials later progressed to a topical formulation to minimize any systemic interaction or side effects, and over the decades there have been numerous papers attempting to understand the nature of phenytoin's action to improve wound healing and how reliably it can be done.[115] It has been shown to have many actions on the wound environment, including increased fibroblast proliferation, increased collagen production, enhancement of granulation tissue formation, and reduced inflammatory response.[116] There is negligible systemic absorption from topical application, even in very large wounds requiring 3 to -6 times the lethal daily oral dose.[117] Multiple case series and randomized controlled clinical trials have shown phenytoin to have a positive effect on wound healing, but even the randomized trials had methodological issues precluding a confident meta-analysis of phenytoin's efficacy.[118,119] Despite this, it is commonly available in compounding pharmacies that work with hospice agencies and is frequently used off-label to encourage healing of recalcitrant wounds.[120] Phenytoin is applied to wounds as powder from opened capsules in a thin layer over the entire wound base. Given minimal systemic absorption, the dosing windows are less critical, but if dosing is of concern there are a small number of studies using 20 mg/cm^2 without any adverse effects.[121,122]

Radiation Damage

Another category of wound frequently encountered in the palliative care setting is the iatrogenic radiation injury. At least 50% of all patients with cancer undergoing treatment will have radiation therapy, and up to 95% of those will have some degree of radiation dermatitis.[123] Skin is uniquely vulnerable to radiation damage because of its rapid cell turnover and continuously self-renewing nature, with up to 10% of basal membrane keratinocytes undergoing mitosis each day.[124] Ionizing radiation damages skin in numerous ways. Initially the high-energy photons cause cell membrane and DNA damage in the generative basal layer with direct production of reactive oxygen species.[125,126] This is rapidly followed by inflammatory mediators such as prostaglandins and leukotrienes that cause capillary vasodilation, which leads to the transient erythema that can develop at the site within the first 24 hours.[127] The first-dose injury leads the undamaged basal keratinocytes to proliferate in response, but because modern radiotherapy is given over time in fractions the repeated injury to the remaining basal layer leads to a disruption of the normal balance of cell production and shedding.[66] This continued cycle of keratinocyte stimulation followed by repeated cell death leads to the various kinds of desquamation seen as a radiation side effect. Initially there is dry desquamation, which is the shedding of the overstimulated keratinocytes that have cornified faster than normal. This usually occurs no sooner than 10 to 14 days after the first fraction, corresponding to the time it takes the injured basal cell to migrate to the epidermal surface. With continued damage the injury will progress to moist desquamation when the basal layer can no longer renew itself and is completely denuded, leading to exposed dermis with overt wounding requiring reepithelialization.[128] Although many metrics have been developed, one of the original and most commonly used tools to grade radiation skin injury is still the Radiation Therapy Oncology Group (RTOG) toxicity criteria, seen in **Box 1**.

RTOG has the advantage of simplicity, but many newer scales have since been developed that have finer gradation of skin changes and include patient-reported outcomes, which unearthed a discrepancy between clinician evaluation of skin toxicity and actual lived patient experience.[65] In particular, it has been noted that people of color suffer more severe skin side effects (independent of treatment expectation and total radiation exposure), more pain, and have higher likelihood of progressing to moist desquamation.[129,130] This is posited to be related to the melanocytes' increased susceptibility to DNA damage with higher melanin production, and that early signs of skin damage such as erythema are often more difficult to visualize in darker skin.

One of the major evolutions in radiation technology that has reduced toxic side effects in the past decades has been intensity-modulated radiotherapy (IMRT). IMRT involves modulating the fluence (a measure of energy received per unit area, usually measured in J/cm^2) of the radiation beams in addition to their geometry, which allows clinicians the ability to minimize the exposure of organs at risk of damage in the path of the beam to the target.[131] RCTs have shown the IMRT significantly reduces both short- and long-term skin effects and improves quality of life in those undergoing radiation treatment.[132,133]

Many interventions to prevent or treat radiation-related skin damage have been studied, but few high-quality studies exist and the data are frequently

Box 1
Radiation therapy oncology group acute skin toxicity grading system

RTOG Grade	Symptoms and Severity
Grade 0	No observable skin changes
Grade 1	Mild erythema, dry desquamation
Grade 2	Bright or tender erythema, edema, areas of moist desquamation in skin folds
Grade 3	Moist desquamation outside of skin folds, pitting edema
Grade 4	Full-thickness ulceration, necrosis, hemorrhage
Grade 5	Death directly related to radiation effects

Adapted from Cox JD, Stetz J, Pajak TF. Toxicity criteria of the Radiation Therapy Oncology Group (RTOG) and the European organization for research and treatment of cancer (EORTC). Int J Radiat Oncol. 1995;31(5):1341-1346. https://doi.org/10.1016/0360-3016(95)00060-C; with permission.

Table 2
Interventions or prophylactic treatments to prevent or mitigate radiation-associated skin toxicity

Intervention	Outcome	References
Washing skin with lukewarm water and mild soap	Reduced severity of skin reactions with washing—washing recommended	132,133
Using deodorant	No difference in side effects with use of metallic or nonmetallic deodorants, improved symptoms with deodorant use—deodorant use recommended	134–137
Topical steroids	• Mometasone 0.1% topical likely delays onset of radiodermatitis and decreases the severity of skin reaction for doses <60 Gy—recommended • Topical betamethasone, methylprednisolone, hydrocortisone trend toward benefit	138–147
Hyaluronic acid	Mixed results, insufficient to recommend use	148–152
Aloe vera	Mostly negative results, use not recommended	153–158
Oral proteolytic enzymes	Mixed results, insufficient to recommend use	131,159,160
Trolamine	Mostly negative results, use not recommended	161–169

methodologically flawed or at high risk of bias.[134] Some trials have been undertaken to investigate the anecdotal lore about radiation-treated skin (no washing, no deodorant, etc) that patients are frequently concerned about and others to explore what treatments might be of benefit. Interventions that have data supportive or unsupportive of their use are described in **Table 2**.

SUMMARY

As we have seen in this review, one of the most interesting aspects of palliative wound care is how it leverages modern medical technology and yet has spurred the resurgence of historic treatments perhaps previously thought to be consigned to the annals of history. In this regard it is an exciting frontier for further research, because the unique needs of palliative and hospice patients allow the focus to shift away from cutting edge scientific novelty and return to the core dictum of patient-focused care above all else. Modern medicine is driven by the desire to cure, and a major tension of living as a palliative wound patient is knowing that cure is generally not possible. Wounds at this stage are doubly complex because they serve as a constant reminder of either the failure of prior interventions or the failure to seek aid. The near-universal sense of shame experienced by patients living with symptomatic malignant wounds drives some to delay seeking treatment, leading to the tragic scenario described as "an avalanche of ignoring": when patients fail to seek help until the cancer is extremely advanced.[170] The surgeon may often cease to interact with their patient in these stages of advanced illness, but there is tremendous opportunity here to deepen and add meaning to the relationship. Surgeon-patient trust is a unique entity; it is often faster-forged but in some ways stronger than in any other part of medicine, as the need for trust escalates in parallel with the risks of the intervention.[171] Tending to the physical and psychological distress of patients with palliative needs means confronting difficult realities, but the indelible bond of surgeon to wound means that we as surgeons are uniquely positioned to help patients navigate this vulnerable time.

REFERENCES

1. Broughton G, Janis JE, Attinger CE. A brief history of wound care. Plast Reconstr Surg 2006;117(7 Suppl):6S–11S.
2. Shah JB. The history of wound care. J Am Coll CertifWound Spec 2012; 3(3):65–6.
3. Lo S-F, Hu W-Y, Hayter M, et al. Experiences of living with a malignant fungating wound: a qualitative study. J Clin Nurs 2008;17(20):2699–708.
4. Probst S, Arber A, Faithfull S. Coping with an exulcerated breast carcinoma: an interpretative phenomenological study. J WoundCare 2013;22(7):352–4, 356-358, 360.
5. Probst S, Arber A, Faithfull S. Malignant fungating wounds – the meaning of living in an unbounded body. Eur J Oncol Nurs 2013;17(1):38–45.
6. Piggin C, Jones V. Malignant fungating wounds: an analysis of the lived experience. J WoundCare 2009;18(2):57–8, 60-64.
7. Maida V, Corbo M, Dolzhykov M, et al. Wounds in advanced illness: a prevalence and incidence study based on a prospective case series. Int Wound J 2008;5(2):305–14.
8. Alexander S. Malignant fungating wounds: epidemiology, aetiology, presentation and assessment. J WoundCare 2009;18(7):273–4, 276-278, 280.
9. Maida V, Ennis M, Corban J. Wound outcomes in patients with advanced illness. Int Wound J 2012;9(6):683–92.
10. Maida V, Ennis M, Kuziemsky C, et al. Symptoms associated with malignant wounds: a prospective case series. J PainSymptomManage 2009;37(2):206–11.
11. Probst S, Arber A, Trojan A, et al. Caring for a loved one with a malignant fungating wound. Support Care Cancer 2012;20(12):3065–70.
12. Alexander SJ. An intense and unforgettable experience: the lived experience of malignant wounds from the perspectives of patients, caregivers and nurses. Int Wound J 2010;7(6):456–65.
13. Ribeiro MDC, Joel SP, Zeppetella G. The bioavailability of morphine applied topically to cutaneous ulcers. J PainSymptomManage 2004;27(5):434–9.
14. Farley P. Should topical opioid analgesics be regarded as effective and safe when applied to chronic cutaneous lesions? J Pharm Pharmacol 2011;63(6): 747–56.
15. Graham T, Grocott P, Probst S, et al. How are topical opioids used to manage painful cutaneous lesions in palliative care? A critical review. Pain 2013; 154(10):1920–8.
16. Bowler PG, Davies BJ, Jones SA. Microbial involvement in chronic wound malodour. J WoundCare 1999;8(5):216–8.
17. Fromantin I, Seyer D, Watson S, et al. Bacterial floras and biofilms of malignant wounds associated with breast cancers. J Clin Microbiol 2013;51(10):3368–73.
18. Ramasubbu DA, Smith V, Hayden F, et al. Systemic antibiotics for treating malignant wounds. CochraneDatabase Syst Rev 2017;(8):CD011609.
19. Watanabe K, Shimo A, Tsugawa K, et al. Safe and effective deodorization of malodorous fungating tumors using topical metronidazole 0.75 % gel (GK567): a multicenter, open-label, phase III study (RDT.07.SRE.27013). Support Care Cancer 2016;24(6):2583–90.
20. Paul JC, Pieper BA. Topical metronidazole for the treatment of wound odor: a review of the literature. Ostomy Wound Manage 2008;54(3):18–27 [quiz: 28–9].

21. Akhmetova A, Saliev T, Allan IU, et al. A comprehensive review of topical odor-controlling treatment options for chronic wounds. J WoundOstomyContinence Nurs 2016;43(6):598–609.
22. Lyvers E, Elliott DP. Topical metronidazole for odor control in pressure ulcers. Consult Pharm 2015;30(9):523–6.
23. Comprehensive wound malodor management: win the RACE. Cleve Clin J Med 2015;82:535–43. Available at: https://www.mdedge.com/ccjm/article/101411/dermatology/comprehensive-wound-malodor-management-win-race. Accessed November 27, 2018.
24. Durán N, Durán M, de Jesus MB, et al. Silver nanoparticles: a new view on mechanistic aspects on antimicrobial activity. Nanomedicine 2016;12(3):789–99.
25. Kalemikerakis J, Vardaki Z, Fouka G, et al. Comparison of foam dressings with silver versus foam dressings without silver in the care of malodorous malignant fungating wounds. J BUON 2012;17(3):560–4.
26. Adderley UJ, Holt IG. Topical agents and dressings for fungating wounds. CochraneDatabase Syst Rev 2014;(5):CD003948.
27. Tricco AC, Antony J, Vafaei A, et al. Seeking effective interventions to treat complex wounds: an overview of systematic reviews. BMC Med 2015;13(1):89.
28. Norman G, Westby MJ, Rithalia AD, et al. Dressings and topical agents for treating venous leg ulcers. CochraneDatabase Syst Rev 2018;(6):CD012583.
29. Gueltzow M, Khalilpour P, Kolbe K, et al. Budget impact of antimicrobial wound dressings in the treatment of venous leg ulcers in the German outpatient care sector: a budget impact analysis. J MarkAccessHealthPolicy 2018; 6(1). https://doi.org/10.1080/20016689.2018.1527654.
30. Activated carbon. In: Wikipedia. 2018. Available at: https://en.wikipedia.org/w/index.php?title=Activated_carbon&oldid=870549060. Accessed November 29, 2018.
31. Morris C. Wound odour: principles of management and the use of CliniSorb. Br J Nurs 2008;17(6):S38. S40-42.
32. Williams C. CliniSorb activated charcoal dressing for odour control. Br J Nurs 2000;9(15):1016–9.
33. Bhattacharya S. Wound healing through the ages. Indian J Plast Surg 2012; 45(2):177–9.
34. Allen KL, Molan PC, Reid GM. A survey of the antibacterial activity of some New Zealand honeys. J Pharm Pharmacol 1991;43(12):817–22.
35. MEDIHONEY | Derma sciences. Available at: http://www.dermasciences.com/medihoney. Accessed December 3, 2018.
36. Honey: a biologic wound dressing. Wounds Research. Available at: https://www.woundsresearch.com/article/honey-biologic-wound-dressing. Accessed December 2, 2018.
37. Lu J, Carter DA, Turnbull L, et al. The effect of New Zealand Kanuka, Manuka and Clover Honeys on bacterial growth dynamics and cellular morphology varies according to the species. PLoS One 2013;8(2):e55898.
38. Jull AB, Cullum N, Dumville JC, et al. Honey as a topical treatment for wounds. CochraneDatabase Syst Rev 2015;(3):CD005083.
39. Lund-Nielsen B, Adamsen L, Kolmos HJ, et al. The effect of honey-coated bandages compared with silver-coated bandages on treatment of malignant wounds—a randomized study. WoundRepair Regen 2011;19(6):664–70.

40. Levinson D. Comparison of prices for negative pressure wound therapy pumps. Washington, DC: Government Printing Office: US. Dept of Health and Human Services, Office of Inspector General; 2009.
41. Suissa D, Danino A, Nikolis A. Negative-pressure therapy versus standard wound care: a meta-analysis of randomized trials. Plast Reconstr Surg 2011; 128(5). https://doi.org/10.1097/PRS.0b013e31822b675c.
42. Dumville JC, Webster J, Evans D, et al. Negative pressure wound therapy for treating pressure ulcers. CochraneDatabase Syst Rev 2015;(5):CD011334.
43. Liu Z, Dumville JC, Hinchliffe RJ, et al. Negative pressure wound therapy for treating foot wounds in people with diabetes mellitus. CochraneDatabase Syst Rev 2018;(10):CD010318.
44. Janssen AHJ, Mommers EHH, Notter J, et al. Negative pressure wound therapy versus standard wound care on quality of life: a systematic review. J WoundCare 2016;25(3):154–9.
45. V.A.C. Therapy indications and contraindications. Available at: http://www.activactherapy.com/cs/Satellite?c=KCI_General_C&childpagename=KCI1/KCILayout&cid=1229624973260&pagename=KCI1Wrapper. Accessed December 7, 2018.
46. Ford-Dunn S. Use of vacuum assisted closure therapy in the palliation of a malignant wound. Palliat Med 2006;20(4):477–8.
47. Riot S, de Bonnecaze G, Garrido I, et al. Is the use of negative pressure wound therapy for a malignant wound legitimate in a palliative context? “The concept of NPWT ad vitam”: a case series. Palliat Med 2015;29(5):470–3.
48. Makler V, Litt JS, Litofsky NS. Palliative coverage of cranial defect following failed cranial flap for advanced squamous cell carcinoma: case report. J Palliat Med 2018;21(1):109–13.
49. Cai SS, Gowda AU, Alexander RH, et al. Use of negative pressure wound therapy on malignant wounds – a case report and review of literature. Int Wound J 2017;14(4):661–5.
50. Cost-minimization analysis of negative pressure wound therapy in long-term care facilities.Wounds research. Available at: https://www.woundsresearch.com/article/cost-minimization-analysis-negative-pressure-wound-therapy-long-term-care-facilities. Accessed December 7, 2018.
51. Delhougne G, Hogan C, Tarka K, et al. A retrospective, cost-minimization analysis of disposable and traditional negative pressure wound therapy medicare paid claims. Ostomy Wound Manage 2018;64(1):26–33.
52. Aderibigbe BA, Buyana B. Alginate in wound dressings. Pharmaceutics 2018; 10(2). https://doi.org/10.3390/pharmaceutics10020042.
53. Gove J, Hampton S, Smith G, et al. Using the exudate decision algorithm to evaluate wound dressings. Br J Nurs 2014;23(6):S24. S26-29.
54. Dowling MB, Chaturvedi A, MacIntire IC, et al. Determination of efficacy of a novel alginate dressing in a lethal arterial injury model in swine. Injury 2016; 47(10):2105–9.
55. Kakimoto M, Tokita H, Okamura T, et al. A chemical hemostatic technique for bleeding from malignant wounds. J Palliat Med 2010;13(1):11–3.
56. Recka K, Montagnini M, Vitale CA. Management of bleeding associated with malignant wounds. J Palliat Med 2012;15(8):952–4.
57. Yanazume Y, Douzono H, Yanazume S, et al. Clinical usefulness of Mohs' paste for genital bleeding from the uterine cervix or vaginal stump in gynecologic cancer. J Palliat Med 2012;16(2):193–7.

58. Masumoto H, Fujiwara S. Cutaneous metastasis of urotherial carcinoma for which MOHS paste was useful: a case report. Nihon Hinyokika Gakkai Zasshi 2017;108(1):41–4 [in Japanese].
59. Satoh E, Ono S, Uehira D, et al. A case report of continuous bleeding due to severe skin metastases of breast cancer successfully treated using mohs paste. Gan To Kagaku Ryoho 2016;43(12):1553–4 [in Japanese].
60. Satoh E, Osanai T, Tomi Y, et al. A case report of recurrent bleeding and massive malodorous effusion due to skin invasion of advanced breast cancer successfully treated with Mohs' paste. Gan To Kagaku Ryoho 2018;45(13):1997–9 [in Japanese].
61. Kamei R, Yamamoto T, Tokuhisa A, et al. A case of advanced breast cancer with improvement in the quality of life by local treatment using mohs paste and systemic pharmacotherapy. Gan To Kagaku Ryoho 2018;45(13):2099–101 [in Japanese].
62. Katz RI, Hovagim AR, Finkelstein HS, et al. A comparison of cocaine, lidocaine with epinephrine, and oxymetazoline for prevention of epistaxis on nasotracheal intubation. J Clin Anesth 1990;2(1):16–20.
63. Krempl GA, Noorily AD. Use of oxymetazoline in the management of epistaxis. Ann OtolRhinol Laryngol 1995;104(9 Pt 1):704–6.
64. Womack JP, Kropa J, Stabile MJ. Epistaxis: outpatient management. Am FamPhysician 2018;98(4):240–5.
65. Phillips CB, Huang CC. Topical oxymetazoline hydrochloride 0.05% as a strategy to reduce intraoperative wound oozing in mohs micrographic surgery. Dermatol Surg 2015;41(6):749–50.
66. Cherny N, Fallon M, Kaasa S, et al. Oxford textbook of palliative medicine. Oxford, United Kingdom: Oxford University Press; 2015.
67. Bellew SD, Johnson KL, Nichols MD, et al. Effect of intranasal vasoconstrictors on blood pressure: a randomized, double-blind, placebo-controlled trial. J Emerg Med 2018;55(4):455–64.
68. Langemo DK, Brown G. Skin fails too: acute, chronic, and end-stage skin failure. Adv SkinWoundCare 2006;19(4):206–12.
69. Pischke SE, Haugaa H, Haney M. A neglected organ in multiple organ failure –'skin in the game'? ActaAnaesthesiol Scand 2017;61(1):5–7.
70. Levine JM. Skin failure: an emerging concept. J Am Med Dir Assoc 2016;17(7): 666–9.
71. Sibbald RG, Krasner DL, Lutz J. SCALE: skin changes at life's end: final consensus statement: October 1, 2009. Adv SkinWoundCare 2010;23(5): 225–36 [quiz: 237–8].
72. Edsberg LE, Langemo D, Baharestani MM, et al. Unavoidable pressure injury: state of the science and consensus outcomes. J WoundOstomyContinence Nurs 2014;41(4):313–34.
73. Levine JM. Historical perspective on pressure ulcers: the decubitus ominosus of Jean-Martin Charcot. J Am Geriatr Soc 2005;53(7):1248–51.
74. Kennedy KL. The prevalence of pressure ulcers in an intermediate care facility. Decubitus 1989;2(2):44–5.
75. Alvarez OM, Brindle CT, Langemo D, et al. The Vcu pressure ulcer summit: the search for a clearer understanding and more precise clinical definition of the unavoidable pressure injury. J WoundOstomyContinence Nurs 2016;43(5):455–63.
76. Kennedy terminal ulcer information and warning signs. Available at: http://www.kennedyterminalulcer.com/. Accessed January 13, 2019.

77. Maida V, Ennis M, Kesthely C. Clinical parameters associated with pressure ulcer healing in patients with advanced illness. J PainSymptomManage 2014; 47(6):1035–42.
78. Artico M, D'Angelo D, Piredda M, et al. Pressure injury progression and factors associated with different end-points in a home palliative care setting: a retrospective chart review study. J PainSymptomManage 2018;56(1):23–32.
79. Hendrichova I, Castelli M, Mastroianni C, et al. Pressure ulcers in cancer palliative care patients. Palliat Med 2010;24(7):669–73.
80. Goldstein NE, Cohen LM, Arnold RM, et al. Prevalence of formal accusations of murder and euthanasia against physicians. J Palliat Med 2012;15(3):334–9.
81. Good P, Cavenagh J, Mather M, et al. Medically assisted hydration for palliative care patients. CochraneDatabase Syst Rev 2008;(2):CD006273.
82. Good P, Richard R, Syrmis W, et al. Medically assisted nutrition for adult palliative care patients. CochraneDatabase Syst Rev 2014;(4):CD006274.
83. Langer G, Fink A. Nutritional interventions for preventing and treating pressure ulcers. CochraneDatabase Syst Rev 2014;(6):CD003216.
84. Dev R, Dalal S, Bruera E. Is there a role for parenteral nutrition or hydration at the end of life? Curr Opin Support Palliat Care 2012;6(3):365–70.
85. Kostakioti M, Hadjifrangiskou M, Hultgren SJ. Bacterial biofilms: development, dispersal, and therapeutic strategies in the dawn of the postantibiotic era. ColdSpringHarb Perspect Med 2013;3(4):a010306.
86. Wilkins RG, Unverdorben M. Wound cleaning and wound healing: a concise review. Adv SkinWoundCare 2013;26(4):160–3.
87. Georgiadis J, Nascimento VB, Donat C, et al. Dakin's solution: "One of the most important and far-reaching contributions to the armamentarium of the surgeons. Burns 2018. https://doi.org/10.1016/j.burns.2018.12.001.
88. Mangum LC, Franklin NA, Garcia GR, et al. Rapid degradation and nonselectivity of Dakin's solution prevents effectiveness in contaminated musculoskeletal wound models. Injury 2018;49(10):1763–73.
89. Barsoumian A, Sanchez CJ, Mende K, et al. In vitro toxicity and activity of Dakin's solution, mafenide acetate, and amphotericin B on filamentous fungi and human cells. J Orthop Trauma 2013;27(8):428–36.
90. Cardile AP, Sanchez CJ, Hardy SK, et al. Dakin solution alters macrophage viability and function. J Surg Res 2014;192(2):692–9.
91. Ueno CM, Mullens CL, Luh JH, et al. Historical review of Dakin's solution applications. J Plast Reconstr Aesthet Surg 2018;71(9):e49–55.
92. Carrell A, Dehelly G. The treatment of infected wounds. New York: Paul Hoeber; 1917.
93. Yang C, Goss SG, Alcantara S, et al. Effect of negative pressure wound therapy with instillation on bioburden in chronically infected wounds. Wounds 2017; 29(8):240–6.
94. Anghel EL, Kim PJ. Negative-pressure wound therapy: a comprehensive review of the evidence. Plast Reconstr Surg 2016;138(3 Suppl):129S–37S.
95. Robson MC, Payne WG, Ko F, et al. Hypochlorous acid as a potential wound care agent. J BurnsWounds 2007;6. Available at: https://www.ncbi.nlm.nih.gov/pmc/articles/PMC1853324/. Accessed January 27, 2019.
96. Armstrong DG, Bohn G, Glat P, et al. Expert recommendations for the use of hypochlorous solution: science and clinical application. Ostomy Wound Manage 2015;61(5):S2–19.
97. Bigliardi PL, Alsagoff SAL, El-Kafrawi HY, et al. Povidone iodine in wound healing: A review of current concepts and practices. Int J Surg 2017;44:260–8.

98. Woo KY. Management of non-healable or maintenance wounds with topical povidone iodine. Int Wound J 2014;11(6):622–6.
99. Vermeulen H, Westerbos SJ, Ubbink DT. Benefit and harm of iodine in wound care: a systematic review. J Hosp Infect 2010;76(3):191–9.
100. Fitzgerald DJ, Renick PJ, Forrest EC, et al. Cadexomer iodine provides superior efficacy against bacterial wound biofilms in vitro and in vivo. WoundRepair Regen 2017;25(1):13–24.
101. Estimating the clinical outcomes and cost differences between standard care with and without cadexomer iodine in the management of chronic venous leg ulcers using a Markov model.Wound Management and Prevention. Available at: https://www.o-wm.com/article/estimating-clinical-outcomes-and-cost-differences-between-standard-care-and-without. Accessed January 27, 2019.
102. Malone M, Johani K, Jensen SO, et al. Effect of cadexomer iodine on the microbial load and diversity of chronic non-healing diabetic foot ulcers complicated by biofilm in vivo. J Antimicrob Chemother 2017;72(7):2093–101.
103. Sibbald RG, Elliott JA. The role of Inadine in wound care: a consensus document. Int Wound J 2017;14(2):316–21.
104. Cadexomer iodine: an effective palliative dressing in chronic critical limb ischemia.Wounds research. Available at: https://www.woundsresearch.com/content/cadexomer-iodine-an-effective-palliative-dressing-chronic-critical-limb-ischemia. Accessed January 28, 2019.
105. Phillips I, Lobo AZ, Fernandes R, et al. Acetic acid in the treatment of superficial wounds infected by Pseudomonas aeruginosa. Lancet 1968;1(7532):11–4.
106. Kerr KG, Snelling AM. Pseudomonas aeruginosa: a formidable and ever-present adversary. J Hosp Infect 2009;73(4):338–44.
107. Madhusudhan VL. Efficacy of 1% acetic acid in the treatment of chronic wounds infected with Pseudomonas aeruginosa: prospective randomised controlled clinical trial. Int Wound J 2016;13(6):1129–36.
108. Kumara DUA, Fernando SSN, Kottahachchi J, et al. Evaluation of bactericidal effect of three antiseptics on bacteria isolated from wounds. J WoundCare 2015;24(1):5–10.
109. Halstead FD, Rauf M, Moiemen NS, et al. The antibacterial activity of acetic acid against biofilm-producing pathogens of relevance to burns patients. PLoS One 2015;10(9):e0136190.
110. Gao X, Jin Z, Chen X, et al. Advances in the progress of anti-bacterial biofilms properties of acetic acid. Zhonghua Shao Shang Za Zhi 2016;32(6):382–4 [in Chinese].
111. Williams RL, Ayre WN, Khan WS, et al. Acetic acid as part of a debridement protocol during revision total knee arthroplasty. J Arthroplasty 2017;32(3):953–7.
112. Hughes G, Webber MA. Novel approaches to the treatment of bacterial biofilm infections. Br J Pharmacol 2017;174(14):2237–46.
113. Kimball OP, Horan TN. The use of dilantin in the treament of epilepsy. Ann Intern Med 1939;13:787–93.
114. Shapiro M. Acceleration of gingival wound healing in non-epileptic patients receiving diphenylhydantoin sodium (dilantin, epanutin). Exp Med Surg 1958; 16(1):41–53.
115. Keppel Hesselink JM. Phenytoin repositioned in wound healing: clinical experience spanning 60 years. Drug Discov Today 2018;23(2):402–8.
116. Bansal NK, Mukul. Comparison of topical phenytoin with normal saline in the treatment of chronic trophic ulcers in leprosy. Int J Dermatol 1993;32(3):210–3.

117. Anstead GM, Hart LM, Sunahara JF, et al. Phenytoin in Wound Healing. Ann Pharmacother 1996;30(7–8):768–75.
118. Hao XY, Li HL, Su H, et al. Topical phenytoin for treating pressure ulcers. CochraneDatabase Syst Rev 2017;(2):CD008251.
119. Shaw J, Hughes CM, Lagan KM, et al. The clinical effect of topical phenytoin on wound healing: a systematic review. Br J Dermatol 2007;157(5):997–1004.
120. McNulty JP, Muller G. Compounded drugs of value in outpatient hospice and palliative care practice. Int J Pharm Compd 2014;18(3):190–200.
121. Lodha SC, Lohiya ML, Vyas MCR, et al. Role of phenytoin in healing of large abscess cavities. BJS 1991;78(1):105–8.
122. Dubhashi SP, Sindwani RD. A comparative study of honey and phenytoin dressings for chronic wounds. Indian J Surg 2015;77(Suppl 3):1209–13.
123. Ryan JL. Ionizing radiation: the good, the bad, and the ugly. J Invest Dermatol 2012;132(3, Part 2):985–93.
124. McQuestion M. Evidence-based skin care management in radiation therapy: clinical update. Semin Oncol Nurs 2011;27(2):e1–17.
125. Riley PA. Free radicals in biology: oxidative stress and the effects of ionizing radiation. Int J Radiat Biol 1994;65(1):27–33.
126. Williams JP, McBride WH. After the bomb drops: a new look at radiation-induced multiple organ dysfunction syndrome (MODS). Int J Radiat Biol 2011;87(8):851–68.
127. Hegedus F, Mathew LM, Schwartz RA. Radiation dermatitis: an overview. Int J Dermatol 2017;56(9):909–14.
128. Radiation dermatitis: recognition, prevention, and management | cancer network. Available at: http://www.cancernetwork.com/oncology-journal/radiation-dermatitis-recognition-prevention-and-management. Accessed December 9, 2018.
129. Ryan JL, Bole C, Hickok JT, et al. Post-treatment skin reactions reported by cancer patients differ by race, not by treatment or expectations. Br J Cancer 2007;97(1):14–21.
130. Wright JL, Takita C, Reis IM, et al. Racial variations in radiation-induced skin toxicity severity: data from a prospective cohort receiving postmastectomy radiation. Int J Radiat Oncol 2014;90(2):335–43.
131. Webb S. The physical basis of IMRT and inverse planning. Br J Radiol 2003;76(910):678–89.
132. Donovan E, Bleakley N, Denholm E, et al. Randomised trial of standard 2D radiotherapy (RT) versus intensity modulated radiotherapy (IMRT) in patients prescribed breast radiotherapy. Radiother Oncol 2007;82(3):254–64.
133. Pignol J-P, Olivotto I, Rakovitch E, et al. A multicenter randomized trial of breast intensity-modulated radiation therapy to reduce acute radiation dermatitis. J Clin Oncol 2008;26(13):2085–92.
134. Chan RJ, Webster J, Chung B, et al. Prevention and treatment of acute radiation-induced skin reactions: a systematic review and meta-analysis of randomized controlled trials. BMC Cancer 2014;14(1):53.
135. Campbell IR, Illingworth MH. Can patients wash during radiotherapy to the breast or chest wall? A randomized controlled trial. Clin Oncol 1992;4(2):78–82.
136. Roy I, Fortin A, Larochelle M. The impact of skin washing with water and soap during breast irradiation: a randomized study. Radiother Oncol 2001;58(3):333–9.
137. Théberge V, Harel F, Dagnault A. Use of axillary deodorant and effect on acute skin toxicity during radiotherapy for breast cancer: a prospective randomized noninferiority trial. Int J Radiat Oncol 2009;75(4):1048–52.

138. Hardefeldt PJ, Edirimanne S, Eslick GD. Deodorant use and the risk of skin toxicity in patients undergoing radiation therapy for breast cancer: a meta-analysis. Radiother Oncol 2012;105(3):378–9.
139. Watson LC, Gies D, Thompson E, et al. Randomized control trial: evaluating aluminum-based antiperspirant use, axilla skin toxicity, and reported quality of life in women receiving external beam radiotherapy for treatment of stage 0, I, and II breast cancer. Int J Radiat Oncol 2012;83(1):e29–34.
140. Lewis L, Carson S, Bydder S, et al. Evaluating the effects of aluminum-containing and non-aluminum containing deodorants on axillary skin toxicity during radiation therapy for breast cancer: a 3-armed randomized controlled trial. Int J Radiat Oncol 2014;90(4):765–71.
141. Ho AY, Olm-Shipman M, Zhang Z, et al. A randomized trial of mometasone furoate 0.1% to reduce high-grade acute radiation dermatitis in breast cancer patients receiving postmastectomy radiation. Int J Radiat Oncol 2018;101(2):325–33.
142. Sio TT, Atherton PJ, Birckhead BJ, et al. Repeated measures analyses of dermatitis symptom evolution in breast cancer patients receiving radiotherapy in a phase 3 randomized trial of mometasone furoate vs placebo (N06C4 [alliance]). Support Care Cancer 2016;24(9):3847–55.
143. Hindley A, Zain Z, Wood L, et al. Mometasone furoate cream reduces acute radiation dermatitis in patients receiving breast radiation therapy: results of a randomized trial. Int J Radiat Oncol 2014;90(4):748–55.
144. Miller RC, Schwartz DJ, Sloan JA, et al. Mometasone furoate effect on acute skin toxicity in breast cancer patients receiving radiotherapy: a phase III double-blind, randomized trial from the North Central Cancer Treatment Group N06C4. Int J Radiat Oncol 2011;79(5):1460–6.
145. Boström Å, Lindman H, Swartling C, et al. Potent corticosteroid cream (mometasone furoate) significantly reduces acute radiation dermatitis: results from a double-blind, randomized study. Radiother Oncol 2001;59(3):257–65.
146. Zenda S, Yamaguchi T, Yokota T, et al. Topical steroid versus placebo for the prevention of radiation dermatitis in head and neck cancer patients receiving chemoradiotherapy: the study protocol of J-SUPPORT 1602 (TOPICS study), a randomized double-blinded phase 3 trial. BMC Cancer 2018;18(1):873.
147. Wong RKS, Bensadoun R-J, Boers-Doets CB, et al. Clinical practice guidelines for the prevention and treatment of acute and late radiation reactions from the MASCC Skin Toxicity Study Group. Support Care Cancer 2013;21(10):2933–48.
148. Omidvari S, Saboori H, Mohammadianpanah M, et al. Topical betamethasone for prevention of radiation dermatitis. Indian J Dermatol Venereol Leprol 2007;73(3):209.
149. Schmuth M, Wimmer MA, Hofer S, et al. Topical corticosteroid therapy for acute radiation dermatitis: a prospective, randomized, double-blind study. Br J Dermatol 2002;146(6):983–91.
150. Meghrajani CF, Co HS, Arcillas JG, et al. A randomized, double-blind trial on the use of 1% hydrocortisone cream for the prevention of acute radiation dermatitis. Expert Rev Clin Pharmacol 2016;9(3):483–91.
151. Liguori V, Guillemin C, Pesce GF, et al. Double-blind, randomized clinical study comparing hyaluronic acid cream to placebo in patients treated with radiotherapy1This study was sponsor by the Institut Biochimique (IBSA), Via al Ponte 13, CH-6903 Lugano, Switzerland.1. Radiother Oncol 1997;42(2):155–61.
152. Primavera G, Carrera M, Berardesca E, et al. A double-blind, vehicle-controlled clinical study to evaluate the efficacy of MAS065D (XClair™), a hyaluronic

acid-based formulation, in the management of radiation-induced dermatitis. Cutan Ocul Toxicol 2006;25(3):165–71.
153. Leonardi MC, Gariboldi S, Ivaldi GB, et al. A double-blind, randomised, vehicle-controlled clinical study to evaluate the efficacy of MAS065D in limiting the effects of radiation on the skin: interim analysis. Eur J Dermatol 2008;18(3):317–21.
154. Kirova YM, Fromantin I, De Rycke Y, et al. Can we decrease the skin reaction in breast cancer patients using hyaluronic acid during radiation therapy? Results of phase III randomised trial. Radiother Oncol 2011;100(2):205–9.
155. Pinnix C, Perkins GH, Strom EA, et al. Topical hyaluronic acid vs. standard of care for the prevention of radiation dermatitis after adjuvant radiotherapy for breast cancer: single-blind randomized phase III clinical trial. Int J Radiat Oncol 2012;83(4):1089–94.
156. Williams MS, Burk M, Loprinzi CL, et al. Phase III double-blind evaluation of an aloe vera gel as a prophylactic agent for radiation-induced skin toxicity. Int J Radiat Oncol 1996;36(2):345–9.
157. Richardson J, Smith JE, McIntyre M, et al. Aloe vera for preventing radiation-induced skin reactions: a systematic literature review. Clin Oncol 2005;17(6):478–84.
158. Haddad P, Amouzgar-Hashemi F, Samsami S, et al. Aloe vera for prevention of radiation-induced dermatitis: a self-controlled clinical trial. Curr Oncol 2013;20(4):345–8.
159. Hoopfer D, Holloway C, Gabos Z, et al. Three-arm randomized phase III trial: quality aloe and placebo cream versus powder as skin treatment during breast cancer radiation therapy. Clin BreastCancer 2015;15(3):181–90.e4.
160. Rao S, Hegde SK, Baliga-Rao MP, et al. An aloe vera-based cosmeceutical cream delays and mitigates ionizing radiation-induced dermatitis in head and neck cancer patients undergoing curative radiotherapy: a clinical study. Medicines (Basel) 2017;4(3):44.
161. Ahmadloo N, kadkhodaei B, Omidvari S, et al. Lack of prophylactic effects of aloe vera gel on radiation induced dermatitis in breast cancer patients. Asian Pac J Cancer Prev 2017;(4). https://doi.org/10.22034/APJCP.2017.18.4.1139.
162. Kaul R, Mishra BK, Sutradar P, et al. The role of Wobe-Mugos in reducing acute sequele of radiation in head and neck cancers–a clinical phase-III randomized trial. Indian J Cancer 1999;36(2–4):141–8.
163. Dörr W, Herrmann T, on Behalf of the Study Group. Efficacy of Wobe-Mugos® E for Reduction of Oral Mucositis after Radiotherapy. Strahlenther Onkol 2007;183(3):121–7.
164. Fisher J, Scott C, Stevens R, et al. Randomized phase III study comparing best supportive care to biafine as a prophylactic agent for radiation-induced skin toxicity for women undergoing breast irradiation: radiation therapy oncology group (RTOG) 97-13. Int J Radiat Oncol 2000;48(5):1307–10.
165. Fenig E, Brenner B, Katz A, et al. Topical Biafine and Lipiderm for the prevention of radiation dermatitis: a randomized prospective trial. Oncol Rep 2001;8(2):305–9.
166. Pommier P, Gomez F, Sunyach M p, et al. Phase III randomized trial of calendula officinalis compared with trolamine for the prevention of acute dermatitis during irradiation for breast cancer. J Clin Oncol 2004;22(8):1447–53.
167. Abbas H, Bensadoun R-J. Trolamine emulsion for the prevention of radiation dermatitis in patients with squamous cell carcinoma of the head and neck. Support Care Cancer 2012;20(1):185–90.

168. Elliott EA, Wright JR, Swann RS, et al. Phase III trial of an emulsion containing trolamine for the prevention of radiation dermatitis in patients with advanced squamous cell carcinoma of the head and neck: results of radiation therapy oncology group trial 99-13. J Clin Oncol 2006;24(13):2092–7.
169. de Menêses AG, dos Reis PED, Guerra ENS, et al. Use of trolamine to prevent and treat acute radiation dermatitis: a systematic review and meta-analysis. Rev Lat Am Enfermagem 2018;26.
170. Lund-Nielsen B, Midtgaard J, Rørth M, et al. An avalanche of ignoring–a qualitative study of health care avoidance in women with malignant breast cancer wounds. Cancer Nurs 2011;34(4):277–85.
171. Axelrod DA, Goold SD. Maintaining trust in the surgeon-patient relationship: challenges for the new millennium. Arch Surg 2000;135(1):55–61.

Image-Guided Palliative Interventions

Jay A. Requarth, MD

KEYWORDS

- Surgical palliative care • Recurrent pleural effusion • Percutaneous cholecystostomy
- Bleed stomal varices

KEY POINTS

- Surgeons practice surgical palliative care every day.
- Image-guided procedures, commonly performed by interventional radiologists, can be added to a surgeon's armamentarium to improve the surgeon's palliative care skills.
- Fibrinothorax (trapped lung) is a common cause of recurrent pleural effusion and failed pleural symphysis.
- Percutaneous cholecystostomy is easily performed at the beside with duplex ultrasound.
- Transjugular intrahepatic portosystemic shunts is an advanced palliative care procedure that can treat bleeding esophageal varices, cirrhotic ascites, and bleeding stomal varices.

INTRODUCTION

All surgeons practice surgical palliative care whether we do it well or poorly. According to the Merriam-Webster Dictionary, the word "palliate" means "to ease (symptoms) without curing the underlying disease" and "to moderate the intensity of" disease or pain.[1] Nowhere in the definition is the word palliate restricted to end-of-life care. The most current version (2005) of the American College of Surgeons Principles of Palliative Care statement specifically states that palliative care is not synonymous with, or restricted to, end-of-life (EOL) care.[2] Despite this, the word palliate is often euphemistically used in reference to end-of-life and hospice care. For example, the National Palliative Care Registry includes patients with life-limiting illnesses.[3] Because of this confusion, there are perceived tensions and a palpable resistance to consulting palliative care services by patients and colleagues and too many equate palliative care with EOL care. Indeed, just changing from "palliative care" to "supportive care" results in significantly more referrals.[4] While we are on the terminology topic, hospice and palliative medicine physicians always practice aggressive care, we aggressively treat distressing symptoms to reduce suffering.

Disclosure Statement: No conflicts of interest.
1959 North Peacehaven Road, #118, Winston Salem, NC 27106, USA
E-mail address: jrequarth@icloud.com

Surg Clin N Am 99 (2019) 921–939
https://doi.org/10.1016/j.suc.2019.06.003

Surgeons also need to understand that hospice is a Medicare benefited program with an interdisciplinary team approach to EOL care, but unfortunately not all dying patients receive hospice services. Hospice is palliative care during the last 6 months of life and focuses on improving the quality of life for terminally ill patients. Ironically, published studies looking at length of life during hospice enrollment suggests that most patients within a given diagnosis often live longer when enrolled in hospice.[5] For Medicare beneficiaries, hospice organizations are compensated with Medicare Part A on a fixed daily rate. Practically, this means that hospice organizations cannot afford high-priced aggressive symptom ameliorative care like hemodialysis for renal failure or angiography and embolotherapy for bleeding tumors. Where that line is drawn is not yet defined as demonstrated by the fact that some hospice organizations pay for dialysis maintenance therapy to optimize quality of life, whereas most do not. For a patient to activate their hospice benefit, the certifying physician must attest that the patient is not expected to live longer than 6 months if their "disease runs its normal course."[6] If a patient wants more aggressive palliative treatments, like embolotherapy, he or she only need to revoke their hospice benefit. After the intervention, hospice benefits can be reactivated. Ideally, any intervention that is deemed indicated for improved quality of life would be covered by the patient's hospice benefits so that revocation would not be necessary.

In this article, the term "surgical palliative care" is used to differentiate it from routine general surgical care, much like vascular surgeons consider vascular surgery to be distinct from general surgery. Surgery training programs gradually adopted a 2-tiered training system so that general surgery residents were prepared to perform certain simple vascular procedures, but a vascular surgery fellowship was needed to gain the experience to perform more complex vascular surgery procedures.[7] Surgeons of all specialties provide routine and/or primary palliative care because many diseases we deal with are not curative. But, just like vascular surgery, surgical palliative care can be much more advanced. Indeed, if more surgeons adopted image-guided palliative therapies that have been devised by interventional radiology, just like vascular surgeons, they would have many new surgical palliative care therapies to offer their patients.

In addition, this article differentiates surgical palliative care from primary palliative care; surgical palliative care is palliative care that is uniquely provided by surgeons, and primary palliative care is the palliative care provided by all physicians (surgeons included) without the need for a knife. Thus, talking to your patient when giving informed consent, discussing treatment options, and establishing goals of care is primary palliative care. All surgeons provide primary palliative care – every day. We just happen to do it juxtaposed to something involving a knife.

This article highlights a few selected image-guided therapeutic options that surgeons could perform in the service of their patients. Although often considered in the realm of interventional radiology, surgeons with minimal additional training can perfect performing these procedures (personal experience of the author). Indeed, the fact that these image-guided palliative care procedures have migrated away from surgery to other specialties has resulted in decreased general surgery case volumes. Rosemurgy and colleagues[8] asked the same question about the surgical palliation of cirrhosis and portal hypertension when they noted that, in Florida, between 1988 and 2012, hospital admissions for portal hypertension complications increased 563%, but surgical decompression decreased to less than 4% of all portal vein decompression procedures. The vast majority of portal hypertension decompression procedures are now performed by interventional radiologists using image-guided transjugular intrahepatic portosystemic shunts (TIPS). General surgeons have not learned how to perform TIPS and thus most of the surgical palliative care associated with portal hypertension has been lost to interventional radiology.

RECURRENT PLEURAL EFFUSIONS

Recurrent pleural effusions, either malignant or benign, cause dyspnea by creating a ventilation/perfusion (V/Q) mismatch (**Fig. 1**). Malignant pleural effusions (MPEs) are a commonly encountered problem in patients dying of advanced malignancy, with approximately 15% of patients having them in one of many postmortem series.[9,10] Although some pleural effusions cause pain, most do not. Usually, patients with recurrent pleural effusions are referred for treatment because of dyspnea. Removal of the fluid is not the goal of treatment, correcting the V/Q mismatch is. Unfortunately, most physicians think removing the pleural fluid equates to correcting the V/Q mismatch, but that is not always the case. In fact, a significant number of patients will continue to have a V/Q mismatch after the pleural effusion is evacuated because of airway obstruction or fibrinothorax. Successful treatment requires removal of all of the pleural fluid, complete expansion of the lung, and visceral and parietal pleural apposition and fibrosis so that there is no place for the fluid to recur.[11]

How drainage is best performed is a matter of debate, and no definitive randomized controlled trials (RCCs) have been performed to determine the best treatment. Different proceduralists prefer different drainage catheters, sclerosing agents, different imaging and tube removal timing. But nonthoracic surgeons generally use small-diameter tubes, which do not drain viscus material well, and thoracic surgeons tend to opt for larger tubes and pleurectomy, which can be more painful but more efficacious (**Fig. 2**).

Percutaneous small-diameter chest tubes are now placed at the bedside or even in the clinic with premade kits. Because atelectatic lung looks the same on radiographic imaging as a pleural effusion, I recommend that chest tubes be placed with Duplex ultrasound (**Fig. 3**). At least 3 different small-diameter thoracostomy kits are now available with different external containers. Unfortunately, small-diameter thoracostomy often fails to treat the pleural effusion complications and

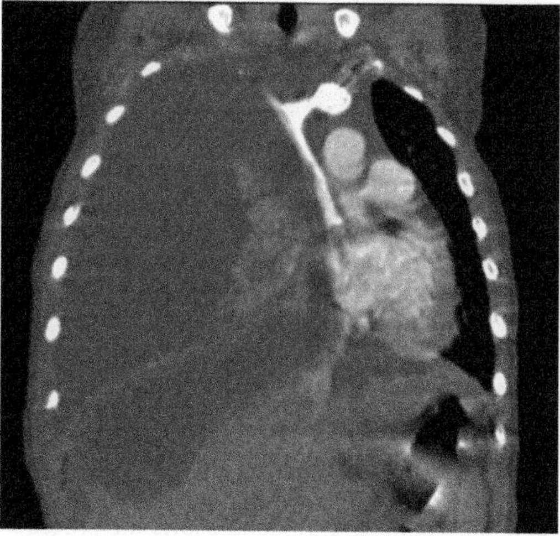

Fig. 1. Tension pleural effusion.

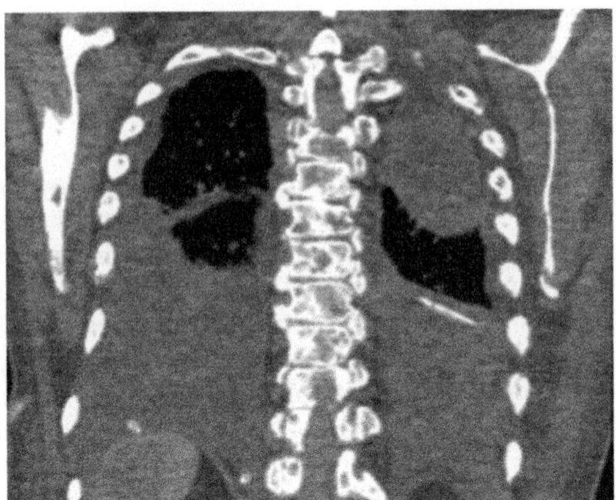

Fig. 2. Coronal sections of a noncontrasted CT of the chest showing a successfully placed small-bore left thoracostomy tube and a persistent pleural effusion. In this case, the fluid was very viscus and this small tube offered just too much resistance. A 36-French chest tube was subsequently placed with removal of all of the fluid.

patients are referred to interventional radiology for follow-up. But, by then, the pleural space is contaminated and the interventional radiologist is now dealing with an empyema.

After tube thoracostomy, with or without chemical pleurodesis, approximately 40% of patients develop recurrent pleural effusions.[12,13] A study by Warren and colleagues[12] found that most pleural effusions that do recur do so because of incomplete reexpansion of the lung (**Fig. 4**). Thus, accurate cross-sectional imaging after a complete thoracentesis is key to determining if the lung can be fully expanded. In my experience, a chest radiograph (CXR) is inadequate to rule out a posterior loculated pleural effusion. The key issue that predicts unsuccessful pleural sclerosis is an unrecognized fibrinothorax (also known as trapped lung) whereby the lung is trapped underneath a

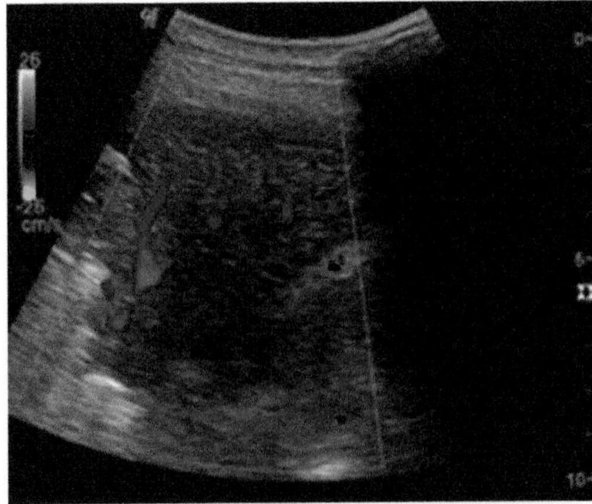

Fig. 3. Atelectatic lung looks the same as a pleural effusion, but it is easily differentiated with Duplex ultrasound. Furthermore, ultrasound allows the proceduralists to accurately identify the location of the diaphragm.

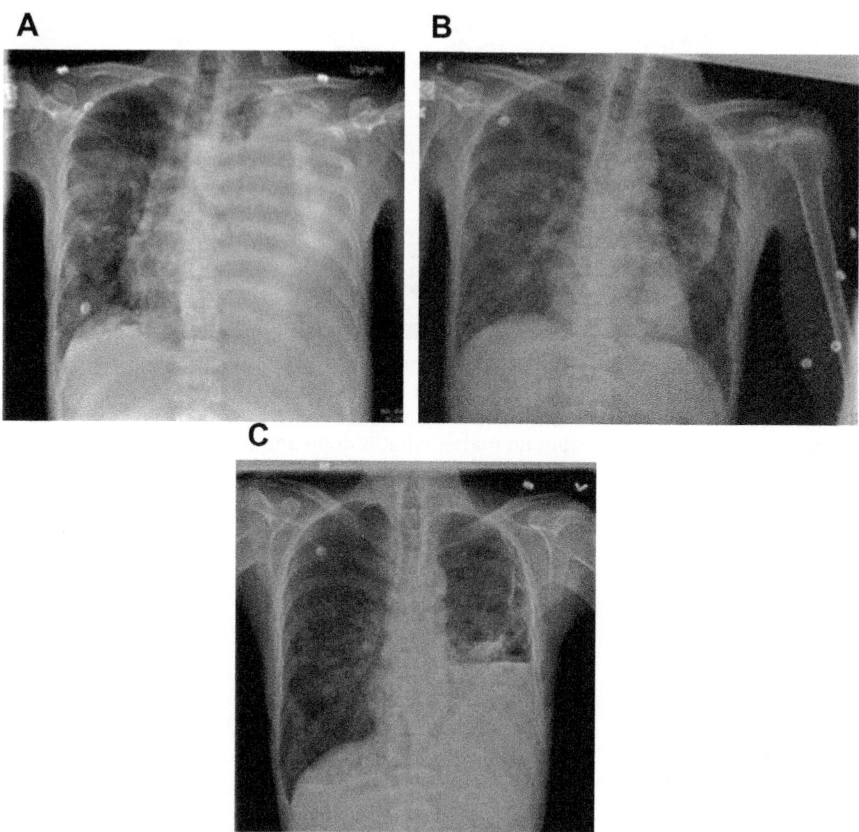

Fig. 4. (*A*) Left pleural effusion. (*B*) After complete thoracentesis, the fibrinothorax (also known as trapped lung) is easily seen on chest radiograph. Sometimes this pocket is located posteriorly, especially in recumbent patients, so I usually recommend a non–contrast-enhanced CT of the chest after complete thoracentesis and before placement of a tube thoracostomy and/or performance of a pleural sclerosis. This is not a pneumothorax, but the radiologist will always call it a pneumothorax. The key difference is whether air was obtained during the thoracentesis. (*C*) Most of the pleural effusion has recurred within 7 days. The body abhors a vacuum and fluid will eventually fill the space. You could drain this pocket a million times and the lung will never reexpand. You could also put in a chest tube and attach it to the most powerful suction device and it will just laugh at you (and not reexpand).

thick peel of fibrin and/or tumor such that the lung will not expand even when the pleural fluid is removed. A fibrinothorax can occur within just 6 weeks even in benign conditions like heart failure.

Early-stage fibrinothoraces can be treated with fibrinolytics, but, in my experience, the results are often incomplete, as shown in **Fig. 5**.

Reexpansion pulmonary edema (**Fig. 6**) is a potential problem after large-volume thoracentesis, but who is at risk and what volume of fluid removal causes the problem is unknown; however, it is associated with a pleural pressure that decreases below -20 cm H_2O.[14] Many physicians have a 1-L limit, but I have removed 3 L many times without trouble. The treatment of reexpansion pulmonary edema is symptom management; diuretics are rarely helpful.

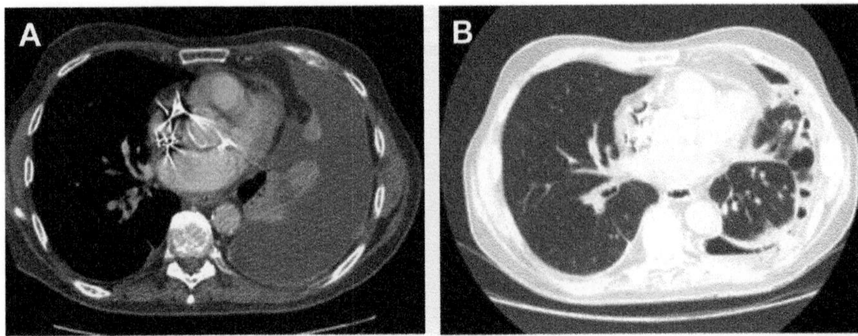

Fig. 5. (*A*) Contrast-enhanced CT of the chest (mediastinal windows) showing a left pleural effusion. (*B*) Contrast-enhanced CT of the chest (lung windows) showing incomplete lung expansion after tube thoracostomy and TPA installation. This patient will continue to develop recurrent pleural effusions no matter what is done and sclerosis will be ineffective.

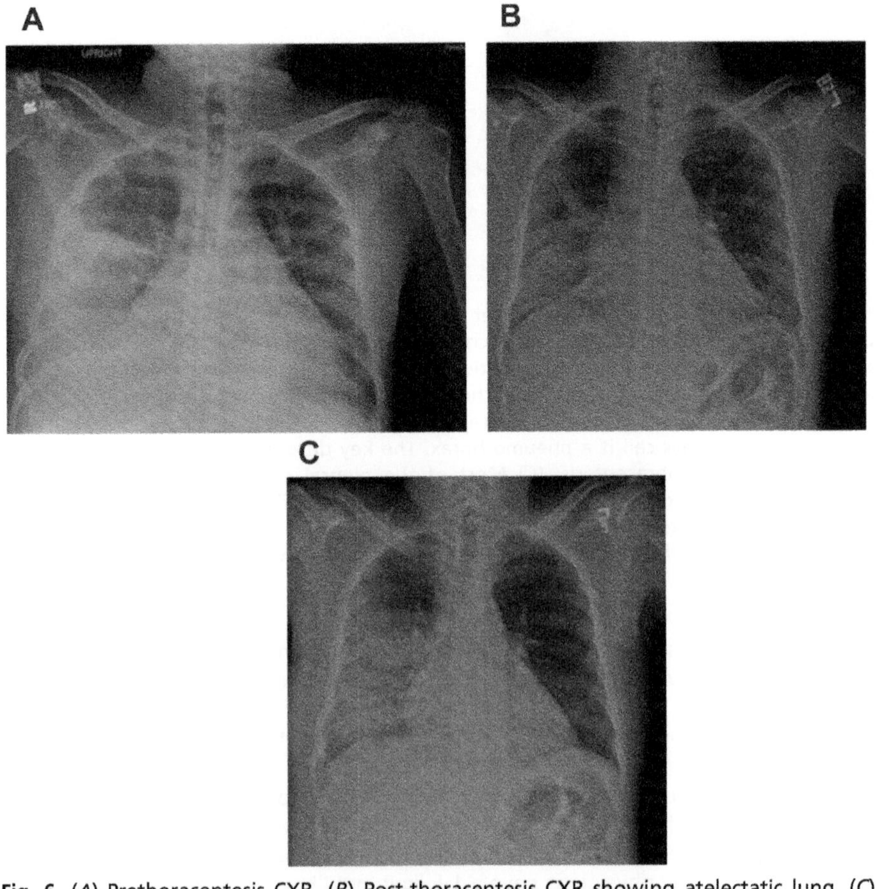

A

B

C

Fig. 6. (*A*) Prethoracentesis CXR. (*B*) Post-thoracentesis CXR showing atelectatic lung. (*C*) CXR approximately 4 hours after thoracentesis was performed for increasing dyspnea. The CXR shows increased pulmonary infiltrates consistent with reexpansion pulmonary edema.

As with all surgical palliative care procedures, surgeons need to consider the treatment burden of chest tubes. Tube thoracostomy is an extremely painful procedure, with 46% of patients rating the pain at a 9 or 10 on a pain scale of 1 to 10.[15] Most physicians limit their pain therapies to oral medications, but intercostal nerve neurolysis (also known as rib block) will significantly reduce chest wall (somatic) pain.[16] A rib block can be temporary (with lidocaine) or last 1 to 3 months (with phenol or absolute alcohol). Visceral pain can be treated with intrapleural lidocaine or bupivacaine.

FEEDING TUBES

Surgical palliative care also includes the insertion, care, and maintenance of feeding and decompression catheters. A complete review of the gastrostomy, gastrojejunostomy, and jejunostomy tubes is beyond the scope of this review; however, I would like to discuss the surgical and image-guided palliative care associated with gastrostomy tubes as an example. In general, feeding gastrostomy tubes are not recommended for the dysphagia associated with dementia.[17] In a prospective study comparing dementia patients with and without gastrostomy tube insertion, Gillick[18] found that the 6-month survival was not significantly different in the feeding tube group versus the non–feeding tube group (195 days vs 189 days).

Nonoperative insertion techniques are broadly divided into percutaneous endoscopic gastrostomy (PEG) and percutaneous radiologic gastrostomy (PRG); the former being performed by gastroenterologists and surgeons and the latter being performed almost exclusively by interventional radiologists. A recent Cochrane Database Systematic Review in 2016 found no prospective randomized trials comparing the 2 techniques, but concluded that both can be performed safely in selected individuals.[19] Clayton and colleagues[20] compared the 30-day outcomes of PRG with PEG in a group of 297 patients (150 with PRG and 147 with PEG) and found that the complication rate was not statistically different; 8% versus 6.8% in PRG and PEG, respectively.

A basic understanding of the patient's pathophysiology and the reason the patient needs either gastric decompression or artificial nutrition and hydration (ANH) is critical to alleviating patients' distressing symptoms. The patient pictured in **Fig. 7** came to see me because of chronic leakage around his gastrostomy tube and the resulting painful skin burn. He had seen several physicians for this problem and his past

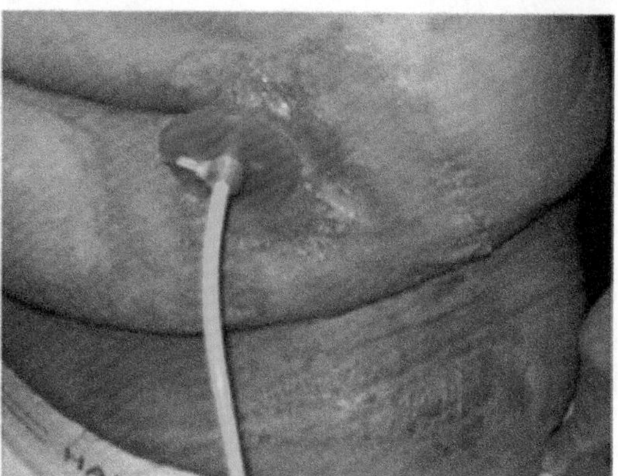

Fig. 7. A patient with a chronic G-tube for ANH. Continued gastric juice leakage and the resultant skin burn were extremely distressing and painful for this patient.

treatments included tube upsizing and topical agents, but the leakage and dermal injury continued.

Using fluoroscopy and iodinated contrast injected through the gastrostomy tube, we diagnosed gastric outlet obstruction (GOO) probably due to radiation-induced vagal nerve dysfunction. Obviously, some of his tube feedings managed to get through the pylorus, but his pyloric obstruction was accentuated when he lay on his back for the fluoroscopic procedure. Because gastric juices had difficulty passing through the pylorus, the gastric juices accumulated in the stomach and eventually found the path of less resistance and leaked out around his gastrostomy tube. It is not physiologic that gastrostomy tubes cause gastrostomy tracts to enlarge allowing gastric juices to ooze around the feeding tube. Under normal circumstances, scars contract and wounds heal around drains; they do not expand.

Using fluoroscopy, a 10-French sheath, a 0.038 Berenstein catheter, and a 0.035 hydrophilic wire, we were able to negotiate through the pylorus into the distal duodenum. Because the hydrophilic wire is difficult to exchange over, we exchanged it for a 0.035 braided wire. This patient's GOO was treated with balloon dilation of the pylorus with a high-pressure 28-mm balloon. Everything except the 28-mm balloon is readily available to any surgeon who performs even minor vascular surgery, and the skills are easily mastered. After the balloon dilation, we also added some creams and powders that were recommended by the ostomy team to treat his skin burn. On follow-up, the patient reported that the gastric leak had stopped and the skin burn was healing.

GOO can also be mechanical in origin. Patient 2 is a middle-aged woman who was dependent on a G-tube for ANH because of esophageal dysmotility. She was seen in the emergency department for aspiration and intermittent crampy abdominal pain. A contrast-enhanced abdominal computed tomography (CT) (**Fig. 8**) was performed and interpreted as a normally placed gastrojejunostomy tube. Because of leakage around her gastrostomy tube, she was referred for gastrojejunostomy tube upsizing.

Fig. 9 shows the normal and migrated positioning of a prototypical balloon-retention gastrostomy tube. The right side of the figure shows the G-tube migrated into the antrum causing a GOO. Because the gastrostomy tube tracts offer a low-pressure

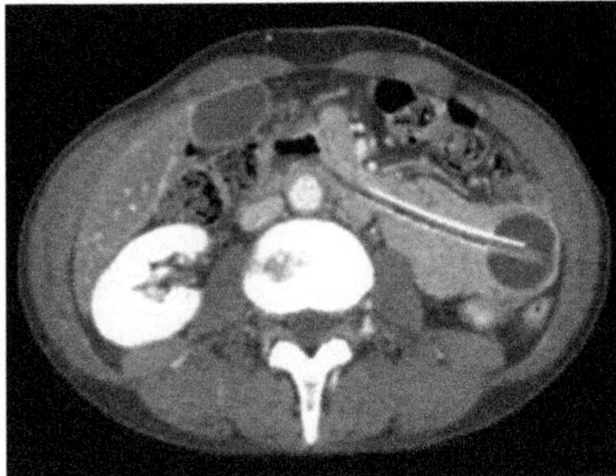

Fig. 8. Contrast-enhanced abdominal CT showing a migrated gastrostomy tube. Gastrojejunostomy tubes do not have a balloon located at the tip of the catheter. Also notice the intussuscepted small bowel proximal to the retention balloon that is causing at least a partial small bowel obstruction.

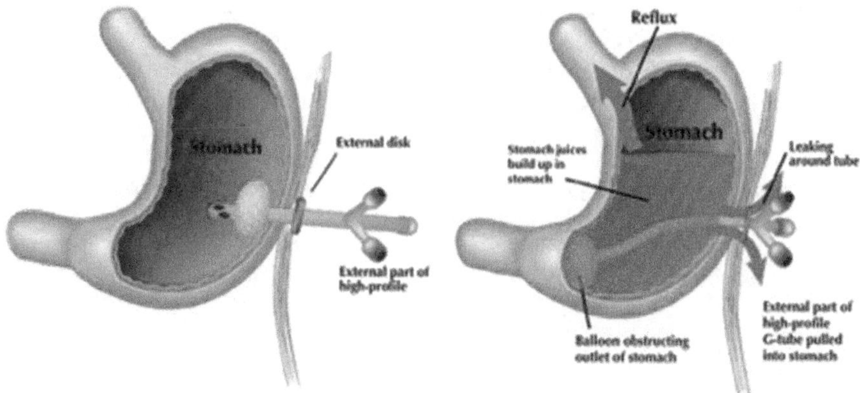

Fig. 9. Diagrams of a well-positioned gastrostomy tube and a migrated gastrostomy tube. G-tubes are used in people with dysphagia who have normal gastric motility. The retention balloon acts like a food bolus and can be pushed through the gastric outlet with gastric peristalsis. (*From* MyCareLibary.com; and *Courtesy of* Jay Requarth.)

decompression route, some or all of the gastric juices will decompress onto the abdominal wall.

G-tubes should be pulled on and the external disc should be pushed down on the skin every day. The mannequin in **Fig. 10**A shows the likely positioning of the external part of a migrated gastrostomy tube for the patient in **Fig. 8**. In this case, the retention balloon should be deflated before pulling back the G-tube, then re-inflated in the stomach. The G-tube is secured when the balloon is pulled against the anterior wall of the

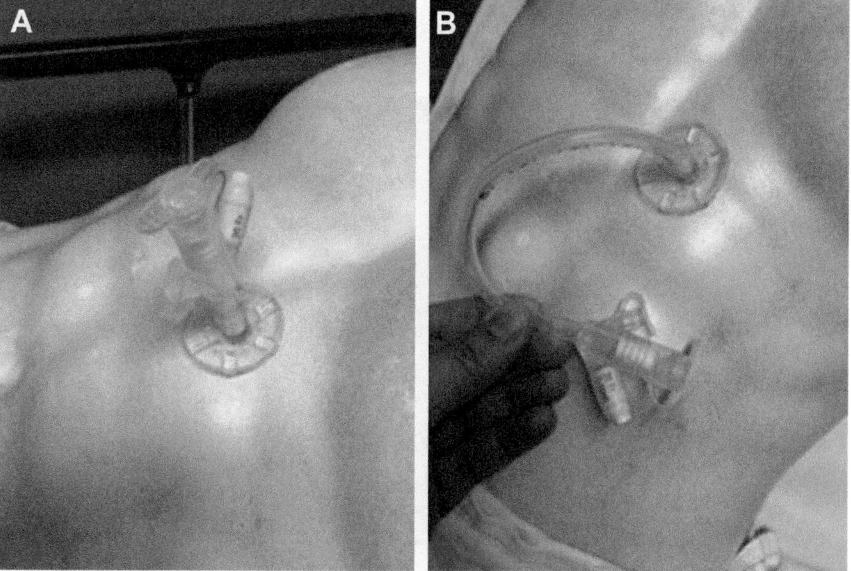

Fig. 10. (*A*) Teaching mannequin showing the external part of a migrated G-tube. No imaging is necessary for this diagnosis or treatment. (*B*) Properly positioned G-tube.

stomach and the external disk is pushed down against the skin of the anterior abdominal wall (**Fig. 10**B).

Percutaneous transesophageal G-tubes are now available for patients with abdominal anatomy that is not conducive to surgical or percutaneous G-tube placement.[21] The procedure uses a rupture-free balloon that is placed in the cervical esophagus. Using duplex ultrasound and fluoroscopy, a needle is inserted through the skin anterior to the sternal head of the sternocleidomastoid muscle into the balloon and the needle is removed over a guidewire. After the balloon and wire are advanced into the stomach, a dilator and sheath are placed over the wire. Eventually, a 15-French catheter is placed into the stomach.

CHOLECYSTITIS

Calculous and acalculous cholecystitis are 2 very different entities, especially when surgical palliative care is considered. Percutaneous drainage of the gallbladder is increasingly being used when patients are too frail and/or too unstable for immediate cholecystectomy. Zarour and colleagues[22] found that percutaneous drainage is a safe and effective procedure as either a bridge to elective cholecystectomy (40%) or as definitive therapy (54%). Interestingly, if percutaneous cholecystostomy was delayed more than 24 hours after admission, patients were more likely to need cholecystectomy. So, if percutaneous cholecystostomy is being considered, it may be better to do it sooner rather than later. Kirkegard and colleagues[23] found that when acalculous cholecystitis was studied independently, percutaneous cholecystostomy was the definitive treatment in 80.4% of patients. Percutaneous cholecystostomy is the prototype of procedures that should be in the armamentarium of a palliative care surgeon.

Placement of a percutaneous cholecystostomy tube can be performed under local anesthesia with or without mild intravenous sedation. The procedure can be performed at the bedside with duplex ultrasound. Identification of the gallbladder with an 8 to 10 MHz curvilinear probe is seen in **Fig. 11**.

I prefer a transhepatic route if possible because it keeps the drainage catheter from looping outside the gallbladder. As demonstrated in **Fig. 12**, the first step is

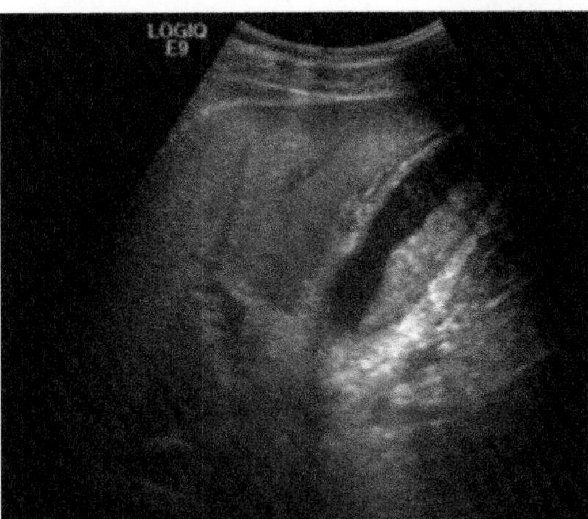

Fig. 11. Sagittaly oriented Duplex ultrasound of the right upper quadrant showing an inflamed gallbladder. The curved appearance of the overlying skin indicates that a curvilinear probe was used for imaging.

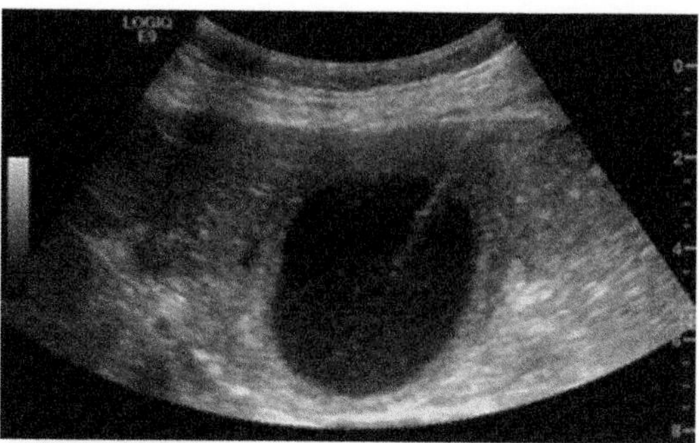

Fig. 12. Long-axis view of a needle being inserted into the gallbladder.

to insert a 22-G × 15-cm needle along the long axis of the duplex ultrasound image. Using the Seldinger technique, a mandrill wire is inserted into the gallbladder through the needle; seeing the mandrill wire curve confirms placement in the gallbladder. Under fluoroscopy, serial dilators are placed over guidewires to develop a tract. I prefer placing at least a 10-French pigtail catheter because the 8-French catheters are apt to kink at the skin suture site. I generally avoid a cholecystogram at the time of percutaneous cholecystostomy because, in my experience, the more the gallbladder is pressurized, the more likely the patient will become septic (personal experience of the author). The gallbladder is aspirated for culture and a gravity drainage bag is attached.

After a few days, a transcatheter cholangiogram is performed to assess the gallbladder, patency of the cystic duct, and check on the catheter's position. **Figs. 13** and **14** show cholecystograms of patients with calculous and acalculous cholecystitis, respectively.

If the cholecystostomy tube is being considered as definitive treatment, the catheter should not be removed until the tract around the catheter is mature (usually by 2 weeks). I do this by removing the catheter over a guidewire and placing a vascular sheath that just engages the abdominal wall. Contrast, injected through the sheath,

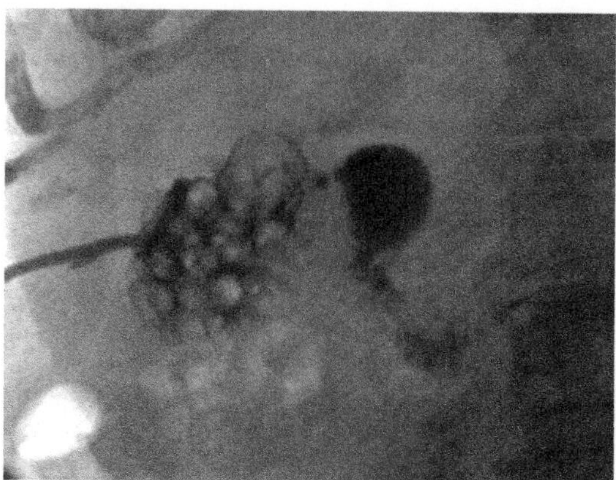

Fig. 13. Cholecystogram of a patient with calculous cholecystitis. The cystic duct is not seen and a cholecystoduodenal fistula decompresses the gallbladder.

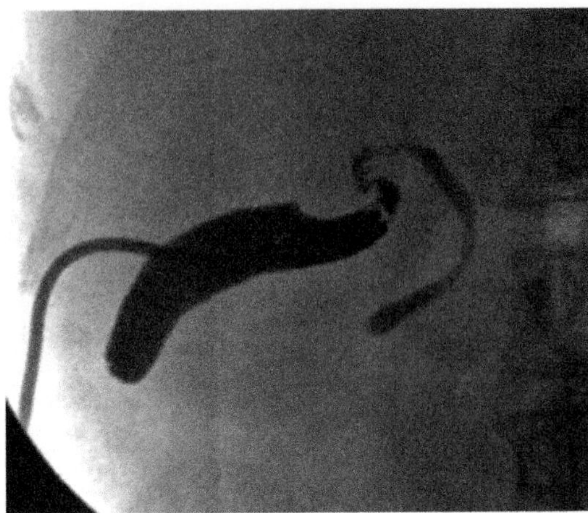

Fig. 14. Cholecystogram of a patient with resolving acalculous cholecystitis. The image shows a functioning valve at the neck of the gallbladder, a patent cystic duct, and no stones in the common bile duct. The serpentine cystic duct is normal in appearance.

should flow directly into the gallbladder; if any contrast flows into the intraperitoneal space, the tract is not mature. Replace the cholecystostomy tube and wait another 2 weeks and check for tract maturity again.

PORTAL HYPERTENSION WITH BLEEDING STOMAL VARICES

As most general surgeons know, surgical decompression of the portal vein is no longer commonly performed.[8] If the gastroenterologists cannot stop the variceal bleeding (or if ascites is recalcitrant to medical therapy), portal vein decompression is now performed by interventional radiologists with TIPSs. The advantages of TIPS are that it is a nonsurgical procedure and the diameter of the shunt is limited to the maximum diameter of the covered stent. The TIPS procedure still requires general endotracheal anesthesia. TIPS is safe and effective in 95% of patients when treating esophageal bleeding and 60% of patients when treating cirrhotic ascites.[24] Because the procedure does not cure the cause of portal hypertension, TIPS is a surgical palliative care procedure; it just happens to be currently performed by interventional radiologists. However, in my experience, the skills are easily attainable by any general surgeon with access to fluoroscopy. Adding intravascular ultrasound makes the procedure almost as easy as ultrasound-guided cannulation of the internal jugular vein.

Modern-day TIPS procedures use a partly covered stent that connects the portal vein and the right hepatic vein. The stent, placed through the liver parenchyma, is then dilated with increasingly larger balloons. Harrod-Kim and colleagues[25] found the mortality of TIPS to be correlated with the preoperative Child-Pugh class C and a Model of End Stage Liver Disease (MELD) score of greater than 25. The higher the MELD score, the higher the mortality. The post-procedural mortality increases with a portosystemic gradient of less than 8 mm Hg, because these shunts divert too much blood away from the liver parenchyma.

Assuming the blood flow through the TIPS is laminar, the post-TIPS pressure gradient is determined by the Hagen-Poisseuille equation, where μ is the fluid viscosity, L is the length of the shunt, Q is the volumetric flow rate, and r is the radius of the shunt.[26] Because μ, L, and Q are constant, ΔP is inversely proportional to the radius to the fourth power.

$$\Delta P = \frac{8\mu LQ}{\pi r^4}$$

For example, if the TIPS is initially dilated to 6 mm and the resulting portosystemic gradient is found to be 20 mm Hg, then dilating the stent to 8 mm will result in dropping the gradient to only 6 mm Hg. This will be great for stopping bleeding or ascites, but the risk of post-TIPS liver failure is too great. Thus, the second balloon dilation should be limited to 7 mm.

Ostomy bleeding can also be due to portal hypertension and treatment depends on whether the veins in the ostomy have developed systemic collaterals. If systemic collaterals have not developed, a TIPS is the only option to decompress the ostomy veins (**Fig. 15**). However, if systemic collaterals have developed, embolization of the draining vein will isolate the stomal veins to a systemic (and lower) pressure. Venous embolization can be performed in an antegrade fashion via a TIPS or retrograde via a stomal vein (**Fig. 16**).

CELIAC PLEXUS NEUROLYSIS

In the 2011 Cochrane Review of celiac plexus block (CPB) versus standard opiate therapy in patients with unresectable pancreatic cancer–related pain, Arcidiacono and colleagues[27] found 6 studies with 358 participants. A meta-analysis showed that at 4 weeks, the CPB group had significantly lower pain scores than those treated with opioids. Although statistical evidence is minimal, the fact that CPB causes fewer adverse effects than opioids is important to patients. Although they could not recommend CPBs, they suggested further studies and randomized controlled trials. A

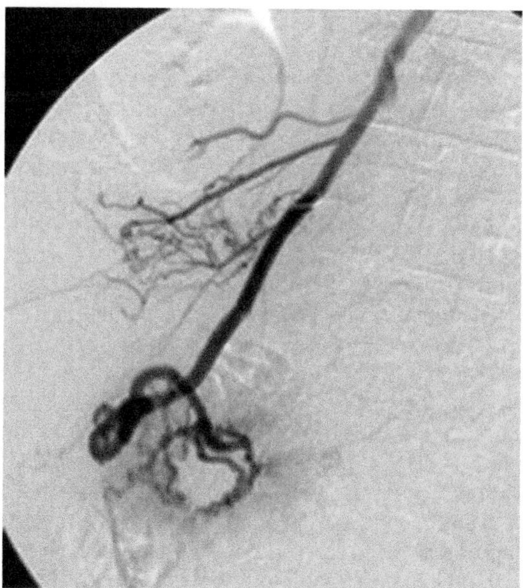

Fig. 15. Superior mesenteric vein (SMV) venogram via a catheter placed through a TIPS. No significant SMV to systemic collaterals are seen.

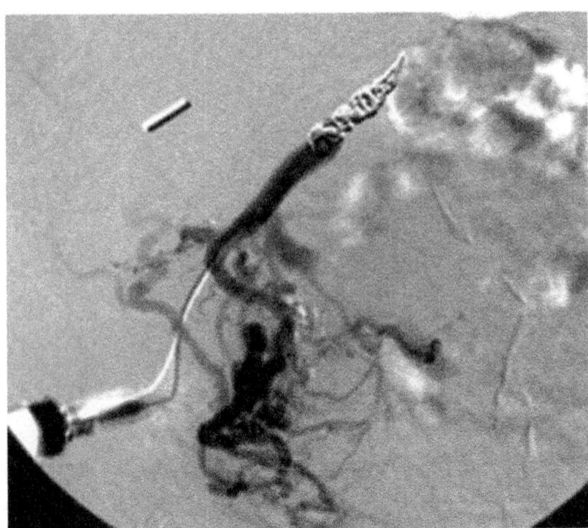

Fig. 16. SMV venogram via a stomal vein. Significant systemic collaterals are seen, so retrograde embolotherapy will isolate the stomal veins without risking viability.

systematic review of publications on the treatment of upper abdominal pain due to cancer by Nagels and colleagues[28] found that CPBs were effective, but that robust evidence for endoscopic ultrasound-guided CPBs is lacking.

CPBs are generally performed by interventional radiologists, anesthesia pain specialists, and gastroenterologists, not surgeons.[27–30] If surgeons have access to the abdomen, they should consider performing a CPB especially if resection is not indicated.

Understanding the anatomy of the upper abdomen is part of all surgical training, but the anatomy of the celiac plexus may not be common knowledge. Kambadakone and colleagues[31] have written an excellent review of the anatomy and indications for CPBs. The celiac ganglion is actually 2 ganglia (1 right and 1 left) located anterior to the aorta and inferior to the celiac artery. Zhang and colleagues[32] reported that 94% of celiac ganglia are located at the level of T12 or L1. The right celiac ganglion is frequently located between the inferior vena cava and the right crus of the diaphragm.

Complications of CPBs are rare, but include transient orthostatic hypotension, mild diarrhea, and peritonitis. Rare but devastating complications include paralysis, occurring in fewer than 0.15%, which may be due to the neurolytic agent (commonly absolute alcohol and 5% phenol) being injected under the nerve sheath and flowing back into the subarachnoid space where it desiccates the spinal cord.[33,34] Another major complication is acute pulmonary hypertension and right heart failure when a bolus is injected intravenously.

BILIARY DRAINS

Obstructive jaundice is occasionally treated with percutaneous drains when endoscopic drainage is not possible. The indications for percutaneous drainage include jaundice (serum bilirubin >5 mg/dl, because above that level the risk of liver failure with chemotherapy increases), pruritis, cholangitis, liver failure, and neurologic changes.[35–37] Placement of the biliary catheter is generally performed by interventional radiologists using Duplex ultrasound and fluoroscopy. After cannulating a peripheral bile duct, wires and catheters are serially increased in size until at least an 8-French pigtail biliary catheter is placed across the obstruction into the duodenum

(**Fig. 17**). Placing the pigtail in the duodenum is key because if the pigtail is placed in a dilated bile duct, it will eventually pull through the liver.[38] It is very important not to cross the hepatic arteries or portal veins; doing so results in bleeding or bile emboli. Do not cross the pleural space either, because bile can drain around the catheter into pleural space causing a biliary empyema.

If the biliary obstruction is in the common bile duct, drainage via the left or right hepatic lobe will equally treat the jaundice; however, in patients with hilar obstruction or large tumors, the best location of the biliary drain will be defined by the patient's anatomy. For right-handed individuals, it is easier for the proceduralists to place the drain through the right intercostal space. The right-sided insertion and subsequent drain changes keep the proceduralists hands out of the X-ray beam. However, the location of the drain influences the treatment burden. Drains placed through the right intercostal space are more painful than those placed through the sub-xyphoid space. For right-sided drains, an intercostal nerve block will decrease the chest wall pain.

These pigtail drains have 2 sets of holes, with the upper set designed to drain the intra-hepatic biliary system and the lower set, located in the pigtails, designed to empty the bile into the duodenum. Of course, the drains can be attached to external bags, but this creates an iatrogenic duodenal fistula, so internalization is best for the patient. Inspissation of the bile is common, especially after the drains are colonized, and the drainage catheters obstruct frequently. Thus, leakage around the catheter into the abdomen or onto the skin is a common occurrence. Patients should be discharged with the appropriate external attachments to treat

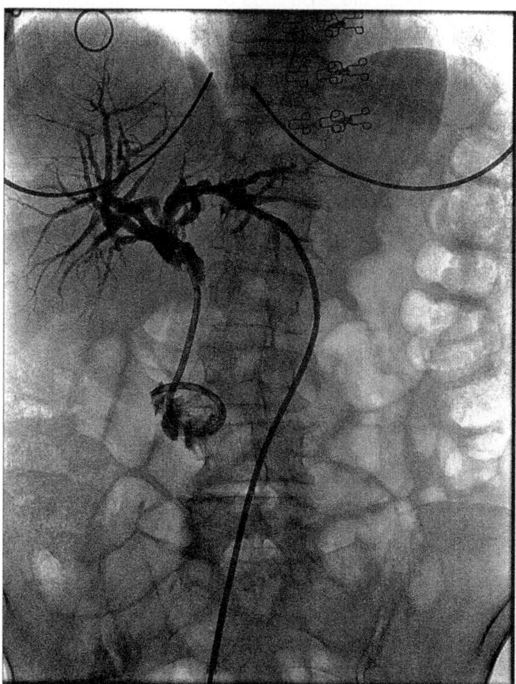

Fig. 17. Right hepatic biliary drain with the tip of the pigtail fixed in the duodenum. Contrast injected through the biliary drain exits the upper catheter holes to fill the intrahepatic biliary drain. Contrast exiting the lower pigtail holes fills the duodenum.

this eventuality. The drain(s) should be exchanged when leakage occurs or every 6 to 9 weeks.

A biliary drain is high-maintenance palliative care, probably not suitable for hospice; physicians providing this care need access to a fluoroscopic operating room to exchange these catheters. However, this care may, paradoxically, provide a longer life expectancy than endoscopically placed drains or stents because the percutaneous drain malfunction can be easily diagnosed and the drain exchanged without anesthesia.

Flushing the catheter will not necessarily keep the catheter open because the flush will just flow out the upper set of holes. The lower part of the catheter will not see any of the flush and can be totally occluded.

ABSCESS DRAINS

With the advent of 3-dimensional imaging, abscesses are commonly treated with percutaneous drainage (**Fig. 18**). Percutaneous abscess drains are also pigtail drains but usually have only one set of holes located in the pigtail part of the catheter. They can be placed using CT or Duplex-ultrasound guidance. Sometimes, the catheter and antibiotics cure the abscess, but can also serve as palliative therapy. Like biliary drains, abscess catheters occlude frequently. If pus drains around the catheter, the drain is occluded. If the catheter stops draining, the abscess may be gone, but more likely, the drain is occluded. Consider 3-dimensional imaging such as CT, MRI, or Duplex ultrasound to rule out residual abscess before removing the catheter. Flushing the catheter is diagnostic only if the catheter will not flush, as many obstructions are one-way. As a general rule, abscess catheters need to be changed every 6 to

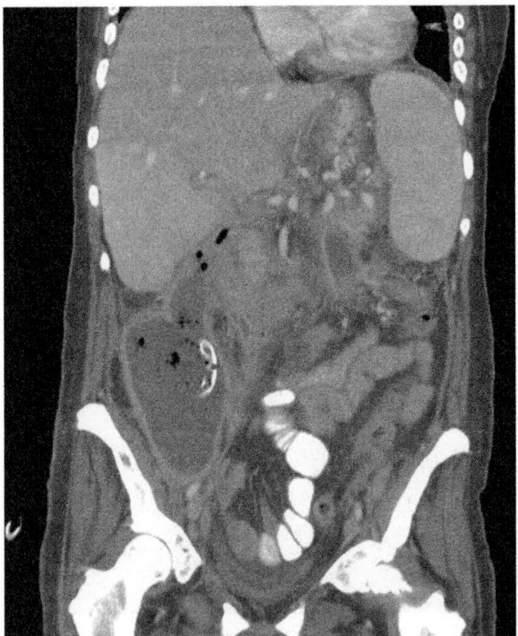

Fig. 18. A coronal section of a contrast-enhanced CT showing an extraperitoneal pig-tail abscess drain.

9 weeks. Flushing these catheters may keep the tube open, but forceful flushing may result in sepsis.

Unlike biliary drains, abscess drains are always attached to external drainage. The drains can be attached to gravity drainage systems or suction devices.

SUMMARY

All surgeons practice surgical palliative care probably on a daily basis. Advanced surgical palliative care practice is contemporaneously performed by interventional radiologists. These skills are easily obtainable by general surgeons with access to fluoroscopy and duplex ultrasonography.

REFERENCES

1. Available at: https://www.merriam-webster.com/dictionary/palliate. Accessed January 15, 2019.
2. Bulletin of the American College of Surgeons. Statement of Principles of Palliative Care August 2005, Vol 90, No 8. Available at: https://www.facs.org/about-acs/statements/50-palliative-care. Accessed July 10, 2019.
3. National Palliative Care Registry. Available at: https://registry.capc.org. Accessed January 30, 2019.
4. Dalal S, Palla S, Hui D, et al. Association between a name change from palliative to supportive care and the timing of patient referrals at a comprehensive cancer center. Oncologist 2011;16:105–11.
5. Temel JS, Greer JA, El-Jawahri A, et al. Effects of early integrated palliative care in patients with lung and GI cancer: a randomized clinical trial. J Clin Oncol 2017; 35:834–41.
6. Electronic Code of Federal Regulations 42 CFR 418.20. Available at: https://www.ecfr.gov/cgi-bin/text-idx?rgn=div5;node=42%3A3.0.1.1.5#se42.3.418_120. Accessed May 4, 2019.
7. Mills JL. Vascular surgery training in the United States: a half-century of evolution. J Vasc Surg 2008;48:90S–7S.
8. Rosemurgy A, Raitano O, Srikumar T, et al. Portal hypertension over the last 25 years: where did it go? J Am Coll Surg 2016;222:1164–70.
9. Rodriguez-Panadero F, Borderas Naranjo F, Lopez-Mejjas J. Pleural metastatic tumours and effusions: frequency and pathogenic mechanisms in a post-mortem series. Eur Respir J 1989;2:366–9.
10. American Thoracic S. Management of malignant pleural effusions. Am J Respir Crit Care Med 2000;162:1987–2001.
11. Suzuki K, Servais EL, Rizk NP, et al. Palliation and pleurodesis in malignant pleural effusion: the role for tunneled pleural catheters. J Thorac Oncol 2011;6: 762–7.
12. Warren WH, Kalimi R, Khodadadian LM, et al. Management of malignant pleural effusions using the PleurX catheter. Ann Thorac Surg 2008;85:1049–55.
13. Walker-Renard P, Vaughan LM, Sahn SA. Chemical pleurodesis for malignant pleural effusions. Ann Intern Med 1994;120:56–64.
14. Light RW, Jenkinson SG, Minh V, et al. Observations on pleural pressures as fluid is withdrawn during thoracentesis. Am Rev Respir Dis 1980;121:799–804.
15. Luketich JD, Kiss M, Hershey J, et al. Chest tube insertion: a prospective evaluation of pain management. Clin J Pain 1998;14:152–4.
16. Gulati A, Shah R, Puttanniah V, et al. A retrospective review and treatment paradigm of interventional theerapies for patients suffering from intractable

thoracic chest wall pain in the oncologic population. Pain Med 2015;16: 802–10.

17. Goldberg LS, Altman KW. The role of gastrostomy tube placement in advanced dementia with dysphagia: a critical review. Clin Interv Aging 2014; 9:1733–9.
18. Gillick M. When the nursing home resident with advanced dementia stops eating: what is the medical director to do? J Am Med Dir Assoc 2001;2: 259–63.
19. Yuan Y, Zhao Y, Xie T, et al. Percutaneous endoscopic gastrostomy versus percutaneous radiological gastrostomy for swallowing disturbances. Cochrane Database Syst Rev 2016;(2):CD009198.
20. Clayton S, DeClue C, Lewis T, et al. Radiologic versus endoscopic placement of gastrostomy tube: comparison of indications and outcomes at a tertiary referral center. South Med J 2019;112:39–44.
21. Mackey R, Chand B, Oishi H. Percutaneous transesophageal gastrostomy tube for decompression of malignant obstruction: report of the first case and our series in the US. J Am Coll Surg 2005;201:695–700.
22. Zarour S, Iman A, Kouniavsky G, et al. Percutaneous cholecystostomy in the management of high-risk patients presenting with acute cholecystitis: Timing and outcome at a single institution. Am J Surg 2017;214:456–61.
23. Kirkegard J, Horn T, Christensen SD, et al. Percutaneous cholecystostomy is an effective definitive treatment option for acute acalculous cholecystitis. Scan J Surg 2015;104:238–43.
24. Fidelman N, Kwan SW, LaBerge JM, et al. The transjugular intrahepatic portosystemic shunt: an update. AJR Am J Roentgenol 2012;199:746–55.
25. Harrod-Kim P, Wael S, Waldman D. Predictors of early mortality after transjugular intrahepatic portosystemic shunt creation for the treatment of refractory ascites. J Vasc Interv Radiol 2006;17:1605–10.
26. Bird RB, Stewart WE, Lightfoot EN. Transport phenomena. New York: John Wiley & Sons, Inc.; 1960. p. 46.
27. Arcidiacono PG, Calori G, Carrara S, et al. Celiac plexus block for pancreatic cancer pain in adults. Cochrane Database Syst Rev 2011;16(3):CD007519.
28. Nagels W, Pease N, Bekkering G, et al. Celiac plexus neurolysis for abdominal cancer pain: a systematic review. Pain Med 2013;14:1140–63.
29. Yasuda I, Wang HP. Endoscopic ultrasound-guided celiac plexus block and neurolysis. Dig Endosc 2017;29:455–62.
30. Strong VE, Dalal KM, Malhotra VT, et al. Initial report of laparoscopic celiac plexus block for pain relief in patients with unresectable pancreatic cancer. JACS 2006; 203:129–31.
31. Kambadakone A, Thabet A, Gervais DA, et al. CT-guided celiac plexus neurolysis: a review of anatomy, indications, technique, and tips for successful treatment. Radiographics 2011;31:1599–621.
32. Zhang XM, Zhao QH, Zeng NL, et al. The celiac ganglia: anatomic study using MRI in cadavers. AJR Am J Roentgenol 2006;186:1520–3.
33. Wang ZJ, Webb EM, Westphalen AC, et al. Multi-detector row computed tomographic appearance of celiac ganglia. J Comput Assist Tomogr 2010;34(3): 343–7.
34. Gallapalli L, Muppuri R. Paraplegia after intercostal neurolysis with phenol. J Pain Res 2014;7:665–8.
35. Shankar A, Taylor I. Clinical examination and investigation in surgery of the liver and biliary tract. 3rd edition. Philadelphia: Saunders; 2000.

36. Covey AM, Brown KT. Percutaneous transhepatic biliary drainage. Tech Vasc Interv Rad 2008;11:11–20.
37. Brown KT, Covey AM. Management of malignant biliary obstruction. Tech Vasc Interv Rad 2008;11:43–50.
38. Saad WE, Wallace MJ, Wojak JC, et al. Quality improvement guidelines for percutaneous transhepatic cholangiography, biliary drainage, and percutaneous cholecystostomy. J Vasc Interv Radiol 2010;21:789–95.

Palliative Care and the Pregnant Surgical Patient

Epidemiology, Ethics, and Clinical Guidance

Benjamin P. Brown, MD, MS[a,*], Roxane Holt, MD[b]

KEYWORDS

- Pregnancy • General surgery • Palliative care • Surgery in pregnancy
- Reproductive justice • Surgical ethics
- Perioperative diagnostic evaluation of the pregnant patient
- Perioperative pain and symptom management during pregnancy

KEY POINTS

- Ensuring pregnant patients have high-quality surgical care is an ethical imperative. If a pregnant patient requires a surgical intervention, providers have a duty to facilitate that care.
- To avoid missed diagnoses and to assure equitable treatment and the best possible outcomes, providers should maintain a high index of suspicion for surgical disease in pregnancy.
- Risks and benefits of planned interventions should be discussed with patients, although many imaging tests, medications, and procedures are acceptable in pregnancy, when indicated.
- Providers and patients should expect that they can obtain a thorough evaluation, definitive treatment, and adequate symptomatic control for almost all pregnant patients with surgical disease.

INTRODUCTION

Surgical disease is a common reason for pregnant patients to present for care. Obstetricians and general surgeons whose practice includes reproductive-age women frequently have to navigate the challenges of providing high-quality surgical care that also is mindful of the unique physiologic, logistical, and ethical circumstances

---

The authors have no financial conflicts to disclose.

[a] Division of Emergency Obstetrics and Gynecology, Alpert Medical School of Brown University, Women and Infants Hospital of Rhode Island, 101 Dudley Street, Providence, RI 02905, USA; [b] Section of Maternal-Fetal Medicine, University of Chicago, University of Chicago Medicine, 5841 South Maryland Avenue, Chicago, IL 60637, USA

* Corresponding author.

E-mail address: benjamin_brown@brown.edu

Surg Clin N Am 99 (2019) 941–953
https://doi.org/10.1016/j.suc.2019.06.004

of pregnancy. This article reviews the epidemiology of various types of surgical disease in pregnancy, provides a framework for unpacking some of the ethical issues related to surgical treatment of pregnant patients, and provides clinical guidance for surgical teams who care for pregnant patients.

EPIDEMIOLOGY

Nonobstetric surgery occurs in 0.5% to 2% of pregnancies.[1] The most common surgical indication in pregnancy is appendicitis,[2] with incidence estimates ranging from approximately 1 in 800 births[3] to 1 in 1500 pregnancies.[4] Although conservative management is a growing trend for treatment of appendicitis in the nonpregnant population, nonoperative management is associated with adverse outcomes in the pregnant patient.[5]

Cholecystectomy is the second most common surgical procedure performed in pregnancy, typically due to cholelithiasis, which affects 0.2% of pregnant patients.[6] Gallstone disease seems associated with an increased risk of preterm birth,[6] although cholecystectomy itself does not seem associated with greater risks in pregnancy.[7] Unsurprisingly, when required in pregnancy, cholecystectomy by a high-volume surgeon is associated with a lower complication risk.[8]

Bowel obstruction represents another common indication for surgical treatment in pregnancy, affecting 1 in 1500 to 1 in 3000 pregnancies.[9] The causes of bowel obstruction in the pregnant patient are multifactorial, including pelvic anatomic shifts due to the growing gravid uterus and adhesions from prior surgery or infection. Rarely, volvulus and intussusception occur in pregnancy as well.[9] Aggressive intervention is warranted for suspected bowel obstruction in pregnancy, because maternal mortality can be as high as 20% and fetal mortality as high as 40%.[9]

The risk of any adnexal surgical emergency in pregnancy is approximately 1 in 1800.[10] The classic adnexal surgical emergency is ovarian torsion. Presumably due to the attendant anatomic shifts, pregnancy also is a risk factor specifically for adnexal torsion (the broad category that includes torsion of the ovaries, fallopian tubes, and other adnexal masses, such as cysts and fibroids): 22% of torsions occur in pregnancy.[11,12] The risk of torsion is greatest with an adnexal mass greater than or equal to 4 cm in size. With a mass of that size, the risk of torsion may be as high as 15%[13] (although other estimates put it lower, at 1%–6%[14,15]). Ovulation induction—which may precede in vitro fertilization or may be combined with timed intercourse or intrauterine insemination—also is a risk factor for torsion, presumably due to the ovarian enlargement it produces.[12,16] Torsion is most likely to occur between 10 weeks'and 17 weeks' gestation, although it can occur throughout pregnancy.[13] When it occurs in the second or third trimester, torsion is more likely associated with normal-appearing ovaries.[16] Establishment of ovarian Doppler blood flow does not rule out torsion in any patient—pregnant or not. That said, false-positive ovarian Doppler flow is more common among pregnant than nonpregnant patients.[12] Given the higher risk in pregnancy and the higher risk of torsion with normal ovaries, work-up for adnexal torsion in pregnancy begins with a high index of suspicion.

Finally, trauma is common in pregnancy: domestic violence affects pregnant patients in 8307 of 100,000 live births, motor vehicle crashes affect 207 of 100,000 live births, and falls affect 48.9 of 100,000 live births.[17] Thorough evaluation, diagnosis, and treatment are indicated, regardless of pregnancy status. Fracture is common among patients presenting for evaluation of traumatic injury: 6% of a series of 1682 pregnant patients evaluated at 1 trauma unit had an orthopedic injury.[18] Orthopedic trauma, therefore, is a common cause for surgical intervention for pregnant patients.

Pregnancy should not preclude surgical treatment if indicated, even of pelvic and acetabular fractures.[19] Many subacute and chronic orthopedic issues, however, can be managed nonsurgically in pregnancy.[20]

ETHICS

The concept of reproductive justice can serve as an ethical framework to guide surgical care for the pregnant patient. Just as palliative care represents an integrated approach to patient well-being, reproductive justice is a holistic concept that arose from the work of women of color in advocacy and academic communities. Its basic tenet is that all people should have the ability to decide if, when, and how to have and raise children and to be able to do so in ways that ensure their own health as well as that of their families.[21] Reproductive justice also is intersectional, meaning that it recognizes that an individual's identity is influenced by multiple factors, for example, race, ethnicity, place of birth, language spoken, gender, sexuality, age, and family and pregnancy status. Each of the innumerable aspects of a person's identity contributes to the ways in which access to health care may be facilitated or impeded in the medical system and to the ways in which providers interact with the person seeking health services.

If pregnant patients are unable to access surgical care for surgical disease, the resultant risks to their health and that of their fetuses represent a systemic reproductive injustice. In short, in such a circumstance, pregnant patients are unable to ensure their own health through their reproductive lives. Likewise, if pregnant patients receive inadequate pain control or palliative treatment because of their pregnancy, this, too, represents a systemic injustice, for the same reason. Finally, through its intersectional approach, the reproductive justice model also is a reminder that people of color, trans men who are bearing children, lesbian, gay, bisexual, trans/nonbinary, queer and intersex patients, and adolescent parents also may face intersecting barriers to care that compound systemic injustices related to pregnancy itself.

Because of the profound ethical hazard of inadequate surgical treatment in pregnancy, the American College of Obstetricians and Gynecologists (ACOG) has specifically endorsed ensuring access to comprehensive surgical treatment when indicated for pregnant patients.[22]

Although a full discussion of the ethics of consent in pregnancy is outside the scope of this article, the authors strongly recommend that providers caring for pregnant patients be well versed in this field. To summarize, the standard for decisional capacity is identical for pregnant and nonpregnant patients. Pregnancy or active labor should never be used in and of itself to disqualify a patient from providing or withholding consent. In cases of truly diminished decisional capacity in a pregnant patient, providers should seek a surrogate decision maker with standing to provide informed consent according to a substituted judgment standard, just as they would for a nonpregnant patient.[23]

CLINICAL GUIDANCE

Normal Pregnancy Physiology

Hemodynamics

Hemodynamic changes of pregnancy begin as early as 5 weeks' gestational age. The overall physiologic rationale for the shifts seen is to maximize oxygen delivery to the maternal and fetal tissues. Because of the increased physiologic demands of pregnancy, the target oxygen saturation in pregnancy is greater than or equal to 95%, higher than the typical target in nonpregnant patients. The most marked cardiac change associated with pregnancy is increased cardiac output, peaking at approximately 20 weeks' to 24 weeks' gestation, at 7 L/min to 8 L/min. This increased flow relies significantly on preload, so cardiac output can be highly positional in pregnancy, with compression of the inferior vena cava associated with dramatic drops in cardiac output. Heart rate also increases through pregnancy, peaking in the third trimester, at approximately 90 beats per minute to 100 beats per minute. Although this is an increase over baseline, a heart rate of 110 beats per minute or higher still qualifies as tachycardia and is abnormal in pregnancy. Due to changes in systemic vascular resistance, the blood pressure actually drops in the first trimester, nadirs at approximately 18 weeks' to 20 weeks' gestational age, and then climbs again to a peak at approximately 36 weeks to 40 weeks.[24]

Respiratory

The entire respiratory tract is affected by pregnancy. Upper airway changes are notable for increased soft tissue edema and vascularity. For example, Mallampati score can change dramatically in pregnancy due to soft tissue edema. Upper airway/upper gastrointestinal tract procedures in pregnancy also may be associated with more bleeding than expected (eg, nasogastric [NG] tube placement or intubation).[24]

Lower airway changes in pregnancy are partially due to physical accommodations to pregnancy: upward displacement of the diaphragm by the growing uterus decreases residual volume. Tidal volume increases, however, through pregnancy. There is a resultant chronic hyperventilation with a consequent respiratory alkalosis, seen as early as 8 weeks' gestation. Overall, vital capacity and respiratory rate remain stable in pregnancy. Despite the physiologic changes of pregnancy, spirometry remains stable in pregnancy and, therefore, is a valid and important measure of pulmonary function and treatment response of pulmonary disease.[24] Due to these respiratory accommodations to pregnancy, incentive spirometry may be particularly helpful postoperatively in pregnant patients to assist in return to preoperative baseline and minimize the risk of pulmonary complications.

Hematologic

During pregnancy, plasma volume increases steadily, beginning as early as 4 weeks' to 8 weeks' gestation and peaking at approximately 32 weeks. Red blood cell mass lags behind plasma volume somewhat but should reach its peak by the week 36. Platelets may decrease mildly due to dilution or destruction. In terms of hemostasis, there is a 5-fold to 6-fold increased risk of thrombosis in pregnancy due to multiple changes to the coagulation cascade, resulting in increased procoagulant factor levels.[24]

Urinary

During the first trimester, glomerular filtration rate increases by 50%, resulting in a drop of mean creatinine from 0.8 in nonpregnant women to 0.5 in pregnancy. Standard creatinine clearance estimation formulae underestimate creatinine clearance in the pregnant patient and should not be used in this population. In dosing renally cleared drugs, providers should review drug-specific and indication-specific recommendations. A consult to a clinical pharmacist or obstetrician may be necessary for less common medications. Reflecting the higher filtration burden, the kidneys increase in size by approximately 1 cm in pregnancy. Mild physiologic calyceal and ureteral dilation begin by 8 weeks' gestation, with right dilation often greater than left.[24]

Clinical Examination and Laboratory Values in Pregnancy

Because the presenting symptom of surgical disease in pregnancy often is abdominal pain, it is helpful to consider this chief complaint as an example of the type of surgical management decision that may arise for the pregnant patient. The differential diagnosis of abdominal pain in pregnancy is largely the same as that outside of pregnancy. The authors typically think in terms of the systems potentially involved, primarily the gastrointestinal, genitourinary, and gynecologic ones. Additionally, for pregnant patients, the authors consider a pregnancy-specific differential diagnosis, including ectopic pregnancy, spontaneous abortion, labor, placental abruption, preeclampsia, acute fatty liver of pregnancy, and chorioamnionitis. Providers must have a high index of suspicion for surgical disease in the pregnant patient, because presentations can vary compared with those in a nonpregnant patient. That said, a surgical abdomen is never normal. Peritoneal signs, fever of 100.4° or higher, intractable nausea and vomiting, and other signs that are red flags in a nonpregnant patient should likewise prompt thorough evaluation in the pregnant patient.

There are a variety of ways in which surgical disease may differ between pregnant and nonpregnant patients. First and foremost, physical examination findings may differ between pregnant and nonpregnant patients. A retrocecal or otherwise displaced appendix may make typical signs, such as McBurney point tenderness, less likely. A retrocecal appendix also may provoke flank pain. In the second trimester or third trimester, the appendix may be displaced superiorly, causing right midquadrant or even right upper quadrant pain.[25,26] Rovsing sign, obturator sign, and psoas sign seem to be rare in pregnancy,[2] although their noninvasive nature and the ability to elicit them at the bedside mean clinicians should still consider performing them. The Murphy sign likewise should be reliable in pregnancy because no significant displacement of the gallbladder is expected.

Additionally, laboratory values may be altered by the normal physiology of pregnancy (**Table 1** for a summary of normal laboratory cutoffs for pregnant patients). Normal transaminase and bilirubin values do not change in pregnancy.

Imaging Modalities in Pregnancy

Although choosing an imaging modality in pregnancy involves different risk-benefit considerations than for the nonpregnant patient, it is almost always feasible to obtain good imaging to evaluate surgical disease in pregnancy. Ultrasound is safe in

Table 1
Selected normal upper and lower test values in pregnancy

Component	First Trimester	Second Trimester	Third Trimester
Liver function tests			
Alkaline phosphatase (IU/L)	17–88	25–126	38–229
Lipase (U/L)	21–76	26–100	41–112
Kidney function test			
Creatinine (mg/dL)	0.4–0.7	0.4–0.8	0.4–0.9
Hematologic tests			
White blood cell count (1000 cells/μL)	5.7–13.6	5.6–14.8	4.9–16.9
Hemoglobin (g/dL)	11.6–13.9	9.7–14.8	9.5–15.0
Platelet count (1000 cells/μL)	174–391	155–409	146–429
International normalized ratio	0.86–1.08	0.83–1.02	0.80–1.09
Fibrinogen (mg/dL)	244–510	291–538	301–696

Data from Cunningham et al., eds. Williams Obstetrics. 23rd ed. New York, NY: McGraw-Hill, 2010. 1259-1261.

pregnancy, so when ultrasound is part of the diagnostic work-up, providers should feel comfortable using it as indicated. As anatomy shifts in pregnancy, ultrasound may be more challenging or less reliable in some circumstances, particularly when evaluating the appendix. When evaluating for gallbladder pathology, however, a right upper quadrant ultrasound is reliable in pregnancy[27]; sludge or delayed emptying may be normal, but evidence of cholecystitis, suggested by wall thickening or pericholecystic fluid, is not.

Magnetic resonance imaging (MRI) also is safe and is generally the imaging test of choice for evaluating intra-abdominal processes not amenable to ultrasound (appendicitis is the classic example). MRI in pregnancy should be performed, however, without gadolinium. Gadolinium passes to the fetus and then is excreted by the fetus into the urine, which forms the amniotic fluid. This is subsequently reingested by the fetus, leading to persistence of gadolinium in the fetal circulation. Moreover, because pure gadolinium is toxic, it is administered with a chelation agent. The longer time in fetal circulation provides additional time to unbind from the chelator. Animal data suggest gadolinium is a possible teratogen, presumably due to this time-dependent chelation-unbinding effect. Specific fetal effects in humans are controversial, but it is possible that gadolinium increases the risk of inflammatory and rheumatic conditions in the fetus that may persist into extrauterine life. Gadolinium also is linked to stillbirth and neonatal death. Gadolinium should be used only if it significantly improves the diagnostic power of the test, which is unusual.[28,29]

Contrary to common belief, radiographs frequently are a safe test to use in pregnancy. Although it is true that radiation can be toxic to the fetus, the response is dose dependent and timing dependent. In very early pregnancy (less than 4 weeks' gestational age), the response is all or nothing, resulting in either loss of the pregnancy or no effect. Between 4 weeks' and 10 weeks' gestational age, structural anomalies are possible. Between 10 weeks' and 25 weeks' gestational age, risks of radiation include intellectual disability and microcephaly. The threshold dose for complications throughout these time periods ranges from 50 mGy to 250 mGy fetal dose. With regard to risk of carcinogenesis, the data are somewhat incomplete, but one helpful estimate is that a fetal exposure of 10 mGy to 20 mGy raises the fetus' eventual leukemia risk by 1.5 times to 2 times over a background risk of 1 in 3000. To put these risks in perspective, a 2-view chest radiograph with fetal shielding has a fetal absorbed dose of approximately 0.0005 mGy to 0.01 mGy. Even CT angiography to evaluate for pulmonary embolism has a relatively low fetal absorbed dose of 0.01 mGy to 0.66 mGy.[28] In short, all patients should be appropriately counseled about the risks and benefits of any radiograph test, but if radiograph or CT angiography is indicated, it is an appropriate test to use, especially in the later second trimester and beyond.

Risks of Surgery in Pregnancy

All surgical procedures carry risks, such as bleeding, infection, and injury to adjacent structures, which do not change with pregnancy. The shifting anatomy of the pregnant abdomen, however, may make dissection and tissue plane identification more challenging. It also is important for surgeons to be mindful of avoiding injury to the uterus during abdominal surgery. Older data suggested a risk of spontaneous abortion as high as 12% in first-trimester surgeries and preterm labor as high as 40% in the third trimester. More recent data, however, suggest laparoscopy in any trimester is unassociated with increased maternal or fetal risks.[30] The baseline risk of spontaneous abortion in the first trimester is approximately 7%, so these older data may well represent a background population risk.[31]

Surgical Approach in Pregnancy

With regard to surgical approach, the choice for laparoscopy versus laparotomy for abdominal surgery in pregnancy should be based largely on the skills and resources of the surgeon and their team. Laparoscopy is reasonable in any trimester, with the same indications and contraindications that apply outside of pregnancy, as long as the surgeon has a reasonable expectation of being able to obtain adequate exposure. The benefits of laparoscopy to the pregnant patient are similar to those for the nonpregnant patient, namely, shorter recovery time, less pain, fewer wound complications, and so forth.[30] Endoscopic procedures, too, are reasonable in pregnancy when indicated (endoscopic retrograde cholangiopancreatography for symptomatic choledocholithiasis, for example).[32]

Nonurgent surgery is ideal in the second trimester due to the potential for a lower risk of spontaneous abortion or preterm labor.[22] For truly elective procedures, the team may consider either timing surgery to coincide with the second trimester or postponing the procedure until after delivery. These decisions should be individualized, however, and consider that delaying a surgery until the postpartum period may cause impediments to caring for a newborn. Pregnancy itself should not delay an indicated procedure when that delay carries a meaningful risk of a worse outcome for the pregnant patient.

Fetal monitoring plans should be individualized, and the plan should be discussed in a multidisciplinary manner between the patient, obstetrician, surgeon, anesthesiologist, and other relevant team members. In general, previable fetuses (earlier than 24 weeks at most institutions) may receive documentation of fetal heart tones before and after the procedure. Viable fetuses should typically receive a nonstress test and tocometry before and after surgery. Rarely, intraoperative fetal monitoring may be used in the setting of a particularly high-risk surgery or when the fetus has some known compromise. If using fetal monitoring intraoperatively, the team should be prepared and able to interrupt the ongoing nonobstetric procedure, reposition the patient if necessary, and perform an emergent cesarean delivery. Preoperative preparations in cases with intraoperative fetal monitoring should also include obtaining consent for cesarean, having the necessary operating room setup for delivery and neonatal resuscitation, and having obstetric and neonatal providers available.

General Perioperative Considerations

Extrapolating from American Society of Anesthesiologists and Society of Obstetric Anesthesia and Perinatology guidelines, preoperative laboratory evaluation should be individualized.[33] In the authors' practice, in addition to laboratory tests relevant to the suspected pathology, a type and screen and a complete blood cell count routinely are obtained prior to surgical intervention on any pregnant patient.

Pregnant patients are at higher risk of aspiration, in part due to progestin-mediated relaxation of the lower esophageal sphincter as well as to the mechanical effect of the gravid uterus. American Society of Anesthesiologists guidelines recommend pregnant patients undergoing elective surgery have no clear liquids within the 2 hours prior to surgery and no solid food in the 6 hours to 8 hours prior to surgery (with the exact timing based on fat content and additional risk factors for delayed gastric emptying). Providers also should consider nonparticulate antacid medication to minimize aspiration risk (eg, sodium citrate/citric acid suspension).[33] Decisions about the timing of emergent or urgent surgery based on nothing-by-mouth status should be individualized in collaborative conversation between the surgeon, anesthesiologist, and obstetrician.

There is no specific standard of care for perioperative NG tube placement or urinary catheterization in the pregnant population. In the authors' practice, NG tube decompression is reserved for the same indications as for those in nonpregnant patients, recognizing that NG tubes also may contribute to aspiration risk, localized pain, and epistaxis if used routinely. Likewise, the authors reserve Foley catheters for the same indications as for nonpregnant patients and seek to minimize urinary catheterization for all patients to reduce the risk of catheter-associated infections.

While anesthetic management is outside the scope of this article, although no randomized trial data are available to guide specific anesthetic choices in pregnancy, no anesthetic agent is associated with teratogenic effects in humans at any gestational age.[22] During surgery, patients should be placed into left lateral uterine displacement if possible, because this improves blood return from the inferior vena cava, maximizing preload and therefore cardiac output.[30] Capnography should be used to monitor gas exchange, particularly if using carbon dioxide insufflation for laparoscopy.[30]

Postoperative Issues in Pregnancy

Pain

The goal of acute postoperative pain control for pregnant patients is the same as that for nonpregnant patients: to achieve a level of pain that minimizes distress and maximizes a patient's ability to participate in postoperative recovery. Pregnancy should not alter the patient or provider expectation of functional pain control. The mainstay of pain control in the pregnant patient is acetaminophen, because it is safe for the fetus and has no risk for dependency, with dosing guidelines similar to those for nonpregnant patients. Nonsteroidal anti-inflammatory drugs (NSAIDs) generally are contraindicated in pregnancy due to the risk of alterations in fetal renal blood flow in early pregnancy and premature closure of the ductus arteriosus in later pregnancy. Short courses of NSAIDs may be used if needed, however, prior to 32 weeks' gestation. Initiation of NSAIDs should be done in consultation with a patient's obstetrician. For musculoskeletal pain, a 1-week to 2-week course of cyclobenzaprine is a reasonable choice in pregnancy as an adjunct to acetaminophen, physical therapy, warm compresses, and other supportive measures. If gabapentin is required by a pregnant patient, the authors recommend consultation with a maternal-fetal medicine specialist and a patient-centered risk-benefit discussion. Small human studies do not show an increased risk of fetal malformations, although there are animal data to suggest a potential association between gabapentin and birth defects.[34–36]

For more severe pain, opioids are an appropriate medication choice in pregnancy. Setting reasonable pain management expectations preoperatively can help providers use the shortest and lowest-dose course possible to minimize the risk of opioid use disorder and of neonatal abstinence syndrome for the fetus/neonate. As in nonpregnant patients, those with opioid use disorder often require higher doses of opioids to obtain therapeutic effect. Providers should avoid under-dosing opioid treatment in the perioperative setting for those with chronic opioid use. Under-dosing patients in this population is likely to result in significant untreated pain. Medication-assisted treatment of opioid use disorder also has become increasingly common in pregnancy, and providers will likely care for many patients who are using buprenorphine, buprenorphine/naloxone, or methadone. Buprenorphine is a partial opioid receptor agonist and, therefore, may interfere with the therapeutic effect of other opioids as well as cause withdrawal symptoms if initiated in a patient who is a chronic opioid user. The authors recommend consulting a palliative medicine or pain control specialist to help optimize pain medication management in complex patients, such as those with opioid use disorder, especially if they are not achieving adequate pain control.

Anticoagulation

Nonobstetric surgery in pregnant patients carries at least moderate risk for venous thromboembolism. Sequential compression devices and early ambulation strategies should be used for all pregnant patients who undergo hospitalization or surgical intervention. Providers also may consider heparin, 5000 units twice daily or 3 times daily, or enoxaparin, 40 units once daily, in patients with additional risk factors for thrombosis.[30,37]

Diet and gastrointestinal symptoms

In general, although no society guidelines are available, postoperative nutritional status for pregnant patients should be managed like that of nonpregnant patients. Pregnant patients have higher basal metabolic needs and are at higher risk of ketosis, so early feeding seems particularly appropriate in this group. There are some data from the cesarean delivery literature to support the assertion that early feeding may shorten hospital stay and time to first bowel movement.[38,39]

Gastrointestinal upset is a common symptom of pregnancy, and it can be exacerbated by perioperative stressors, such as anesthetic medications, antibiotics, prolonged nothing-by-mouth status, and infection. First-line medications for nausea and vomiting in pregnancy are vitamin B_6 and doxylamine. These work best as daily controller medications. For acute nausea and vomiting, additional medications often are necessary. Safety data are reassuring for metoclopramide, prochlorperazine, and promethazine, and, in the authors' practice, one of these medicines frequently is begun as a first-line intervention for acute perioperative nausea and vomiting. Diphenhydramine also may provide some antinausea effect as well as being a useful sleep aid. Data on ondansetron are inconsistent; some data suggest an increased risk of cleft palate and possibly cardiac anomalies with first trimester use, but these data come from small studies. More research is needed on this association. If ondansetron is required by a patient, it is reasonable to use this medicine after patient-centered counseling about risks and benefits.[40]

For opioid-induced constipation and ileus, human data are lacking on the safety of peripherally acting μ-opioid receptor antagonists (PAMORAs) in pregnancy, although animal data are reassuring. The authors do not routinely use PAMORAs, although care may be individualized, particularly for surgeries with a high risk of prolonged postoperative ileus. The authors' typical practice for managing ileus is NG tube decompression if required for control of severe postoperative nausea and vomiting, diet advancement as tolerated, supportive care for nausea, close monitoring to maintain the minimal dose of opioids that achieves functional pain control, and early ambulation.

For gastroesophageal reflux, H_2-receptor antagonists and proton pump inhibitors are reasonable and safe interventions. Mechanical interventions, such as elevating the head of the bed and eating while fully seated, also may improve patient symptoms and comfort. For diarrhea, unfortunately, symptomatic treatments in pregnancy are limited. Loperamide has conflicting data but may be associated with teratogenicity, and bismuth subsalicylate has the risk of early closure of the ductus arteriosus.

Pruritis

If pruritis is believed histamine mediated (or the exact cause is unclear), antihistamines, such as diphenhydramine or hydroxyzine, are a low-risk and cost-effective intervention. In the setting of opioid-induced pruritis, butorphanol may be considered, bearing in mind that it increases the risk of sedation and other, rarer opioid-related side effects, such as respiratory depression and hypotension.

Insomnia and anxiety

The first-line treatment of insomnia in the perioperative setting should be an evaluation for provoking factors, such as poorly controlled pain, unnecessary bedside procedures or evaluations overnight, anxiety, and so forth. In particular, providers should consider whether overnight vital sign checks, nursing evaluations, and other interventions may be spaced out to allow longer interruption-free time for sleep. If management of these factors does not improve sleep quality, a trial of a sedating antihistamine, such as diphenhydramine or doxylamine, is reasonable. The authors prefer to avoid other sedative-hypnotics, such as zolpidem, in pregnancy and the perioperative period, due to the potential for delirium and behavioral disinhibition as well as the potential for neonatal respiratory depression if given close to delivery. If required by a patient, zolpidem may be considered, after a patient-centered risk-benefit discussion. There are few data on melatonin use in pregnancy, but it is reasonable to consider a short course of the medication if required by the patient.

Anxiety should first be managed by nonpharmacologic care (social work intervention, music or art therapy, engagement of family members, reassurance about specific concerns, and so forth). If these interventions are inadequate to obtain symptomatic improvement, medication is a reasonable choice, with a first-line medication being a mildly sedating/anxiolytic antihistamine, such as diphenhydramine or hydroxyzine. Benzodiazepines may be used in pregnancy if indicated, particularly in the second and third trimesters. There are some conflicting data to suggest risk of teratogenicity at doses higher than typically administered if benzodiazepines are used in the first trimester. There also is a risk of neonatal withdrawal syndrome if benzodiazepines are given in repeated doses in the third trimester or within hours of delivery. The authors recommend involvement of the obstetrician and, ideally, a psychiatrist with expertise in pregnancy and the peripartum period if benzodiazepines are being initiated.

Enhanced Recovery Pathways and the Pregnant Patient

Overall, enhanced recovery after surgery (ERAS) recommendations are appropriate for pregnant patients as well as for nonpregnant patients. The ERAS guidelines from ACOG do not include specific recommendations for pregnant patients.[41] Key potential ERAS pathway deviations related to pregnancy include

- Potentially stricter nothing-by-mouth requirements.
- Use of acetaminophen and avoidance of celecoxib or gabapentin for perioperative prophylactic pain medication. Gabapentin is a reasonable perioperative medication in breastfeeding patients.
- Avoidance of NSAIDs in pregnancy. NSAIDs are safe for breastfeeding patients.
- Individualization of transdermal scopolamine use. Scopolamine is considered safe in pregnancy, though providers should balance the potential benefit of reduced nausea/vomiting with the risk of worsening the already-delayed gastrointestinal transit of pregnancy.

SUMMARY

In summary, notwithstanding the unique challenges of evaluating surgical disease in pregnancy, providers and patients should expect that they can obtain a thorough evaluation and adequate symptomatic control in almost all cases. Moreover, ensuring pregnant patients have high-quality surgical care is an ethical imperative. A reproductive justice lens is a reminder that surgical disease is surgical disease, regardless of pregnancy status. If a pregnant patient requires an urgent or emergent surgery, providers have a duty to facilitate that care.

REFERENCES

1. Balinskaite V, Bottle A, Sodhi V, et al. The risk of adverse pregnancy outcomes following nonobstetric surgery during pregnancy: estimates from a retrospective cohort study of 6.5 million pregnancies. Ann Surg 2017;266(2):260.
2. Tamir IL, Bongard FS, Klein SR. Acute appendicitis in the pregnant patient. Am J Surg 1990;160(6):571–6.
3. Andersen B, Nielsen TF. Appendicitis in pregnancy: diagnosis, management and complications. Acta Obstet Gynecol Scand 1999;78(9):758–62.
4. Mourad J, Elliott JP, Erickson L, et al. Appendicitis in pregnancy: new information that contradicts long-held clinical beliefs. Am J Obstet Gynecol 2000;182(5): 1027–9.
5. Abbasi N, Patenaude V, Abenhaim HA. Management and outcomes of acute appendicitis in pregnancy-population-based study of over 7000 cases. BJOG 2014;121(12):1509–14.
6. Ibiebele I, Schnitzler M, Nippita T, et al. Outcomes of gallstone disease during pregnancy: a population-based data linkage study. Paediatr Perinat Epidemiol 2017;31(6):522–30.
7. Silvestri MT, Pettker CM, Brousseau EC, et al. Morbidity of appendectomy and cholecystectomy in pregnant and nonpregnant women. Obstet Gynecol 2011; 118(6):1261–70.
8. Kuy S, Roman SA, Desai R, et al. Outcomes following cholecystectomy in pregnant and nonpregnant women. Surgery 2009;146(2):358–66.
9. Coleman MT, Trianfo VA, Rund DA. Nonobstetric emergencies in pregnancy: trauma and surgical conditions. Am J Obstet Gynecol 1997;177(3):497–502.
10. Johnson TR, Woodruff JD. Surgical emergencies of the uterine adnexae during pregnancy. Int J Gynaecol Obstet 1986;24(5):331–5.
11. Tsafrir Z, Hasson J, Levin I, et al. Adnexal torsion: cystectomy and ovarian fixation are equally important in preventing recurrence. Eur J Obstet Gynecol Reprod Biol 2012;162(2):203–5.
12. Hasson J, Tsafrir Z, Azem F, et al. Comparison of adnexal torsion between pregnant and nonpregnant women. Am J Obstet Gynecol 2010;202:536.e1-6.
13. Yen C-F, Lin S-L, Murk W, et al. Risk analysis of torsion and malignancy for adnexal masses during pregnancy. Fertil Steril 2009;91(5):1895–902.
14. Bromley B, Benacerraf B. Adnexal masses during pregnancy: accuracy of sonographic diagnosis and outcome. J Ultrasound Med 1997;16(7):447–52 [quiz: 453–4].
15. Schmeler KM, Mayo-Smith WW, Peipert JF, et al. Adnexal masses in pregnancy: surgery compared with observation. Obstet Gynecol 2005;105(5 Pt 1): 1098–103.
16. Smorgick N, Pansky M, Feingold M, et al. The clinical characteristics and sonographic findings of maternal ovarian torsion in pregnancy. Fertil Steril 2009;92(6): 1983–7.
17. Mendez-Figueroa H, Dahlke JD, Vrees RA, et al. Trauma in pregnancy: an updated systematic review. Am J Obstet Gynecol 2013;209(1):1–10.
18. Cannada LK, Hawkins JS, Casey BM, et al. Outcomes in pregnant trauma patients with orthopedic injuries. Submitted for Fall meeting of American Academy of Orthopedic Surgeons. Dallas, TX, October 2008.
19. Desai P, Suk M. Orthopedic trauma in pregnancy. Am J Orthop 2007;36(11): E160–6.

20. Ritchie JR. Orthopedic considerations during pregnancy. Clin Obstet Gynecol 2003;46(2):456–66.
21. SisterSong. Reproductive justice. Available at: https://www.sistersong.net/reproductive-justice/. Accessed January 22, 2019.
22. American College of Obstetricians and Gynecologists, American Society of Anesthesiologists. Nonobstetric surgery during pregnancy (committee opinion 696). Obstet Gynecol 2017;129:777–8.
23. American College of Obstetricians and Gynecologists. Refusal of medically recommended treatment during pregnancy (committee opinion 664). Obstet Gynecol 2016;127:e175–82.
24. Gabbe SG, Niebyl JR, Simpson JL, editors. Obstetrics: normal and problem pregnancies. 5th edition. Philadelphia: Churchill Livingstone; 2002. p. 57–71.
25. Pates JA, Avendiano TC, Zaretsky MV, et al. The appendix in pregnancy: confirming historical observations with a contemporary modality. Obstet Gynecol 2009; 114(4):805–8.
26. Mahmoodian S. Appendicitis complicating pregnancy. South Med J 1992;85(1): 19–24.
27. Parangi S, Levine D, Henry A, et al. Surgical gastrointestinal disorders during pregnancy. Am J Surg 2007;193(2):223–32.
28. American College of Obstetricians and Gynecologists. Guidelines for diagnostic imaging during pregnancy and lactation (committee opinion 723). Obstet Gynecol 2017;130:e210–6.
29. Expert Panel on MR Safety, Kanal E, Barkovich AJ, Bell C, et al. ACR guidance document on MR safe practices: 2013. J Magn Reson Imaging 2013;37(3): 501–30.
30. Society of American Gastrointestinal and Endoscopic Surgeons. Guidelines for diagnosis, treatment, and use of laparoscopy for surgical problems during pregnancy. Surg Endosc 2008;22:849–61.
31. Wang X, Chen C, Wang L, et al. Conception, early pregnancy loss, and time to clinical pregnancy: a population-based prospective study. Fertil Steril 2003; 79(3):577–84.
32. Cappell MS, Stavropoulos SN, Friedel D. Systematic review of safety and efficacy of therapeutic endoscopic-retrograde-cholangiopancreatography during pregnancy including studies of radiation-free therapeutic endoscopic-retrograde-cholangiopancreatography. World J Gastrointest Endosc 2018;10(10): 308–21.
33. American Society of Anesthesiologists, Society for Obstetric Anesthesia and Perinatology. Practice guidelines for obstetric anesthesia. Anesthesiology 2016; 124(2):1–31.
34. Holmes LB, Hernandez-Diaz S. Newer anticonvulsants: lamotrigine, topiramate and gabapentin. Birth Defects Res A Clin Mol Teratol 2012;94(8):599–606.
35. Fujii H, Goel A, Bernard N, et al. Pregnancy outcomes following gabapentin use: results of a prospective comparative cohort study. Neurology 2013;80(17): 1565–70.
36. Prakash, Prabhu LV, Rai R, et al. Teratogenic effects of the anticonvulsant gabapentin in mice. Singapore Med J 2008;49(1):47–53.
37. American College of Obstetricians and Gynecologists. Prevention of deep vein thrombosis and pulmonary embolism (committee opinion 84). Obstet Gynecol 2007;110:429–40.
38. Soriano D, Dulitzki M, Keidar N, et al. Early oral feeding after cesarean delivery. Obstet Gynecol 1996;87(6):1006–8.

39. Patolia DS, Hilliard RLM, Toy EC, et al. Early feeding after cesarean: randomized trial. Obstet Gynecol 2001;98(1):113–6.
40. American College of Obstetricians and Gynecologists. Nausea and vomiting of pregnancy (practice bulletin 189). Obstet Gynecol 2018;131:e15–30.
41. American College of Obstetricians and Gynecologists. Perioperative pathways: enhanced recovery after surgery (committee opinion 750). Obstet Gynecol 2018;132:e120–30.

Tracheostomies and PEGs

When Are They Really Indicated?

Melissa Red Hoffman, MD, ND*

KEYWORDS

• Tracheostomy • Feeding tube • PEG • Goals of care

KEY POINTS

- Tracheostomies, both percutaneous and open, may be performed in patients with neurodegenerative disorders, severe brain injury, head and neck cancers, and an inability to wean from mechanical ventilation.
- Percutaneous endoscopic gastrostomies (PEGs) may be performed in patients with neurodegenerative disorders, severe brain injury, and head and neck cancers, as well as for management of symptoms secondary to malignant bowel obstructions.
- Before performing a tracheostomy or a PEG, the surgeon is responsible for determining whether the procedure is appropriate given the patient's prognosis and goals of care.

INTRODUCTION

In the United States, more than 100,000 tracheostomies are performed on adult patients each year.[1] According to Healthcare Cost and Utilization Project data from 2015, tracheostomy was associated with the longest length of stay of 231 procedures, as well as the third highest cost of stay and the fifth highest in-hospital mortality, indicating the critical nature of this patient population.[2] More than 215,000 percutaneous endoscopic gastrostomy (PEG) tubes are also placed each year.[3] Although the 2015 cost of stay was much less for these patients, this population still ranked in the top 10% for in-hospital mortality.[2]

Beyond discussing the appropriate patient population, the correct timing, and the potential risks and benefits of both tracheostomies and PEGs, it is also important to acknowledge and consider the meaning of these tubes to both patients and their families. Most of these procedures are performed in response to or in anticipation of the loss of a vital function. The presence of such tubes serves as a concrete reminder not only of the loss of function but also of a potential loss of independence. Further, in some (but not all) disease states, the need for such tubes portends a poor

Disclosure: The author has nothing to disclose.
Department of Surgery, Mission Hospital, Asheville, NC, USA
* 509 Biltmore Avenue, Asheville, NC 28801.
E-mail address: redhoffman@gmail.com

Surg Clin N Am 99 (2019) 955–965
https://doi.org/10.1016/j.suc.2019.06.009

prognosis. Given this, the decision to place either a tracheostomy or a PEG should always be made in the context of both the patient's prognosis and the patient's goals of care.

TRACHEOSTOMY IN NEUROLOGIC DISORDERS

In patients with neurodegenerative diseases, particularly amyotrophic lateral sclerosis (ALS), progressive muscle paralysis leads to respiratory failure secondary to both diaphragmatic weakness and an inability to manage respiratory secretions. Although median survival for patients with ALS is 3 to 5 years, many patients have chronic hypoventilation long before death.[4] Most patients choose to use only noninvasive ventilation (NIV) to manage their symptoms, but a small subset (between 2% and 10%) undergo tracheostomy.[5] Given the progressive nature of ALS, respiratory failure should be anticipated and the options for treatment as well as the preferences of the patient and the family should be discussed long before a tracheostomy is ever considered.[5]

Multiple studies have addressed tracheostomy in patients with ALS. Albert and colleagues[6] prospectively followed a group of 118 patients with ALS for a median of 12 months; 93 (78.8%) patients had been diagnosed within the past year and were considered recently diagnosed, whereas 25 (21.2%) patients had been diagnosed more than 1 year before the study inception and were considered long-term patients. By the last follow-up, only 4 (4.3%) recently diagnosed patients had undergone tracheostomy, compared with 5 (20%) of the long-term patients, with a 53.8% mortality in the recently diagnosed group and a 32% mortality in the long-term group. The investigators concluded that tracheostomy offered a survival benefit, as shown by the lower mortality of the long-term patients. A 10-year population-based study of 1260 Italian patients with ALS found that 134 (10.6%) patients underwent tracheostomy, and median survival after the procedure was 253 days; younger age, enteral nutrition, marital status, and follow-up at a multidisciplinary ALS center were all independently associated with increased survival.[7] In a 12-year retrospective study of 316 Norwegian patients with ALS, 79 (25%) underwent tracheostomy. The median survival was 15.4 months for those using NIV and 74.8 months for those with tracheostomy.[8]

In patients with severe brain injury caused by stroke, trauma, or cardiac arrest, a tracheostomy may be indicated because of an inability to manage respiratory secretions secondary to either muscle weakness or altered mental status. Although prognostication is difficult in brain-injured patients, it must be a key component of any tracheostomy discussion and should include not only the likelihood of survival but also the possible cognitive and functional outcomes.[9]

The 30-day mortality of patients with stroke requiring mechanical ventilation ranges from 46% to 75%.[9] The Stroke-related Early Tracheostomy Versus Prolonged Orotracheal Intubation in Neurocritical Care trial (SETPOINT) randomized 60 patients with severe ischemic or hemorrhagic stroke and an estimated need for at least 2 weeks of mechanical ventilation to either early (1–3 days) or standard (7–14 days) tracheostomy. Although there was no difference in the primary outcome of intensive care unit (ICU) length of stay between the two groups, the early group did have a lower use of sedatives as well as lower ICU and 6-month mortality, although the investigators caution that the study was not powered to investigate these secondary outcomes.[10] In a retrospective study of 240 patients with hemorrhagic stroke (113 with subarachnoid hemorrhage and 127 with intracerebral hemorrhage), timing of tracheostomy was not associated with mortality, but, in patients surviving to discharge, earlier tracheostomy was associated with a shorter ICU length of stay.[11] The possible benefits of early tracheostomy in patients with stroke must be balanced with the benefit of allowing a time-limited trial of mechanical ventilation during which time prognosis and goals of care may be clarified.[9]

TRACHEOSTOMY IN TRAUMA AND CRITICAL ILLNESS

A 2013 study compared a propensity-matched cohort of 1514 adults with isolated traumatic brain injury (TBI) and found that early (<8 days) tracheostomy was associated with shorter duration of mechanical ventilation, decreased ICU length of stay, and decreased hospital length of stay. There was no difference in mortality between the early and late (>8 days) groups.[12] A retrospective study of 152 patients with TBI in Iran also found that early (<6 days) tracheostomy was associated with decreased ICU length of stay and decreased hospital length of stay. Again, there was no mortality difference between the early and the late (>6 days) groups.[13] In addition, a retrospective study of 583 adult patients with trauma with TBI compared those patients who received tracheostomy with those who did not; the 2 groups were similar in terms of age; gender; race; Glasgow Coma Scale score; Abbreviated Injury Score Head, Face, and Chest scores; as well as Injury Severity Score. In this study, although tracheostomy was associated with both longer duration of mechanical ventilation and longer ICU length of stay, the tracheostomy group did have a higher rate of survival to discharge.[14]

Patients with trauma without TBI are another group that may require prolonged mechanical ventilation. A prospective, randomized, intention-to-treat trial of 60 patients with trauma without head injury compared tracheostomy before postinjury day 8 with tracheostomy after day 28 and found no differences in duration of mechanical ventilation, frequency of pneumonia, or ICU length of stay.[15] A prospective, randomized, intention-to-treat trial of 44 patients with burns compared early (postburn day 4) tracheostomy with conventional (postburn day 14) tracheostomy and also reported no differences in duration of mechanical ventilation, incidence of pneumonia, or survival between the two groups.[16] All of these findings suggest that it is reasonable to consider a time-limited trial of mechanical ventilation to allow for clarification of goals of care.

Critically ill patients represent a heterogeneous cohort. The tracheostomy management in critical care (TracMan) trial randomized 909 adults in the United Kingdom, most with pulmonary disorders, to either early (within 4 days of admission) or late (after 10 days) tracheostomy and reported no improvement in median length of stay or 30-day mortality.[17] Of note, overall morality was 41% at discharge, 47% at 1 year, and 53% at 2 years, a testament to the necessity of discussing both prognosis and goals of care before performing any procedure. In chronically critically ill patients, defined as those with a constellation of features, including ventilator dependence, brain dysfunction, neuromuscular weakness, endocrinopathy, and malnutrition, prognostication becomes even more difficult.[18] The ProVent probability model was designed to predict 1-year mortality in patients requiring at least 21 days of mechanical ventilation following acute illness.[19] Bice and colleagues[20] suggest using this model when discussing the potential benefits and limitations of tracheostomy in this group of patients.

TRACHEOSTOMY IN HEAD AND NECK CANCER

Head and neck cancers represent a diverse group of patients, including those with cancers of the skin, oropharynx, larynx, trachea, jaw, and thyroid. Tracheostomy may be indicated in the setting of impending airway compromise. A retrospective review of 109 patients with locoregionally advanced tumors of the base of tongue, larynx, or hypopharynx compared 28 who underwent tracheotomy before chemoradiotherapy with 11 who underwent tumor debulking and found debulking to be a safe alternative to tracheostomy. In patients with at least 2 years of follow-up, none of those who underwent debulking required long-term tracheostomy and all were taking at least some nutrition by mouth, whereas 19% of those who underwent tracheostomy remained tracheostomy dependent and 81% were taking at least some nutrition by mouth. The investigators conclude that, although tracheostomy provides a safe and definitive airway, surgical debulking is a viable alternative in a select group of patients.[21] As discussed earlier, the practice of symptom anticipation, rather than symptom management, invites both providers and patients to discuss whether the placement of a tracheostomy is aligned with the overall goals of care before any sort of emergency occurs.[5]

PERCUTANEOUS ENDOSCOPIC GASTROSTOMIES IN NEUROLOGIC DISORDERS

The progressive muscle paralysis of ALS also leads to choking, aspiration, and dysphagia. In the United States, the rate of PEG placement in patients with ALS ranges from 13% to 40%.[22] Practice guidelines from the American Academy of Neurology summarize 9 studies of enteral nutrition via PEG in patients with ALS and conclude that PEG placement is likely effective in stabilizing body weight.[23] Although the investigators offer a nutrition management algorithm in which patients with ALS are classified as low, moderate, or high risk for PEG placement based on their functional vital capacity (FVC) and note that risk increases when FVC decreases to less than 50%, they conclude that there are insufficient data to support specific timing of PEG. A 2011 Cochrane Review focused on the efficacy of PEGs on survival, nutritional status, and quality of life and found no randomized controlled trials that compared enteral tube feeding with oral intake. The investigators state that, although the evidence suggests a survival advantage associated with tube feeding in some patients with ALS, this conclusion is tentative at best.[22]

Patients with severe brain injury may also require placement of a permanent feeding tube. In patients with stroke, particularly those with cerebral, cerebellar, or brain stem lesions, difficulty swallowing can also lead to the need for feeding access. Further, diminished levels of consciousness secondary to stroke or TBI can lead to decreased volitional consumption of both solids and liquids. In a systematic review of 24 articles, up to 78% of patients with stroke were found to have dysphagia on videofluoroscopic assessment.[24] Evidence suggests that at least 50% of stroke-related dysphagia resolves within 1 to 2 weeks, and the American Heart Association Stroke Council recommends continuing nasogastric tube feeding for 2 to 3 weeks before considering placement of a more permanent gastrostomy tube.[25] As discussed earlier, a time-limited trial (in this case, of nasogastric tube feeding) allows time for both prognosis and goals of care to be clarified. However, tensions exist between these recommendations and the need for treatment teams to facilitate patient discharge to less acute levels of care. Although a retrospective case-matched controlled study of 193 patients with stroke admitted to stroke rehabilitation found that patients with a PEG tube had a higher likelihood of both transfer back to an acute hospital and death, a wide variation exists regarding enteral nutrition–related admission policies in skilled nursing facilities (SNFs).[26] For example, researchers found that SNFs in New York City are much less likely to accept patients with nasogastric feeding tubes than randomly selected SNFs throughout the country.[27]

Much has been written regarding enteral feeding in patients with dementia. As stated earlier, the need for a feeding tube can signal a precipitous decline. The

Choices, attitudes, and strategies for care of advanced dementia at end-of-life (CASCADE) study followed 323 nursing home residents with advanced dementia for a period of 18 months and found that the 6-month adjusted mortality after the development of an eating problem was 38.6%. The median survival for this cohort was 1.3 years.[28] In a review of the literature spanning more than 30 years, Finuacane and colleagues[29] conclude that tube feeds in this patient population do not prevent pneumonia, do not prevent the consequences of malnutrition, do not prolong survival, do not improve functional status, and do not prevent pressure injuries. Cervo and colleagues[30] note the importance of reminding both referring providers and families that advanced dementia is a terminal illness; just like in cancer, these patients die not of starvation but of their underlying disease process. In addition, the American Geriatrics Society specifically states that feeding tubes are not recommend in older patients with advanced dementia, defined as a stage 7 (out of 7) on the Global Deterioration Scale and consistent with an inability to recognize loved ones, minimal to no verbal communication, total functional dependence, incontinence of both urine and stool, and an inability to ambulate independently. The society notes that the presence of feeding tubes leads to an increase in both agitation and health care use, as well as to the development of new pressure injuries.[31] Instead, careful hand feeding as tolerated by the patient is suggested.

PERCUTANEOUS ENDOSCOPIC GASTROSTOMIES IN HEAD AND NECK CANCER

Head and neck cancers can lead to dysphagia and odynophagia either from the tumor or as a result of treatment, including surgery, chemotherapy, and radiation; substantial weight loss is a well-reported issue in this patient population.[32] The National Comprehensive Cancer Network guidelines for head and neck cancers strongly suggests prophylactic feeding tube placement in the following patients: those with severe weight loss before treatment, those with symptoms interfering with their ability to eat or drink, those with comorbidities that may be aggravated by poor nutritional intake, those with severe aspiration, and those who will receive large fields of high-dose radiation to the oral mucosa and adjacent connective tissues.[33] However, the guidelines also encourage oral intake during treatment in order to maintain swallowing function. This possible loss of function is one argument against the placement of a prophylactic feeding tube. In a retrospective study of 445 patients with head and neck cancer, Olson and colleagues[34] found that patients who underwent prophylactic feeding tube placement had a higher rate of feeding tube dependence at 90 days postradiation, but no difference at 1 year. In contrast, a retrospective study of 111 patients with locally advanced head and neck cancer undergoing chemoradiation found that prophylactic PEG placement correlated with less weight loss and no difference in posttreatment tube dependence.[35]

PERCUTANEOUS ENDOSCOPIC GASTROSTOMIES IN MALIGNANT BOWEL OBSTRUCTION

Malignant bowel obstruction is a common complication in patients with advanced gastrointestinal and gynecologic cancers With an average life expectancy of 80 days at the time of presentation, this condition is a poor prognostic indicator and thus the decision to pursue any procedures must be made with this fact in mind.[36] Mobily and Patel[37] reviewed the outcomes of palliative PEG tube placement in patients with gastrointestinal cancer and found that in multiple studies most patients reported improvement in their obstructive symptoms. Rath and colleagues[38] performed a retrospective chart review of 53 patients with ovarian, peritoneal, or fallopian tube cancer who underwent placement of a percutaneous upper gastrointestinal decompressive tube; 2 (3.8%) required large-volume paracentesis before tube placement. Relief of nausea and vomiting was reported by 92.5% of patients, 91% were able to tolerate oral intake, and 50% were discharged to home. Median survival following tube placement was 46 days.

It is common for surgeons to be consulted for PEG placement in patients with cancer and other chronically ill patients. In these instances, it is important to recognize the presence of anorexia-cachexia syndrome. Associated with both weight loss and fat and muscle tissue wasting secondary to disruption of multiple hormones as well as altered carbohydrate, lipid, and glucose metabolism, this syndrome has failed to show any benefit from nutritional support, including hypercaloric feeding.[39]

MORBIDITY, MORTALITY, AND PATIENT EXPERIENCES WITH TRACHEOSTOMIES AND PERCUTANEOUS ENDOSCOPIC GASTROSTOMIES

In a 10-year retrospective study of 1130 consecutive tracheostomies performed at 1 US institution, 49 (4.3%) major complications were reported, including subglottic stenosis, severe hemorrhage, tracheocutaneous fistula, severe infection, decannulation, tension pneumothorax, and tracheoesophageal fistula. Eight (0.7%) patients died as a direct result of the procedure.[40] A 1-year retrospective study of 113,653 US adult patients who underwent tracheostomy in 2006 reported 21,821 (19.2%) in-hospital deaths with only 628 (0.6%) deaths related to the procedure. Patients with neurologic conditions, trauma, and upper airway infections were more likely to survive to discharge. The complication rate was 3.2%; tracheoesophageal fistula, tracheal stenosis, and infection were the most common complications.[1] The TracMan trial reported a 5.5% complication rate in patients undergoing tracheostomy within 4 days and a 7.8% complication rate in those undergoing a tracheostomy after 10 days.[17]

Kaub-Wittemer and colleagues[4] specifically studied quality of life and psychosocial issues of both patients with ALS and of their caregivers in an effort to compare NIV with mechanical ventilation via tracheostomy. All but 1 of the tracheostomy patients was mechanically ventilated 24 h/d. Although there were no differences in quality of life among the NIV and mechanically ventilated patients, there were marked differences in quality of life between the two groups of caregivers. Thirty percent of tracheostomy caregivers rated their quality of life as less than that of the mechanically ventilated patient.

In a 1-year retrospective study of 719 patients who underwent PEG placement in the United Kingdom in 2002, 97% of whom had a neurologic disease, 309 patients (43%) died within 1 week of the procedure.[41] In a second retrospective study of 181,196 patients who underwent PEG placement in the United States in 2006, 19,562 patients (10.8%) died while in the hospital, with 2934 patients (15%) dying within 2 days of placement. Patients with malnutrition as the indication for PEG placement had the highest morality rate, whereas those with head and neck cancer had the lowest rate.[42] A study of 7369 Veterans Affairs patients, most with either neurologic disease or head and neck cancer, reported a 23.5% in-hospital mortality and a median survival of 7.5 months after PEG placement.[43] A 5-year, single-institution, retrospective study of 189 patients with malignancies (excluding head/neck and thoracic) reported a 19.6% in-hospital mortality, a 10.2% major complication rate, and a 11.3% minor complication rate.[44] Given these low complication rates (compared with the in-hospital mortalities quoted in this study and those discussed earlier), it is likely that most mortalities in these studies were related to the underlying disease processes rather than to the procedure itself. Again, this underlies the importance of discussing PEG placement in the context of both prognosis and goals of care.

Schrag and colleagues[45] provide a comprehensive review of PEG-related complications and divide them into 1 of 3 categories: those related to the upper endoscopy, those related to the placement of the PEG, and those occurring after the procedure has been completed. The 3 most common complications are postprocedural and are benign pneumoperitoneum (seen in up to 50% of patients and usually self-limiting), clogged tube (in up to 45% of patients), and wound infection (the rate can be decreased from 18% to as low as 3% with a single dose of periprocedural antibiotics). The most serious complication, esophageal perforation, is related to endoscopy and is extremely rare (incidence of 0.008%–0.04%). A cross-sectional survey of 50 head and neck patients who had undergone PEG placement as part of their treatment reported deficits in multiple quality of life domains, including appearance and activity.[46] Even when PEG placement is reasonable in terms of prognosis and in line with goals of care, patients should be extensively counseled regarding the potential of both complications and negative influence on quality of life.

ETHICAL TENSIONS AND THE SURGEON AS CONSULTANT

Most physicians, including those who consult the surgeons to place either a tracheostomy or a feeding tube, have little formal training in palliative care.[9] Therefore, it may be incorrect to assume that a discussion regarding whether the requested intervention supports the patient's goals of care occurred before the consultation was placed. In a retrospective study of 205 adult patients who underwent gastrostomy tube placement, only 24 (11.7%) had a documented goals of care discussion.[47] Although little has been written to guide the behavior of surgeons acting in the role of consultant, the American College of Surgeons' "Statement on Principles" says that each surgeon is responsible for providing consultation when requested and notes that such consultations "may be for opinion only, to assist with management or for the transfer of care."[48] Thus, the surgeon should inquire whether the referring physician would like the surgeon to address goals of care or to merely act as a technician. However, the "Statement on Principles" also notes that a surgeon must only "recommend surgery when it is the best method of treatment for the patient's problem."[48] The American College of Surgeons' "Statement of Principles of Palliative Care" takes this one step further by declaring that surgeons must recognize their "responsibility to discourage treatments that are unlikely to achieve the patient's goals and encourage patients and families to consider hospice care when the prognosis for survival is likely to be less than a half-year."[49] If the consulting surgeon views the requested intervention as one that may prolong suffering, an ethical tension can arise between the referring physician, the surgeon, and perhaps the patient and the family.[50]

Published in 1983, but still relevant now, the "Ten Commandments for Effective Consultations" offers guidance to surgeons who may find themselves in this situation.[51] Goldman and colleagues[51] suggest consultants "honor thy turf" and state that "although the consultant has a responsibility to the patient, this responsibility should be expressed through discussions with the referring physician and not by competing for the attention and loyalty of the patient." Cohn,[52] writing about the role of the medical consultant, summarizes the 9 ethical principles of consultation as defined by the American Medical Association. Regarding communication, Cohn[52] states that discussions should occur primarily between the referring physician and the consultant and goes on to clarify that discussions between the consultant and the patient should only occur with permission of the referring doctor. Regarding conflicts of opinion, Cohn[52] notes that the consultant has the right to give an opinion to the patient in the presence of the referring physician. The aforementioned "Statement of Principles of Palliative Care" also reminds clinicians to "maintain a collegial and supportive attitude towards others entrusted with care of the patient."[49] In short, when acting as a consultant, the surgeon must balance 2 primary objectives: to determine whether the requested procedure is in the best interest of the patient and to respect and honor the relationship between the referring physician and the patient. If the surgeon deems the requested intervention is not in the patient's best interest, the surgeon should first discuss this with the referring physician to avoid causing undue confusion or suffering to the patient and the family.

In order to guide both referring physicians and consultants through such discussions, Rabeneck and colleagues[53] developed an ethics-based algorithm to assist in determining the appropriateness of feeding tube placement. By posing 2 questions (Will this intervention improve the patient's physiology? Will this intervention improve the patient's quality of life?) the investigators were then able to categorize patients into 1 of 4 groups and offer ethically sound clinical guidance for each group. The first group, those with anorexia-cachexia syndrome, are unable to properly metabolize nutrients, receive no physiologic benefit from nutrition, and are therefore not offered a gastrostomy tube. In a slight modification to this schema, Angus and Burakoff[54] suggest offering a gastrostomy tube to moderately and severely malnourished patients with cancer who are currently undergoing disease-modifying treatment that is expected to last longer than 4 weeks.[54] The second group, those in a permanent vegetative state, may benefit physiologically but have no improvement in quality of life; thus, surgeons recommend against placement of the tube. The third group, those with dysphagia but no other complications, are likely to experience improvement in both physiology and quality of life and are offered tube placement. The fourth group, those with dysphagia and complications, including patients with stroke with multiple deficits, patients with neuromuscular disease with progressive symptoms, and patients with dementia, have an uncertain benefit. This group of patients in particular requires a detailed goals of care discussion in order to clarify exactly what the patient or family hopes to gain from the intervention. The investigators conclude by stating that both the referring physicians and the consultants are responsible for ensuring that patients and families understand the risks and benefits of the proposed procedure.

SUMMARY

Depending on the patient and the diagnosis, a tracheostomy or a PEG can serve as an essential component of recovery, a means to prolong life, or a way to extend suffering. Although the morbidity and mortality directly attributed to either procedure is low, the poor outcomes shown by patients undergoing these procedures serves as a reminder of the critical nature of this population. Given this, it is imperative that the referring providers and the surgeons work together with the patients and their families to ensure that the decision to place a tracheostomy or a PEG tube is appropriate in the context of both prognosis and goals of care.

REFERENCES

1. Shah RK, Lander L, Berry JG, et al. Tracheotomy outcomes and complications: a national perspective. Laryngoscope 2011;122:25–9.
2. HCUPnet. A tool for identifying, tracking, and analyzing national hospital statistics. Available at: https://hcupnet.ahrq.gov. Accessed January 12, 2019.

3. Rosenberger LH, Newhook T, Schirmer B, et al. Late accidental dislodgement of a percutaneous endoscopic gastrostomy tube: an underestimated burden on patients and the health care system. Surg Endosc 2011;25:3307–11.
4. Kaub-Wittemer D, von Steinbüchel N, Wasner M, et al. Quality of life and psychosocial Issues in ventilated patients with amyotrophic lateral sclerosis and their caregivers. J Pain Symptom Manage 2003;26:890–6.
5. Chan T, Devaiah AK. Tracheostomy in palliative care. Otolaryngol Clin North Am 2009;42:133–41.
6. Albert SM, Murphy PL, Del Bene ML, et al. Prospective study of palliative care in ALS: choice, timing, outcomes. J Neurol Sci 1999;169:108–13.
7. Chiò A, Calvo A, Ghiglione P, et al. Tracheostomy in amyotrophic lateral sclerosis: a 10-year population-based study in Italy. J Neurol Neurosurg Psychiatry 2010; 81:1141–3.
8. Indrekvam S, Fondenes O, Gjerdevik M, et al. Longterm mechanical ventilation in ALS – Outcome and perspective. A 12 year national register study of non-invasive and invasive ventilation in Norway. Eur Respir J 2015;46(suppl):59.
9. Creutzfeldt CJ, Robinson MT, Holloway RG. Neurologists as primary palliative care providers. Neurol Clin Pract 2016;6:40–8.
10. Bösel J, Schiller P, Hook Y, et al. Stroke-related early tracheostomy versus prolonged orotracheal intubation in neurocritical care trial (SETPOINT): A randomized pilot trial. Stroke 2013;44:21–8.
11. McCann MR, Hatton KW, Vsevolozhskaya OA, et al. Earlier tracheostomy and percutaneous endoscopic gastrostomy in patients with hemorrhagic stroke: associated factors and effects on hospitalization. J Neurosurg 2019;1–7 [Epub ahead of print].
12. Alali AS, Scales DC, Fowler RA, et al. Tracheostomy timing in traumatic brain injury. J Trauma Acute Care Surg 2014;76:70–8.
13. Khalili H, Paydar S, Safari R, et al. Experience with traumatic brain injury: is early tracheostomy associated with better prognosis? World Neurosurg 2017;103: 88–93.
14. Humble SS, Wilson LD, McKenna JW, et al. Tracheostomy risk factors and outcomes after severe traumatic brain injury. Brain Inj 2016;30:1642–7.
15. Barquist ES, Amortegui J, Hallal A, et al. Tracheostomy in ventilator dependent trauma patients: a prospective, randomized intention-to-treat study. J Trauma 2006;60:91–7.
16. Saffle JR, Morris SE, Edelman L. Early tracheostomy does not improve outcome in burn patients. J Burn Care Rehabil 2002;23:431–8.
17. Young D, Harrison DA, Cuthbertson BH, et al. Effect of early vs late tracheostomy. JAMA 2013;309:2121–9.
18. Nelson JE, Cox CE, Hope AA, et al. Chronic critical illness. Am J Respir Crit Care Med 2010;182:446–54.
19. Carson SS, Kahn JM, Hough CL, et al. A multicenter mortality prediction model for patients receiving prolonged mechanical ventilation. Crit Care Med 2012;40: 1171–6.
20. Bice T, Nelson JE, Carson SS. To Trach or Not to Trach: uncertainty in the care of the chronically critically Ill. Semin Respir Crit Care Med 2015;36:851–8.
21. Langerman A, Patel RM, Cohen EEW, et al. Airway management before chemoradiation for advanced head and neck cancer. Head Neck 2012;34:254–9.
22. Katzberg HD, Benatar M. Enteral tube feeding for amyotrophic lateral sclerosis/ motor neuron disease. Cochrane Database Syst Rev 2011;(1):CD004030.

23. Miller RG, Jackson CE, Kasarskis EJ, et al. Practice parameter update: the care of the patient with amyotrophic lateral sclerosis: drug, nutritional, and respiratory therapies (an evidence-based review). Neurology 2009;73:1218–26.
24. Martino R, Foley N, Bhogal S, et al. Dysphagia after stroke. Stroke 2005;36: 2756–63.
25. Holloway RG, Arnold RM, Creutzfeldt CJ, et al. Palliative and end-of-life care in stroke. Stroke 2014;45:1887–916.
26. Iizuka M, Reding M. Use of percutaneous endoscopic gastrostomy feeding tubes and functional recovery in stroke rehabilitation: a case-matched controlled study. Arch Phys Med Rehabil 2005;86:1049–52.
27. Burgermaster M, Slattery E, Islam N, et al. Regional comparison of enteral nutrition-related admission policies in skilled nursing facilities. Nutr Clin Pract 2016;31:342–8.
28. Mitchell SL, Teno JM, Kiely DK, et al. The clinical course of advanced dementia. N Engl J Med 2009;361:1529–38.
29. Finucane TE, Christmas C, Travis K. Tube feeding in patients with advanced dementia: a review of the evidence. JAMA 1999;282:1365–70.
30. Cervo F, Bryan L, Farber S. To PEG or not to PEG: A review of evidence for placing feeding tubes in advanced dementia and the decision-making process. Geriatrics 2006;61:30–5.
31. American Geriatrics Society Ethics Committee and Clinical Practice and Models of Care Committee. American Geriatrics Society feeding tubes in advanced dementia position statement. J Am Geriatr Soc 2014;62:1590–3.
32. Schoeff SS, Barrett DM, DeLassus Gress C, et al. Nutritional management for head and neck cancer patients. Pract Gastroenterol 2013;37:43–51.
33. National Comprehensive Cancer Network. Head and neck cancers (Version 1.2018). Available at: http://www.nccn.org/professionals/physican_gls/pdf/headandneck.pdf. Accessed January 20, 2019.
34. Olson R, Karam I, Wilson G, et al. Population-based comparison of two feeding tube approaches for head and neck cancer patients receiving concurrent systemic-radiation therapy: is a prophylactic feeding tube approach harmful or helpful? Support Care Cancer 2013;21:3433–9.
35. Rutter CE, Yovino S, Taylor R, et al. Impact of early percutaneous endoscopic gastrostomy tube placement on nutritional status and hospitalization in patients with head and neck cancer receiving definitive chemoradiation therapy. Head Neck 2011;33:1441–7.
36. Chakraborty A, Selby D, Gardiner K, et al. Malignant bowel obstruction: natural history of a heterogeneous patient population followed prospectively over two years. J Pain Symptom Manage 2011;41:412–20.
37. Mobily M, Patel JA. Palliative percutaneous endoscopic gastrostomy placement for gastrointestinal cancer: roles, goals, and complications. World J Gastrointest Endosc 2015;7:364–9.
38. Rath KS, Loseth D, Muscarella P, et al. Outcomes following percutaneous upper gastrointestinal decompressive tube placement for malignant bowel obstruction in ovarian cancer. Gynecol Oncol 2013;129:103–6.
39. Inui A. Cancer anorexia-cachexia syndrome: current issues in research and management. CA Cancer J Clin 2002;52:72–91.
40. Goldenberg D, Ari EG, Golz A, et al. Tracheotomy complications: a retrospective study of 1130 cases. Otolaryngol Head Neck Surg 2000;123:495–500.

41. Johnston SD, Tham TCK, Mason M. Death after PEG: results of the national confidential enquiry into patient outcome and death. Gastrointest Endosc 2008;68: 223–7.
42. Arora G, Rockey D, Gupta S. High In-hospital mortality after percutaneous endoscopic gastrostomy: results of a nationwide population-based study. Clin Gastroenterol Hepatol 2013;11:1437–44.
43. Rabeneck L, Wray NP, Petersen NJ. Long-term outcomes of patients receiving percutaneous endoscopic gastrostomy tubes. J Gen Intern Med 1996;11:287–93.
44. Keung EZ, Liu X, Nuzhad A, et al. In-hospital and long-term outcomes after percutaneous endoscopic gastrostomy in patients with malignancy. J Am Coll Surg 2012;215:777–86.
45. Schrag SP, Sharma R, Jaik NP, et al. Complications related to percutaneous endoscopic gastrostomy (PEG) tubes. a comprehensive clinical review. J Gastrointestin Liver Dis 2007;16:407–18.
46. Rogers SN, Thomson R, O'toole P, et al. Patients experience with long-term percutaneous endoscopic gastrostomy feeding following primary surgery for oral and oropharyngeal cancer. Oral Oncol 2007;43:499–507.
47. McGreevy CM, Pentakota SR, Mohamed, et al. Gastrostomy tube placement: An opportunity for establishing patient-centered goals of care. Surgery 2017;161: 1100–7.
48. Board of Regents of the American College of Surgeons. Statement on Principles. Available at: https://www.facs.org/about-acs/statements/stonprin. Accessed January 12, 2019.
49. Board of Regents of the American College of Surgeons. Statement of principles of palliative care. Available at: https://www.facs.org/about-acs/statements/50-palliative-care. Accessed April 20, 2019.
50. Venkat A. The threshold moment: ethical tensions surrounding decision making on tracheostomy for patients in the intensive care unit. J Clin Ethics 2013;24: 135–43.
51. Goldman L, Lee T, Rudd P. Ten commandments for effective consultations. Arch Intern Med 1983;143:1753–5.
52. Cohn SL. The Role of the Medical Consultant. Available at: https://www.hopkinsmedicine.org/gim/_pdf/Consult_Curric/cohn_con_curr.pdf. Accessed January 12, 2019.
53. Rabeneck L, Mccullough LB, Wray NP. Ethically Justified, clinically comprehensive guidelines for percutaneous endoscopic gastrostomy tube placement. Lancet 1997;349:496–8.
54. Angus F, Burakoff R. The percutaneous endoscopic gastrostomy tube: medical and ethical issues in placement. Am J Gastroenterol 2003;98:272–7.

Beyond the Technical

Determining Real Indications for Vascular Access and Hemodialysis Initiation in End-Stage Renal Disease

Erika R. Ketteler, MD, MA, RPVI, FSVS

KEYWORDS

• Hemodialysis • Vascular access • Renal failure • Communication
• Interventionalists • Medical home

KEY POINTS

- Determining valid indications for vascular access creation and hemodialysis initiation in end-stage renal disease requires utilization of verified prognostication tools and recognition of triggers to initiate serious conversations and implementation of concurrent palliative care and/or hospice care is recommended.
- Establishment of a multidisciplinary team that includes consideration of interventionalists in the predialysis medical home in end-stage renal disease is important.
- A "catheter best" approach may be the most appropriate for some patients to meet goals of care.

VASCULAR ACCESS AND HEMODIALYSIS: REAL INDICATIONS WITH BENEFITS OVER BURDENS

For those with end-stage renal disease (ESRD), renal replacement therapies, such as hemodialysis, are perceived as being beneficial to extend quantity of life—but often at the great expense of quality of life. It is important to recognize the following:

- Approximately 14% of the population of the United States have chronic kidney disease (CKD). Despite numerous advances in understanding the mechanics of progression, the incidence of ESRD remains exceedingly high. As many as 115,000 patients in the United States annually transition from nondialysis-dependent CKD to maintenance dialysis. It is estimated that 70% of patients

Disclosure: The author has nothing to disclose.
Vascular Surgery and Endovascular Therapy, Albuquerque Raymond G. Murphy VAMC, 1501 San Pedro Southeast (112), Albuquerque, NM 87108, USA
E-mail address: erika.ketteler@va.gov

Surg Clin N Am 99 (2019) 967–975
https://doi.org/10.1016/j.suc.2019.06.010
0039-6109/19/Published by Elsevier Inc.

with ESRD are receiving hemodialysis worldwide, and this incidence in the United States is 2160 per million patients.[1]

- Although dialysis patients constitute less than 1% of the Centers for Medicare and Medicaid Services beneficiaries, this population accounts for up to 7% of health care spending and has 1.88 times higher cost of care than those who are afflicted with cancer.[2]
- The morbidities, mortalities, and costs of dialysis are most directly related to dialysis access creation (ie, fistula, graft, or catheter) and maintaining the optimal function of such access.[3]
- Elderly patients (defined as those over 75 years of age) are the most rapidly growing segment of the dialysis population, but dialysis patients younger than 75 years may have a geriatric physiologic age because of complex medical comorbidities (eg, frailty, cognitive impairment, and functional disability).[4]
- Factors that originally prompted hemodialysis initiation (poor cognitive or functional status) may actually worsen with the initiation of hemodialysis.[4,5] For patients 80 years of age and older, the nonmedical aspects of hemodialysis (social support, transportation, and/or financial difficulties) are significantly burdensome.[6]
- Of those on maintenance hemodialysis, 1 in 6 die each year. The highest mortality is typically within the first few months after initiation.[7] Mortality in the first year on dialysis for patients over 75 years old approaches 40%, and even dialysis patients with good function still face a high likelihood for multiple hospitalizations and progressive decline of status.[8]

Acknowledging the above, it is clear that the timing of native vascular access creation and hemodialysis (in that preferred order) is a significant challenge. Whereas hemodialysis was founded as a bridge to transplantation, its evolution into a liberally prescribed therapy among an increasingly large candidacy pool have magnified the burdens in terms of quality of life. The technologically advanced procedure of hemodialysis has clear longevity benefits when applied to patients fit for transplant, but such returns diminish with the application to a population that is more severely ill and aged. The latter is not well perceived by the public, in general, contributing to an unprecedented increase in demand for dialysis therapies.[9] Despite all the factors involved in initiating and maintaining hemodialysis for older and frail populations, renal replacement therapy is considered to be the norm rather than the exception. [10]

ESRD, in the absence of transplant, remains a terminal condition replete with a myriad of palliative issues involving a heavy symptom burden and an intensity of care that rivals the treatment of some advanced cancers. Pain, sleep disturbances, fatigue, and pruritus are extremely common.[11] Managing pain is a real problem as medications require dosages adjusted for renal function and delayed elimination increases the risk of associated side effects. The complex pathophysiology with confluence of cardiovascular disease, chronic inflammation, and bone disease in hemodialysis correlate with malnutrition and medical frailty.[12] Dialysis patients have greater frequencies of intensive care admissions, longer inpatient stays, and hospice referrals only half of that for cancer or heart failure patients.[2]

Although there is a large demand for palliative care, hospice referrals for patients with ESRD are often “too little too late,”[13] with an average length of stay of only 3 days. "Although hospice utilization among Medicare beneficiaries treated with maintenance hemodialysis from 2000 to 2014 more than doubled from 11.0% to 26.7%, almost two-thirds (64.0%) of hemodialysis patients only received 1 week or less of hospice care compared with 39%, 36%, and 34% reported for Medicare hospice beneficiaries with heart failure, colorectal cancer, and dementia, respectively."[10] Directly related to these data is the current inability to provide hospice care for a dialysis patient only for the diagnosis of ESRD, but there is also much to focus on to improve the care and recognition of the suffering in advanced renal disease, especially determining in which patients hemodialysis has undue burden over benefits.

PROGNOSTICATION CONUNDRUM

Accurate prognosis of longevity and timing to the need for renal replacement therapy to aid in vascular access placement and planning for dialysis initiation is sorely needed. Unlike some other conditions, the decline of renal function is not always linear. There are many reasons for this, such as the numerous causes of kidney disease and a poor estimation of glomerular filtration rate in multiple populations, such as the frail and the elderly.[14] In the United States, 80% of patients with ESRD initiate hemodialysis via catheters rather than native access due to urgent medical events. This rate has remained essentially unchanged for over a decade despite aggressive "fistula first" guidelines.[15] Trajectory curves generated by renal disease care providers are more general guides to progression rather than true prediction, because the decline in kidney function is modified by age and unpredictable events, including the competing risk of death. It has been noted among patients with CKD that 13% experience a nonlinear, rapid decline in kidney function in the 2 years preceding initiation of dialysis.[16] Older patients have a slower decline in kidney function than younger patients at a given level of kidney function. The former are more likely to die before meeting the indications for renal replacement therapy.[4]

To assist in the prediction of timing of hemodialysis, several tools have been generated. The French Renal Epidemiology and Information Network risk score[17] uses a 6-month survival probability based on 9 elements. Patients without any elements have a predicted 6-month mortality of 8%. Patients meeting all 9 criteria have an estimated 6-month mortality of 70%. A limitation of this model is that it is based on the French population; among the multiple confounders are the translatability to the United States population because the nationalized French health care system has different quality parameters and metrics and timing, and frequency of dialysis access placements relative to patient symptoms.

Another predictive tool for hemodialysis initiation is the "Surprise Question." The question, "Would I be surprised if this patient died in the next 12 months?"[18] has applicability for estimating 6-month survival. In addition to the question, values for age, serum albumin, presence of dementia, and presence of peripheral vascular disease, are factored into the estimation. This tool is available as an online calculator (https://qxmd.com/calculate/calculator_135/6-month-mortality-on-hd) and is based on a US population demographic. Potential biases in this calculator are the weight given to age (a correlate of increased mortality) and assessment of time-specific comorbidities. Furthermore, laboratory values are required and functional limitations are not factored into the tool—an important aspect of the impact of illness and frailty on mortality risk. Application of these predictive tools may be useful for overall prognosis and can assist providers in focusing on quality of life, which may include avoiding initiation of dialysis.

Adding to the challenge of physiologic prognostication, many nephrologists are reluctant to discuss death from renal failure and instead default to offering dialysis to maintain hope. This certainly has some grounding in the perception that discussions of a patient's prognosis can be interpreted as negative.[19] Naturally, then, providers may tend to avoid engaging in difficult discussions. Paradoxically, most renal failure patients acknowledge the uncertainty of their disease and the limitations of predictions, but they still want to know about the expected course of their kidney disease. As a patient stated, "The unknown is frightening and more knowledge must be better than none." In the study, by Mandel and colleagues,[8] of serious conversations surrounding ESRD, nearly 90% of dialysis patients wanted to have serious discussions to guide their treatments, but less than 10% of the patients report having had such conversations; in addition, less than 50% of the patients had advance directives to outline their preferences, and of those who did complete the documentation, the preferences were related to cardiopulmonary resuscitation and mechanical ventilation and not to dialysis limits. Thus, the following interactions have been recommended to address this gap in discussions of goals of care[20]:

- Provider interactions must avoid mistrust, alienation, abandonment, and isolation.
- Health care system interactions should avoid fragmentation of care and services.
- "Meaning-making" for the patient is necessary to limit the struggle to make sense of the illness, and to avoid blame and responsibility.
- Improving communication skills and increasing comfort in having difficult conversations are important areas to focus on to assist in changing prognostic discussions.

As more providers feel at ease in approaching palliative topics regarding dialysis initiation in a nonthreatening manner, and understanding that hope is not removed in doing so, patient-centered goals may translate into higher satisfaction and more efficient utilization of health care services, such as vascular access and hemodialysis, for true benefit over burden.

IS THERE SOMETHING BETTER THAN HEMODIALYSIS?

Sixty percent of patients on dialysis regret starting dialysis and nearly one-fifth of annual deaths of patients on dialysis result from patient decisions to withdraw.[8] This begs the question: Is something better than hemodialysis as an option for treatment of ESRD? If prolongation of life is the single goal, then hemodialysis will likely prolong survival for elderly patients (age >75 years) who have ESRD by approximately 2 years.[14] The quality of a prolonged life, however, is equally important to patients. In individuals who declined hemodialysis initiation and instead chose maximal conservative management (MCM), they were seen to survive a substantial length of time and achieved similar numbers of hospital-free days compared with patients who initiated hemodialysis.[9] In studies by Murtagh and colleagues,[21,22] patients who chose MCM with ischemic coronary artery disease or more than one other comorbidity had the same survival as patients who started dialysis; it was uncommon for the nondialysis patients to develop uremic symptoms, and when they died they often had nonuremic deaths. This recognition of reasonable survival with quality of life benefits supports the consideration of nondialysis management for patients who meet criteria to initiate hemodialysis. Offering MCM instead of hemodialysis requires, however, proactive prognostic conversations for patients who have relatively stable decline; thus, being comfortable with serious conversations is a necessary skill to be developed for all those involved in dialysis and vascular access management.

THE INTERVENTIONALIST'S ROLE

Proceduralists such as vascular surgeons who create and maintain dialysis access have unique relationships with the population with ESRD. The projected workload for vascular procedures in 2020 is estimated to be greatest for dialysis access, yet there are few evidence-based guidelines for vascular access creation and the planning for interventions to maintain ideal function. In total, this future projection for dialysis access work will create a workload crisis.[23–25] As the aged and frail population increases concomitant with suboptimal outcomes from dialysis access placement, it is important for surgeons and other interventionalists to embrace a partnership role in finding real indications for beneficial vascular access and hemodialysis.

The population with severe CKD is vulnerable due to disease progression, a culmination of comorbidities, and the escalation and transition of care as ESRD approaches. Optimizing outcomes depends on decisions made before dialysis. Frank discussions to aid decision making are ideal well before the creation of vascular access. Anatomic feasibility should only be a part of candidacy for hemodialysis. Honest informed consent through serious conversations about the benefit and burden of dialysis should be highlighted to optimize utilization of hemodialysis access creation and maintenance interventions.

To improve outcomes, it has been proposed to combine the care of patients with CKD and ESRD into an even more multidisciplinary approach, covering primary care, nephrology, palliative care, and the dialysis unit as a "medical home."[12] However, this "home" omits a very important group of providers for treatment of ESRD: the proceduralists, who create and maintain dialysis access. This omission is especially concerning because it is known that patients value the clinical opinions of interventionalists.[19,26] Thus, involvement of proceduralists in decision making surrounding dialysis access and initiation could help patients weigh benefits versus burdens. Surgeons and interventionalists need to embrace their uniquely important roles in dialysis care and should engage in partnering in the "ESRD Life-Plan"[4] algorithm. The proceduralist's role is especially vital in the assessment stage, generating individualized plans taking into consideration "the patient's limited life expectancy, reduced reserves and resistance to stressors, degree of dependence, and personal preferences."[4] Supporting the fact that the "ESRD Life-Plan" needs critical proceduralist input because the delineated hemodialysis plan has factors inherent to the surgeons/interventionalists: estimated life expectancy, likelihood of successful arteriovenous fistula maturation, timing of access placement relative to dialysis initiation, previous vascular access history, and patient preference. With shortened life expectancy, some elderly patients no longer chose a dialysis access because of its favorable long-term outcomes but rather for its short-term aspects that affect their day-to-day quality of life, including the risk of burdensome, invasive, and time-consuming access procedures, cannulation-associated pain, and bleeding and/or bruising; [27] the significance of vascular access interventions voiced by many patients is the core outcome measure for choosing access.[4] The role of the surgeon and/or interventionalist is clearly necessary and they should be accepted and encouraged to be a key partner in the medical home for patients with renal failure, anticipating discussions about dialysis vascular access initiation and on-going maintenance of access.

Many triggers to have serious conversations about ESRD cross directly into the path of the surgeon and/or interventionalist: access referral, access placement, transplant referral, recurrent or prolonged hospitalizations, and access to procedures requested (**Box 1**).[8] A "tincture of time" trial (eg, catheter instead of native vascular access creation) may be beneficial in that a window is provided allowing the determination of how the patient tolerates and adjusts to dialysis. Important input from the proceduralist can guide the type of vascular access based on overall function and prognosis because the trend for arteriovenous graft over arteriovenous fistula for those aged over 70 years with less than 2-year life expectancy is based on $11,000 cost savings to gain 1

Box 1
Triggers for serious conversations with regard to ESRD

- Before dialysis
  - Clinical triggers
    - Not surprised in answer to surprise question
    - High likelihood (Tangri score) of progression to ESRD
    - Dialysis modality teaching referral
    - Access referral
    - Access placement
    - Transplant referral
    - Recurrent or prolonged hospitalizations
    - Changes in function or dependence
    - Sentinel events or indicators (falls, poor appetite, falling albumin, or weight loss)
  - Patient or family request
- After beginning dialysis
  - Clinical triggers
    - Not surprised in answer to surprise question
    - Access procedures
    - Recurrent or prolonged hospitalizations
    - Changes in function or dependence
    - Sentinel events or indicators (falls, poor appetite, falling albumin, weight loss, or change in interdialytic weight gain, or falling BP)
  - Time-based triggers
    - Admission to the dialysis unit
    - After 3 mo on dialysis
    - Annually
  - Patient or family request

From Mandel EI, Bernacki RE, Block SD. Serious illness conversations in ESRD. From Clin J Am Soc Nephrol. 2017 May 8;12(5):854-863. https://doi.org/10.2215/CJN.05760516. Epub 2016 Dec 28; with permission.

quality-adjusted life-year.[28,29] In addition, catheter rather than fistula creation may have value for those patients with life expectancy less than 6 months. Catheter use for dialysis access may offer more benefit over burden as it is now accepted that the historic associations of catheters with increased infections, hospitalizations, malfunction, and mortality was based on poor observational data, and that catheter complications are based on patient comorbidity burden rather than type of access.[2] We suggest a “catheter best” approach, as a novel, but more consistent approach, in how many patients with ESRD value benefit over burden, and that such a model will need to be adopted in dialysis and vascular access guidelines, which currently prefer native access over catheter access.

FINAL RECOMMENDATIONS TO GUIDE VASCULAR ACCESS AND HEMODIALYSIS INDICATIONS

Kidney disease is due to many different causes, and is diagnosed more commonly in older and frail individuals. Therefore, renal functional decline follows many different trajectories. Despite well over a century of study, it is difficult to predict the timing of renal replacement therapy. Clinicians involved in dialysis care also commonly face communication challenges surrounding honest discussions with patients with renal disease. Without involvement by proceduralists—vascular surgeons, interventional radiologists, and interventional nephrologists—in the predialysis planning, multiple gaps exist. Hence, the following criteria should be addressed to assist with decision making regarding placement of vascular access and predialysis planning.

Provide Accurate Information Tailored to the Patient's Comorbidities and Resources

Optimal quality of life discussions that guide informed decision making are founded on accurate information. Objective considerations of conservative medical management instead of hemodialysis need to be adopted by nephrologists. This will help demystify prognostication and should improve quality of life. Patients with kidney disease warrant honest information. Nephrology-focused research needs some directing toward better prognostic tools and communication instruments to provide a means of optimally balancing longevity with quality of life. Embracing and being comfortable with palliative conversational skills is essential for providers who interact with patients with CKD; the emotional and psychological stresses that accompany ESRD, its comorbidities, and concomitant interventions demand clear communication. There are plenty of opportunities to explore interventions permitting quality benefit and burden discussions.

Look for Triggers to Reevaluate the Clinical Situation

A change in patient status offers an opportunity to discuss goals of care. Discussions to guide current and future treatments should be held with each repeat hospitalization, when there are changes in function or dependence, when there is the appearance of sentinel clinical markers for frailty, or when the patient and/or family comment on or question dialysis care. Proceduralists need to be aware of these and similar prompts regarding interventions on current access or new access requests. These are opportunities to reevaluate goals of care and reassess the value of dialysis. Recognizing these events as opportunities to initiate serious conversations is vital to optimizing quality of life and maximizing the value of renal replacement therapy.

Implement Proactive Shared Decision Making for Goals of Care to Include Concurrent Palliative and/or Hospice Care Approaches

There are many potential advantages with early integration of palliative care. This addresses substantial and often-unrecognized symptoms, functional declines, and the caregiving burdens faced by many patients with CKD and their family members, especially for the elderly and/or frail. Concomitant nephrology and palliative care involvement early in the illness will certainly translate to a smooth and appropriately timed transition to hospice care. A future that allows patients with ESRD to simultaneously receive maintenance hemodialysis with hospice benefits after the diagnosis of ESRD will have the greatest promise to improve the quality of care of patients with renal failure while also reducing costs.[13]

Institute a Multidisciplinary Care Team, Including Proceduralists, to Ensure that Dialysis Occurs for the "Right Patient, at the Right Time, for the Right Reasons"

The renal care program needs to include a fully active multidisciplinary team with nephrologists, primary care givers, palliative care givers, and surgeons and/or interventionalists. Proceduralists possess technical expertise and provide a framework for initiating serious informed conversations.[30] Such specialists should be fully engaged partners in the predialysis planning process beyond only a critique on the anatomic and technical aspects of vascular access creation, especially if it is determined that a "catheter best" approach is most appropriate.

These recommendations should be seen to focus on yielding benefits over burdens. The values of patients and their families need to be factored into the indications for vascular access and hemodialysis to insure dialysis occurs for the "right patient, at the right time, for the right reasons.[4] More research is needed to discern the optimal method in acquiring vascular access and delivering dialysis in the framework of the goals enumerated herein. Candid shared decision making among providers and patients should address all aspects of a palliative care approach to encompass the physical, psychological, social, and spiritual elements that plague those with advanced kidney disease, with the goal to find the *real* indications governing decisions regarding vascular access and hemodialysis.

ACKNOWLEDGMENTS

Special acknowledgment to Dr Brent Wagner, Chief of Nephrology, Albuquerque VAMC, for his critical review and formative input to this article.

REFERENCES

1. The United States Renal Data System. USRDS annual data report. 2018. Available at: https://www.usrds.org/2018/view/Default.aspx. Accessed January 31, 2019.
2. Ravani P, Quinn R, Oliver M, et al. Examining the association between hemodialysis access type and mortality: the role of access complications. Clin J Am Soc Nephrol 2017;12:955–64.
3. Chen B, Kuo C, Huang N, et al. Reducing costs at the end of life through provider incentives for hospice care: a retrospective cohort study. Palliat Med 2018;32(8): 1389–400.
4. Viecelli AK, Lok CE. Hemodialysis vascular access in the elderly – getting it right. Kidney Int 2019;95:38–49.
5. Broers NJH, Martens RJH, Canaud B, et al. Health-related quality of life in end-stage renal disease patients: the effects of starting dialysis in the first year after the transition period. Int Urol Nephrol 2018;50:1131–42.
6. Franco MR, Fernandes NM. Dialysis in the elderly patient: a challenge of the XXI century – narrative review. J Bras Nefrol 2013;35(2):132–41.
7. Robinson BM, Zhang J, Morgenstern H, et al. Worldwide, mortality risk is high soon after initiation of hemodialysis. Kidney Int 2013;85:158–65.
8. Mandel EI, Bernacki RE, Block SD. Serious illness conversations in ESRD. Clin J Am Soc Nephrol 2017;12:854–63.
9. Carson RC, Juszczak M, Davenport A, et al. Is maximum conservative management an equivalent treatment option to dialysis for elderly patients with significant comorbid disease? Clin J Am Soc Nephrol 2009;4:1611–9.
10. Wachterman MW, Hailpern SM, Keating NL, et al. Association between hospice length of stay, health utilization, and Medicare costs at the end of life among patients who received maintenance hemodialysis. JAMA Intern Med 2018;178(6): 792–9.
11. Germain MJ, Cohen LM. Maintaining quality of life at the end of life in the end-stage renal disease population. Adv Chronic Kidney Dis 2008;15(2):133–9.
12. Bansal AD, Leonberg-Yoo A, Schnell JO, et al. Ten tips nephrologists wish the palliative care team knew about caring for patients with kidney disease. J Palliat Med 2018;21(4):546–51.
13. Schwarze ML, Schueller K, Jhagroo A. Hospice use and end-of-life care for patients with end-stage renal disease. JAMA Intern Med 2018;178(6):799–801.

14. Sumida K, Kovesdy CP. Disease trajectories before ESRD: implications for clinical management. Semin Nephrol 2016;37:132–43.
15. National Kidney Foundation, Inc. Fistula first catheter last. Available at: https://www.esrdncc.org/en/fistula-first-catheter-last. Accessed January 31, 2019.
16. O'hare AM, Batten A, Burrows NR, et al. Trajectories of kidney function decline in the 2 years before initiation of long-term dialysis. Am J Kidney Dis 2012;59(4):513–22.
17. Couchoud C, Labeeuw M, Moranne O, et al. A clinical score to predict 6-month prognosis in elderly patients starting dialysis for end-stage renal disease. Nephrol Dial Transplant 2009;24:1553–61.
18. Moss AH, Ganjoo J, Sharma S, et al. Utility of the "surprise" question to identify dialysis patients with high mortality. Clin J Am Soc Nephrol 2008;3:1379–84.
19. Schnell JO, Patel UD, Steinhauser KE, et al. Discussions of the kidney disease trajectory by elderly patients and nephrologists: a qualitative study. Am J Kidney Dis 2012;59(4):495–503.
20. O'hare AM, Richars C, Szarka J, et al. Emotional impact of illness and care on patients with advanced kidney disease. Clin J Am Soc Nephrol 2018;13:1–8.
21. Murtagh FEM, Murphy E, Sheerin NS. Illness trajectories: an important concept in the management of kidney failure. Nephrol Dial Transplant 2008;23:3746–8.
22. Murtagh FE, Marsh JE, Donohoe P, et al. Dialysis or not? A comparative survival study of patients over 75 years with chronic kidney disease stage 5. Nephrol Dial Transplant 2007;22:1955–62.
23. Heikkien M, Salenius JP, Auvinen O. Projected workload for vascular service in 2020. Eur J Vasc Endovasc Surg 2000;19:351–5.
24. Argyriou C, Gerorgiadis GS, Lazarides MK. Vascular access guidelines: do we need better evidence? Eur J Vasc Endovasc Surg 2018;56(4):608.
25. Williams K, Schneider B, Lajos P, et al. Supply and demand: will we have enough vascular surgeons by 2030? Vascular 2016;24(4):414–20.
26. Mcnair AG, Mackichan F, Donovan JL, et al. What surgeons tell patients and what patients want to know before major cancer surgery: a qualitative study. BMC Cancer 2016;16:258.
27. Allon M, Lok CE. Dialysis fistula or graft: the role for randomized clinical trials. Clin J Am Soc Nephrol 2010;5(12):2348–54.
28. Hall RK, Myers ER, Rosas SE, et al. Choice of hemodialysis access in older adults: a cost-effectiveness analysis. Clin J Am Soc Nephrol 2017;12(6):947–54.
29. Bylsma LC, Gage SM, Reicher H, et al. Arteriovenous fistulae for haemodialysis: a systematic review and meta-analysis of efficacy and safety outcomes. Eur J Vasc Endovasc Surg 2017;54(4):513–22.
30. Kruser JM, Taylor LJ, Campbell TC, et al. "Best case/worst case"; training surgeons to use a novel communication tool for high-risk acute surgical problems. J Pain Symptom Manage 2017;53:711–9.

Postoperative Recovery and Survivorship After Acute Hospitalization for Serious Life-Limiting Illness

Ann Wilborn Jackson, PT, DPT, MPH*

KEYWORDS

• Discharge planning • Patient-centered care • Palliative care • Serious life-limiting • Life-altering • Communications

KEY POINTS

- Health care team members should provide materials and interactions to improve the health literacy of patients and caregivers.
- When support is provided to patients and primary decision makers, they are better prepared to participate in the creation, implementation and evaluation of customized and meaningful discharge/transition planning.
- Discharge planning should begin early and be flexible.
- Discharge planning must be intentional and can be guided by communication tools.

REFLECTIONS FROM THE ARTICLE AUTHOR

"How will I live?" This profoundly difficult question is asked by millions of people (Appendix 1). Some of these people are aging adults and/or adults living with complex, chronic health conditions who must grapple with relying on others to help them with activities of daily living like personal grooming, bathing, mouth care, toileting, transferring to/from the bed/chair, walking, climbing stairs, eating, and household chores as well as instrumental activities of daily living, like shopping, cooking, managing medication, using the telephone and looking up numbers, performing housework, managing finances, and driving/using public transportation. Other people affected are family members and loved ones who are confronting life-altering events like caring for an adult child permanently incapacitated by a tragic accident, or a parent suffering from the aftermath of a stroke. Regardless of who asks the question, too often, the answer is unsatisfactory and involves myriad limitations that promote feelings of resentment and shame. In a quest to offer informed recommendations for better patient concordant outcomes, I, along with my colleagues, set out on a mission to

MacLean Center for Clinical Medical Ethics, University of Chicago, Flossmoor, IL, USA
* 18860 Hamlin Avenue, Flossmoor, IL 60422.
E-mail address: awjackson@waymaker.biz

Surg Clin N Am 99 (2019) 977–989
https://doi.org/10.1016/j.suc.2019.06.012

empower those who not only want to know how they will live but also want to exercise agency in determining the factors that impact their lives. We understand that, as practitioners, we can share knowledge that will serve as tools for short-term and long-term care planning.

We developed this article, "Postoperative Recovery and Survivorship After an Acute Hospitalization for a Serious Life-Limiting Illness," to serve as a roadmap, with guideposts that provide individuals who are confronting a life-limiting and/or life-altering condition and their caregivers with recommendations on how to create and implement highly customized and effective discharge-transition and long-term care strategies. As health care leaders, we are called upon to recognize the care needs of those entrusted to us not only in a particular moment but also in the days and months to come, up to and including end of life. Our ability, as health care providers, to fulfill this duty is limited by innumerable variables and unanticipated circumstances. With this in mind, this article offers readers instruments that are part of a knowledge-based, patient-centered, and authentic platform designed to present people with an opportunity to exercise greater authority over how they will live up to the time of death. As experts, we outline best practices for introducing difficult conversations and reaching sound decisions in a thoughtful, respectful, and ethical manner.

Because my duties include direct service provider, health care systems navigator, patient advocate, and an engineer of solutions to injustices, serving as author for this article has been a highlight of my career. Given my commitment and passion to help chronically ill and aging people preserve their dignity and improve their quality of life, there were moments when I struggled with ensuring that there was a balance between including the most pertinent information and leaving out content that might only serve to undermine the article's role as an easy-to-use resource. Nevertheless, as a community-based physical therapist who serves chronically ill and aging people and witnesses how they and their families cut back on expenses, work tirelessly around the clock, and limit their time away from home, I am humbled and strengthened to move confidently into unchartered challenges, as they do each day. Their grace, dignity, fearlessness, and joy have encouraged and inspired me to write this article. Today and always, I dedicate my work to the brave individuals who declare, "I will live empowered and proudly, because I am equipped with the knowledge to do so."

INTRODUCTION

American hospitals are discharging patients "quicker and sicker" than ever before.[1,2] Among health care providers, patients, researchers, and advocates, there is a growing concern that these discharges are occurring without proper planning and limited input from patient stakeholders.[3,4] Consequently, there is an urgency to prepare patients and their caregivers/decision makers for discharge through enhanced communication, goal setting, health literacy, and a shared sense of respect to reduce rates of readmission and promote greater patient and caregiver activation and long-term compliance with plans of care.

There is no one-size-fits-all model for transition of care planning. Instead, appropriate transition of care planning depends on health care teams conducting in-depth investigation of individual patient needs, identifying financial, emotional, and spiritual considerations that must be addressed in the transition of care planning process.[2–5] Steinhauser and colleagues[4] in their piece indicate that pain and symptom management, preparation for death, achieving a sense of completion, decisions pertaining to treatment preferences, and being treated as a "whole person" are essential to those facing the end of life.

This urgency is further complicated when patients face conditions that are considered sustained life-limiting conditions.[1,5,6] Sustained life-limiting conditions as described by the International Association of Hospice and Palliative Care, an online Palliative Care Directory, are illnesses or diseases that are progressive and fatal, or a condition from which progression of the condition cannot be reversed.[7] For those living with a serious life-limiting or life-altering diagnosis, the conversation would be slightly different with emphasis on short- and long-term goals of care. The conversational guides listed may guide the team in framing the discharge conversation with the patient and their caregivers[6]:

1. Find out how much information the patient and family have and wish to know.
2. Summarize the medical situation.
3. Ask questions regarding goals, values, and preferences.
4. Incorporate values and preferences information into recommendations for a treatment plan and present possible options.
5. Discuss your recommendations.
6. Review to ensure understanding.

This article is designed to help provide decision makers with guidance as to the best practices associated with patient-centered care like shared decision making with either the patient and/or their surrogate decision maker.

THE NEED FOR PALLIATIVE CARE

The World Palliative Care Alliance estimates that each year approximately 20 million people worldwide are in need of hospice or palliative care.[8] Because inadequate access to hospice and palliative care is documented worldwide and with an aging population that is living longer and presenting with increasingly complex medical histories, the demand for palliative and end-of-life care is only going to increase. One path to palliative care for those at the end of life has been to enroll in hospice. However, trends are beginning to emerge that acknowledge the benefits of palliative care for nonterminal patients with serious life-limiting illness. Individuals who are living with serious life-limiting conditions as well as those who care for them are recognizing the benefits from palliative care support.[8,9] Historically, hospice and palliative care programs directed most of their resources toward the needs of patients with cancer, despite the fact that most patients who have palliative care needs suffer from symptoms related to nonmalignant conditions.[8–10] The recognition of the collective suffering of those with serious life-altering conditions and their caregivers will only reinforce the need for more resources in this area.[8]

According to the definition above, health care providers must be concerned about the needs of the chronically ill and disabled because they are the ones who need palliative care services, not only those who are among the actively dying.[6–11] This article postulates that through an organized process of discovery and implementation, health care systems will be better able to meet the discharge and long-term health care planning needs of this population.

In 2010, the United States Census Bureau estimated that 56.7 million Americans were disabled, reflecting 2 in 10 adults. Disability was defined as “having a physical or mental impairment that can occur at birth or at any point in a person’s life, that affects one or more major life activities, such as walking, bathing, dressing, eating, preparing meals, and/or going outside the home”. The median earnings in the past 12 months for someone with a disability was $20,184.00, with the US Department of Health and Human Services reporting that a family of one is within the poverty guidelines when earnings are $12,490.00 or less, and the number of individuals with disabilities who live below the poverty line was 23%, as compared with those without a disability at 15%[12–14] (**Fig. 1**).

RECIPIENTS OF PALLIATIVE CARE

Definition and Scope in Adults

In adults (anyone 15 or older), palliative care is defined as[4–7,11]

- Palliative care is needed in chronic as well as life-threatening/life-limiting conditions.
- There is no time or prognostic limit on the delivery of palliative care.
- The World Health Organization (WHO) Global Atlas, a WHO organization, with members in more than 90 countries, offers a global perspective on hospice and palliative care, describes the need for palliative care at all levels of care.
- Palliative care is not limited to any one care setting.

The information provided, thus far, establishes the ground work for the complexity of care needs associated with people who have serious life-limiting illnesses. Most often, people are not succumbing to a catastrophic health incident, but rather living longer with more disability.[9,12] According to a study conducted by the National Health Service, "The number of older people who have at least four different medical conditions is set to double by 2035, in a trend that will put huge, extra strain on health services."[15]

Adult Principal Diagnosis List

The following facts and statistics are provided by a 2014 Center to Advance Palliative Care publication[7–9,11,16]:

- Approximately 90 million Americans are living with serious illness, and this number is expected to more than double over the next 25 years with the aging of the baby boomers.

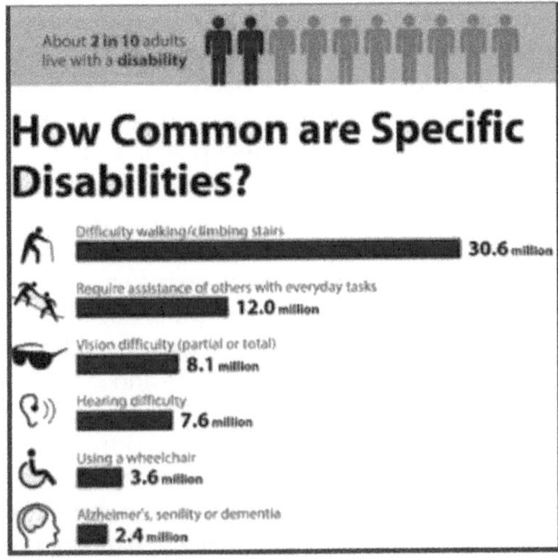

Fig. 1. Functional limitations of a person with a disability in the United States from 2010 US Census Bureau. (*From* US Census Bureau. Available at: https://www.census.gov/newsroom/facts-for-features/2013/cb13-ff15.html.)

- Approximately 6 million people in the United States could benefit from palliative care.
- According to a 2010 study reported in the *New England Journal of Medicine*, patients with lung cancer receiving early palliative care had less depression, improved quality of life, and survived 2.7 months longer.
- Illnesses most commonly treated by palliative care are heart disease, cancer, stroke, diabetes, renal disease, Parkinson disease, and Alzheimer disease.

THE DISCHARGE

Health care systems must begin to manage reasonable expectations after discharge with tailored discharge planning that aligns with patient and caregiver goals and expectations while being sensitive to personal, cultural, spiritual, financial, and disease diversity.[3,4] Discharge preparation should be initiated when an individual enters the health care system and be reassessed on some level by someone who is able to follow the patient across the care continuum; sometimes that person is the patient or a primary caregiver. Ideally, the multidisciplinary care team is involved in a patient's transition of care to ensure that the care will continue to be comprehensive and attend to the whole patient.[3,9] When the discussion of some form of palliative care occurs, it is usually because the patient has

- Been admitted to an acute-care setting with of one the conditions that is acute/chronic and life threatening or life altering
- A deteriorating medical condition that may require symptom and/or pain control
- Greater than a 6-month life expectancy
- Considering enrollment in a Hospice program

Health care providers should be trained and comfortable opening a line of communication with patients and caregivers regarding patient and caregiver goals and preferences at discharge. Obtaining the patient and caregiver's discharge preferences in the most respectful manner preserves a patient's dignity during a clear change in their functional status. Implementing a discharge plan that incorporates a patient's values has the greatest possibility of success. McMurray and colleagues[3] offer a list of questions when transitioning general surgery patients, "General surgical patients' perspectives of the adequacy and appropriateness of discharge planning to facilitate health decision-making at home." The article suggests that creating a systematic conversational flow assists the discussion facilitator, whether it be a social worker, nurse, physician, or some other member of the treatment team to ensure that all stakeholders are given an opportunity to participate in the information discovery and development of the care plan.

Identifying the Patients at Greatest Risk for Adverse Events and Readmissions

Recognizing which patients are at greatest risk for adverse events and/or readmission owing to a poor transition of care is an important aspect of transitional care management.[17] Health care providers and institutions should risk-stratify patients to adjust transitional care planning to accommodate individual patient care needs. To identify which patients are at greatest risk of unsuccessful transitions, initial and high-risk screening tools exist, such as the one found at health.ny.gov or https://www.health.ny.gov/professionals/patients/discharge_planning/discharge_transition.htm, each with a graduated level of discharge complexity warranting different levels of support to satisfy the specific needs of each patient and their caregiver.

Initial discharge screens to determine whether a more comprehensive assessment is indicated

- Was the patient independent before admission?
- Will this current episode of illness change the patient's level of baseline function?
  - Short term? OR
  - Long term?
- Does the patient have adequate informal supports to compensate for functional loss?
- Does the patient have adequate financial and/or insurance benefits to support discharge needs, such as getting discharge medications, durable medical equipment, therapy services, home care services, and provider follow-up?
- If the patient had prior home care services in place, are they still appropriate and adequate?
- Are there any special requirements needed to access the new care setting?
- Is there a different level of care needed, and is there a different payer because of this hospital stay?

Has the patient had multiple hospital admissions in the last 12 months? Compilation of high-risk screening criteria

- Disabled and younger than 65
- Age older than 70
- Multiple diagnoses associated with high readmission rates
- History of readmissions
- Multiple comorbidities and/or chronic illness
- Frailty
- Numerous medications
- Compromised cognitive status
- Language barriers
- Impaired mobility
- Impaired self-care skills
- Catastrophic injury or illness
- Psychosocial and emotional factors
  - Mental health conditions
  - Challenging interpersonal relationships
  - Complex family dynamics
- Substance use disorders
- Other socioeconomic disadvantages
  - Illiteracy
  - Homelessness
- Inadequate social supports
- History of repetitive emergency department care
- History of multiple hospital admissions
- Anticipated long-term health care needs

PLACEMENT OPTIONS

A. *Home Care Services:* Individuals returning to a residential setting following a hospitalization who need part-time nursing services or rehabilitative services, but not yet able to receive services in outpatient setting at this time.

B. *Acute Rehabilitation Care:* A care setting designed to improve an individual's condition/function within a defined set of time or a setting in which patients and caregivers can be trained to maintain the current health status of an individual or reduce risk of health condition becoming worse.
C. *Skilled Nursing Care:* A level of care provided when a patient no longer meets the criteria to be hospitalized but is not able to *return* to home setting, because of some type of medical condition. Often persons are admitted to skilled nursing units to receive extended rehabilitation services.
D. *Respite Care:* A care setting that provides temporary relief for caregivers and families, which provides specialized care to individuals with disabilities, other special needs, or long-term care needs, and to those who are at risk for abuse or neglect.
E. *Long-Term Acute Care Facilities:* A care setting that is a Medicare designated level of acute care services. It is most appropriate for those whose general condition has stabilized yet the patient continues to need acute level care. These centers provide intensive nursing care in addition to rehabilitation services.
F. *Hospice Care:* A unique system to care for someone who is dying. Care can be provided in a home, a hospital, a nursing home, or a dedicated free-standing hospice facility.

CASE STUDY

Clinical History

Ms D is a 35-year-old woman who was involved in a motor vehicle collision and sustained right hand fractures, right fourth through eighth rib fractures, and a significant traumatic brain injury.

Before the injury, Ms D was a healthy single woman without significant past medical history who lived with a roommate in a 2-story condominium. She was employed as a mechanical engineer for a company that is located 40 miles from her home. In her leisure time, she enjoyed traveling and furniture restoration. At the time of her injury, Ms D received her health insurance from her employer.

Clinical Course

Ms D was hospitalized for 32 days during which she underwent a tracheostomy and was vent dependent for 10 days. She had a gastrostomy inserted on hospital day 20 because of a poor swallow reflex. She had neurosurgery on day 2 and again on day 6 to relieve intracranial pressure and evacuate hematomas. Once stabilized, she was transferred to an inpatient rehabilitation center for another 45 days to participate in physical, occupational, and speech therapy. Since the motor vehicle collision, Ms D has been diagnosed with hospital-acquired pneumonia twice and consistently reported a pain level of 4 or higher related to her rib fractures at rest and with structured exercise. At the end of the inpatient rehabilitation experience, Ms D was not independent with self-care needs, ambulated using a wide-base quad cane, demonstrated a high fall risk, and required prompts to fully express thoughts. She was discharged into the care of her parents, who at the time were Ms D's surrogate decision makers. The plan of care after discharge consisted of continuation of therapy services in the outpatient setting and adding vocational services to assess life skills and readiness to return to work and independent living. Over the next 9 months, Ms D participated in therapy services at a frequency of 3, and then 2 visits weekly for all 4 disciplines with a mixture of individual and group settings. At the time of program discharge, Ms D was out from work on long-term disability, receiving approximately two-thirds of her salary and continuing to receive employee group insurance at a modified rate.

Table 1
Outpatient experience for Ms D

Impairments at Time of Admission to Outpatient Therapy Program	Plan of Care to Address Impairment	Functional Outcomes after 9 mo of Outpatient Physical, Occupational, and Speech Therapy
Ms D and family uncertain of potential for" full recovery"	Patient and family education pertaining to findings obtained from rehabilitation team evaluations followed by the establishment of shared potentially obtainable goals for the short and long term. Family participates in therapy sessions when possible and participates in monthly team meeting with rehabilitation providers in person or via telehealth	Patient and family are able to strategize when confronting new challenges and rely on community resources to address limitations still present at conclusion of outpatient therapy treatment
Pain with movement, which progressively decreases	Implementation of pharmacologic and nonpharmacologic strategies to address pain, emphasis on patient and family education regarding all options and potential side effects. Strategies such as guided imagery, acupuncture, yoga, massage, aqua therapy may be implemented either directly by program or identified as a community resource	Ms D has transitioned to community-based yoga and aqua exercise classes and is now a part of monthly neurologic support group. Her pain levels range from 0 to 3 on a 10-point scale depending on activity level and physical demands of activity. She continues to use a combination of over-the-counter medications and supportive therapies to address discomfort
Decreased range of motion of fractured limbs and shortening of corresponding soft tissue with adhesions	Initiate active movement, active exercise based on radiological evidence of healed structures Include joint and soft tissue mobilization techniques into treatment plan	Client demonstrates greater freedom of soft tissue, which has resulted in improved range of motion and improved strength
Decreased strength and endurance	Create individualized therapeutic exercise program that includes various types of strength training, incorporate activities to improve endurance and balance in as many positions as medically available	Client is now able to tolerate 6–10 h of moderately paced activity on 3 d a week, which has resulted in return to part-time work with prior employer
Unable to ambulate without use of an assistive device and moderate assistance	Incorporate activities to promote balance, agility, protective, and self-	Client is now able to ambulate using a wide-base quad cane to

(*continued on next page*)

Table 1
(*continued*)

Impairments at Time of Admission to Outpatient Therapy Program	Plan of Care to Address Impairment	Functional Outcomes after 9 mo of Outpatient Physical, Occupational, and Speech Therapy
from a person, especially for transitional activities	righting responses with variability to setting and type of assistive device used	ambulate in home and community settings up to 50 ft independently. Distances beyond this range are managed by her riding in a motorized mobility system
Decline in fitness level and compromised cardiorespiratory status	Reduction of recurrent cardiorespiratory incidents and progress of individualized cardiorespiratory conditioning program	Client has not experienced upper respiratory infection in 4 mo and is now able to walk around the block at self-paced low intensity for 18 min using single-point cane and close supervision of another

• Patient and family education was embedded in all interventions, so that therapeutic intervention and functional application remained focused on the goals of the primary stakeholders.

Table 1 outlines the challenges and outcomes of this outpatient experience for Ms D and the management guidelines postfracture/postimmobilization.

Considerations at Discharge

1. Will Ms D be able to return to her home? If so, does she have financial, cognitive, and physical functionality to do so? If not, when? What, if any, services/supports will she need to be safe and independent while living at home?
2. Will Ms D be able to return to any type of work? Will her employer be willing to make accommodations for her transition back to work?
3. How does this injury possibly change the trajectory of Ms D's life?

INNOVATIVE IDEAS TO MEET PALLIATIVE CARE NEEDS

- The individualized management for patient centered targets (IMPACT) model: The University of Pennsylvania Health System embeds community health workers into its clinical teams throughout its system to support low-income patients with emotional support and to provide real-time assistance as they navigate through the University's Health system and attempt to identify and receive community-based services and resources.
  Outcome: Increased patient activation, reduced hospital readmissions, and reduced reporting of depression-related symptoms.[18]
- Community-based health coaches and care coordinators: In a program that provides community-based services to the elderly of Merrimack Valley in Northeastern Massachusetts via a mobile technology, trained health coaches visit recently discharged Medicare patients in their homes and monitors them via telephone to identify and address changes in their health status that might lead to a readmission. They used a tablet-based application that provided suggested questions to assess overall health of client and determine if medical intervention was needed, before the development of conditions that would require a hospital readmission.

Outcomes: Reduced readmissions of at-risk Medicare patients, fewer readmissions and enhanced access to postdischarge primary care.[19]

SUMMARY

This article should be looked upon as a road map with guideposts for the discharge planning process for patients with serious life-limiting and life-altering conditions, with its emphasis on a patient-centered approach within a shared decision-making framework.[9,10] The article highlights that the conversations must begin at the time of admission and be adjusted accordingly as more is learned about the short- and long-term needs and goals of each patient and their family and as needs change and evolve over time. This method leads to greater patient and family satisfaction, lower rates of mortality, and fewer hospital readmissions.[9,18–20] People around the world are not succumbing to sudden or insidious health conditions; they are living longer with greater health complications, and they are often in need of palliative care. In the United States, according to the 2010 census, 56.7 million Americans had some type of disability; this designation impacts how people live, work, enjoy leisure, and participate in their communities.[9,12]

Payer sources are also motivated to monitor how discharge planning for this group of patients is done. They are tracking patient progress during hospitalizations, discharge placements, and readmission rates. An individual and shared approach to this patient population has far-reaching ramifications to health care systems and society at large.

Health care providers, no matter the discipline or setting, must use the tools available to create patient-centered discharge plans that will preserve the goals, values, and dignity of those who have entrusted us with their care.

ACKNOWLEDGMENTS

The author would like to acknowledge Michelle M. Thompson, JD and Roberta Kuchler O'Shea, PT, DPT, PhD for their contributions to the completion of this article.

REFERENCES

1. A guide to understanding your discharge options after hospitalization. Lebanon (NH): Darthmouth-Hitchock Medical Center; 2007.
2. Qian X, Russell LB, Viliyeva E, et al. " Quicker and Sicker" under Medicare's prospective payment system for hospitals: new evidence on an old issue from a national longitudinal survey. Bull Econ Res 2011;63:1–27.
3. McMurray A, Johnson P, Wallis M, et al. General surgical patients' perspective of the adequacy and appropriateness of discharge planning to facilitate health decision-making at home. J Clin Nurs 2007;16(9):1602–9.
4. Steinhauser KE, Christakis NA, Clipp EC, et al. Factors considered important at the end of life by patients, family, physicians and other care providers. JAMA 2000;284(19):2476–82.
5. Slatyer S, Toye C, Popescu, et al. Early re-presentation to hospital after discharge from an acute medical unit: perspective of older patients, their family caregivers and health professionals. J Clin Nurs 2013;22:445.
6. Pearce J, Riley J. Communication in life-limiting illness: A practical guide for physicians written. BCMJ 2016;58(5):262–7.
7. Adapted for NCPPC Glossary of Term V2.0 2014. Available at: Pallipedia.org/life-limiting-condition. Accessed June 23, 2016.
8. Global Atlas of Palliative Care at the End of Life. Available at: https;//www.who.int/nmh/Global-_Atlas_of_Palliative_Care.pdf.2014. Accessed October 1, 2018.

9. Favley J, Burke R, Kyle D, et al. Role of physical therapist in reducing hospital readmissions: optimizing outcomes for older adults during care transitions from hospital to community. Phys Ther 2016;96(8):1125–34.
10. Franco B, Dharmakulaseelan L, McAndrew A, et al. The experiences of cancer survivors while transitioning from tertiary to primary care. Curr Oncol 2016; 23(6):378–85.
11. DeLima L, Radbrunch L. The International Association for Hospice and Palliative Care: advancing hospice and palliative care worldwide. J Pain Symptom Manage 2018;55(2):S96–103.
12. Americans with disabilities. Available at: www.census.gov/prod/2012pubs/p70-131.pdf. Accessed October 1, 2018.
13. Fraser LK, Parslow R. Children with life-limiting conditions in paediatric intensive care units: a national cohort, data linkage study. Arch Dis Child 2018;103:540–7.
14. Available at: https://aspe.hhs.gov/poverty-guidelines.Internet. Accessed May 13, 2019.
15. Available at: https://www.theguardian.com/society/2018/jan/23/well-live-longer-but-suffer-more-ill-health-by-2035-says-study. Internet. Accessed May 13, 2019.
16. Available at: https://media.capc.org/filer_public/68/bc/68bc93c7-14ad-4741-9830-8691729618d0/capc_press-kit.pdf Internet. Accessed May 13, 2019.
17. Available at: https://www.health.ny.gov/professionals/patients/discharge_planning/discharge_transition.htm. Accessed November 1, 2018.
18. Kangovi S. Community health workers embedded in inpatient and outpatient clinical teams enhance access to primary care and improve health outcomes for low-income patients. Agency for Healthcare Research and Quality, Innovations Exchange; 2014. Available at: https://innovations.ahrq.gov/profiles/community-health-workers-embedded-inpatient-and-outpatient-clinical-teams-enhance-access. Accessed October 1, 2018.
19. Ostrovsky A. Community-based health coaches and care coordinators reduce readmissions using information technology to identify and support at-risk Medicare patients after discharge. Agency for Healthcare Research and Quality, Innovations Exchange; 2014. Available at: https://innovations.ahrq.gov/profiles/community-based-health-coaches-and-care-coordinators-reduce-readmissions-using-information. Accessed October 1, 2018.
20. Mherekumombe MF. From inpatients to clinic to home to hospice and back: using the "pop-up" pediatric palliative model care. Children (Basel) 2018;5(5) [pii:E55].

GLOSSARY[1]

Acute Hospital Care: When medical needs are met in a hospital and are provided by 24-hour professional staff with daily doctor intervention.

Assisted Living: Residents are generally independent but need help with a small number of tasks, such as cooking, laundry, or housekeeping/maintenance.

Medicare: Medicare is the federal health insurance program for people aged 5 and over and certain disabled persons. It is not based on financial need.

Medicaid: Medicaid is health insurance provided by the state in which you reside. It is a medical assistance program for people with low income and limited financial assets. It is important to know that Medicaid is administered by each individual state, so there may be some variation in coverage.

Skilled Nursing Facility: Skilled nursing facilities provide short-term, rehabilitative, and convalescent care, which is delivered by professional staff hours a day.

APPENDIX 1: NATIONAL ORGANIZATIONS THAT SERVE AS RESOURCES FOR DISCHARGE PLANNING

Agency	Contact Information	Description
Family Caregiving Alliance: National Center on Caregiving	(415) 434-3388 (800) 445-8106 Web site: www.cargiver.org E-mail: info@caregiver.org	Family Caregiver Alliance seeks to improve the quality of life for caregivers through education, services, research, and advocacy
Next Step in Care: United Hospital Fund	Web site: www.nextstepincare.org	Comprehensive information and advice to help family caregivers and health care providers plan transitions for patients
Medicare's Nursing Home Compare	Web site: www.medicare.gov/nursinghomecompare	
Medicare Rights Center	Web site: www.medicarerights.org	The Medicare Rights Center is a national, nonprofit consumer service organization that works to ensure access to affordable health care for older adults and people with disabilities through counseling and advocacy, educational programs, and public policy initiatives
Center for Medicare Advocacy "Hospital Discharge Planning"	Web site: www.medicareadvocacy.org	The Center for Medicare Advocacy's mission is to advance access to comprehensive Medicare coverage and quality health care for older people and people with disabilities by providing exceptional legal analysis, education, and advocacy
Aging Life Care Associations	Web site: www.aginglifecare.org	Leading the community of Aging Life Care Professionals through education, professional development, and the highest ethical standards
Your Discharge Planning Checklist	Website: www.medicare.gov/pubs/pdf/11376-discharge-planning-checklist.pdf	For patients and their caregivers preparing to leave a hospital, nursing home, or other care setting
Area Agencies on Aging and Aging and Disability Resource Centers	Web site: www.eldercare.gov (800) 677-1116	Helping older adults, people with disabilities, and their caregivers
Medicare	Web site: www.medicare.gov	Provides information and support to caregivers of people with Medicare
Long Term Care (LTC) Ombudsman Program	Web site: www.ltcombudsman.org	Advocates for and promotes the rights of residents in LTC facilities

(*continued on next page*)

(continued)

Agency	Contact Information	Description
Senior Medicare Patrol Programs	Web site: www.smpresource.org	Works with seniors to protect themselves from the economic and health-related consequences of Medicare and Medicaid fraud, error, and abuse
Centers for Independent Living	Web site: www.ilru.org/html/publications/directory/index.html	Helps people with disabilities live independently
State Technology Assistance Project	Web site: www.resna.org (703) 524-6686	Has information on medical equipment and other assistive technology
National Long-Term Care Clearinghouse	Web site: www.longtermcare.gov	Provides information and resources to plan for your long-term care needs
National Council on Aging	Web site: www.benefitscheckup.org	Provides information about programs that help pay for prescription drugs, utility bills, meals, health care, and more
State Health Insurance Assistance Programs	Web site: www.shiptacenter.org (800) 633-4227	Offers counseling on health insurance and programs for people with limited income
Medicaid	Web site: www.medicare.gov/contacts (800) 633-4227	Helps with medical costs for some people with limited income and resources
Project BOOST	Web site: www.hospitalmedicine.org/ResourceRoomRedesign/RRCareTransitions/PDFs/TARGET.pdf	The 8 Ps assessing your patient's risk for adverse events after discharge
American Cancer Society	Web site: www.cancer.org	At the American Cancer Society, they're on a mission to free the world from cancer
Christopher & Dana Reeves Foundation	Web site: www.christopherreeve.org	The Reeve Foundation is dedicated to curing spinal cord injury by funding innovative research, and improving the quality of life for people living with paralysis through grants, information, and advocacy
American Heart Association	Web site: www.heart.org	To be a relentless force for a world of longer, healthier lives
United Spinal Association	Web site: https://www.unitedspinal.org/	United Spinal Association is a national 501(c) (3) nonprofit membership organization dedicated to enhancing the quality of life of all people living with spinal cord injuries and disorders, including veterans, and providing support and information to loved ones, care providers and professionals

Navigating the Murky Waters of Hope, Fear, and Spiritual Suffering

An Expert Co-Captain's Guide

Buddy Marterre, MD, MDiv[a,*], Kristel Clayville, MA, PhD[b]

KEYWORDS

- Fear • Hope • Spiritual suffering • Existential suffering • Spiritual history taking
- Emotions • Dying process • Surgery • Chaplaincy

KEY POINTS

- Surgeons must move from their heads and hands to their emotional and spiritual hearts to provide excellent whole-person surgical care.
- Understanding hopes and fears is a key to understanding spiritual suffering and delivering compassionate holistic care.
- Responsibly reframing hope to underlying meanings, and away from specific outcomes or events, is critical to compassionate surgical care.
- A peaceful dying process can be facilitated by surgeons, because surgeons possess a unique set of skills, which include a drive for excellence, pragmatic realism, visualization and creative mental preparation, imagination, and an undying sense of personal hope.
- Surgeons who have the courage to sustain realistic hope for their patients–all the way to the end–will reap rewards of deep professional satisfaction as well as profound personal spiritual growth.

When hope is so strong that it altogether drives out fear, its nature changes and it becomes complacency or confidence.... Likewise, when fear is so extreme that it leaves no room at all for hope, it is transformed into despair....

—René Descartes, The Passions of the Soul, 1649[1]

Disclosure: Neither B. Marterre nor K. Clayville have any direct financial interest in anything discussed in this article.

[a] Surgical Palliative Care, Department of General Surgery, Wake Forest Baptist Health, 5th Floor, Watlington Hall, Medical Center Boulevard, Winston-Salem, NC 27157, USA; [b] Zygon Center for Religion and Science, MacLean Center for Clinical Medical Ethics, 1100 East 55th Street, Chicago, IL 60615, USA

* Corresponding author. Surgical Palliative Care, Department of General Surgery, Wake Forest Baptist Health, 5th Floor, Watlington Hall, Medical Center Boulevard, Winston-Salem, NC 27157.

E-mail address: b.marterre@wakehealth.edu

Surg Clin N Am 99 (2019) 991–1018
https://doi.org/10.1016/j.suc.2019.06.013
surgical.theclinics.com

Surgical palliative care puts surgeons at the intersection of fixing patients and alleviating suffering, but with a different long-term goal: a better dying process. This better living until the end of life comes with the need for engaging and understanding surgeons' and patients' emotions and spirituality, because patients bring their whole selves to end of life care. For surgeons offering holistic care, these are "murky waters" to navigate, bordered by conscious and subconscious fears, with hope and spiritual transcendence in the mix as well.

Surgeons are result-oriented and aim to provide excellent technical care. This intention is a character strength, but, when patients need noncurative therapy for grave illnesses, their result orientation must yield to caring for patients as they die. Because surgeons assume tremendous vicarious agency for patients in the operating room, the process of "giving up" and relying on spiritual resources can be personally daunting. To help navigate these waters, this article offers practical methods for recognizing fear and spiritual distress, incorporating chaplains into patient care, and reframing hope: from cure to comfort to a peaceful dying process.

THE PROBLEM: SURGEONS PREFER TO STAY IN THEIR HEADS AND HANDS

Surgery is a highly rational and technical field, and consequently surgeons are taught early on that they are the captain of the surgical team, or, to run with the metaphor, the surgical ship. Expert surgeons have confidence in their ability to steer the surgical ship particularly in times of crisis in the operating room. They also have an uncanny ability to be calm in the midst of operative maelstroms,[2] and, fortunately, that unwavering calm[3,4] is contagious to the other members of the operative team. In the process, surgeons instill profound existential faith, hope, and an inscrutable transcendent peace into the entire operative theater before taking action. However, in the context of surgical palliative care, when realistic options for cure have been exhausted, the emotional storms of fear and spiritual distress can seep under the surgeon's own skin, making some surgeons wish they were not captains at all.[5]

Almost 2 decades ago, in the essay paralleling this one in *Surgical Oncology Clinics of North America*, Thomas Krizek[6] claimed that, "Surgeons are technicians for whom the spirituality of death and the dying process is terrifying." Surgeons have made strides in emotional intelligence,[7] but navigating through spiritual suffering[8] resists the reductive, algorithmic thinking that surgeons are taught and so readily embrace. Many surgeons are uncomfortable dealing with their patients' spiritual and existential distress,[9] and when surgeons are distracted by issues such as their own fear of the unknown, the entire surgical ship can be in danger of taking on water.[10,11]

How can surgeons support responsible hope in the face of fear?[12] The mysterious waters of hope, fear, and spiritual suffering are every bit as critical to patients' well-being as their surgical results. Like it or not, patients look to the captain of the medical team to help them navigate these murky waters, which include enormously difficult living and dying decisions.[13] Many patients appoint their surgeons to the priest role,[14] just as they expect them to perform the technical aspects of their surgery with excellent care, even to the point of performing miracles.[15] Surgeons can exercise the same excellence in basic spiritual screening and support (while collaborating with their more skilled spiritual coworkers) with which they exercise the technical aspects of their craft.[14,16–19] Surgeons have learned to trust their heads and hands to fix difficult problems, and these skills can be augmented with emotional and spiritual heart.[20]

The First Step: Moving from Head and Hands to Heart

Surgeons can diagnose significant spiritual suffering and offer patients a safe space and engage chaplain co-captains wherein the two can embark on healing together by recognizing and naming patients' hopes and fears, aligning with them emotionally through deep listening (putting data and medical jargon aside), and helping them reframe hope around their values and meaningful relationships.[21] Cognitive knowledge does not empower patients and families; patients report that medical knowledge is a barrier to shared decision-making.[22] Thus, the surgical instinct, which is to rely on facts and figures to help sway or shape the opinions of patients, becomes ineffective because it is incompatible with the psychology of human information processing.[23] Particularly when people are presented with difficult information, they must process the emotion first, before they can even begin to take in data.[24] Emotions are also powerful mediators of memories, influencing meaning-making of traumatic events and losses, and are retriggered by immediately present stimuli,[25,26] such as when people hear a distressing medical report.[27]

Despite the American College of Surgeons' recommendations that surgeons communicate empathically and recognize, assess, discuss, and offer access to services for psychological, social, and spiritual issues,[28] addressing emotions and spiritual pain are skill sets in which surgeons need training.[29–33]

Surgeons need to allow space for patients to express emotions before effectively communicating a shared decision-making plan in order to honor their hopes and goals. Surgeons do this by slowing down,[3] avoiding more data provision or educating them medically,[22–24] allowing silence, not interrupting their emotional flow, and by showing empathy.[33–36] Most surgeons begin their encounters with patients and families by telling them medical news. It is much better, however, to begin by asking what they know and how they feel about their own or their loved ones' condition before relaying information (See **Table 2**).[24,37–42] This approach both reempowers the patient and facilitates active listening on the part of the clinician. Active listening is a basic and very effective form of spiritual care, which anyone, including surgeons, can provide. It helps surgeons spiritually as well. Sue Patton Thoele[43] says, "Deep listening is miraculous for both listener and speaker. When someone receives us with open-hearted, non-judging, intensely interested listening, our spirits expand." After attending to their emotions completely, surgeons may move on to delivering medical news, necessary data, and goal-concordant recommendations (**Table 1**).[27,37,44–48]

There are 3 key elements of spirituality (**Box 1**)[49–51] that all human beings, regardless of individual beliefs and practices, share.[52] These elements are meaning, purpose, and connectedness. In crises of any kind, these are the common elements of humanity that people routinely both fall back on and/or question.[53] They are also key features of a spiritual history.[53–56] Patient's hopes and fears are tied to meaning, goals, and relationships, and are therefore an excellent guide to obtaining a poignant spiritual inquiry.

The Second Step: Understanding Spiritual/Existential Suffering

Relief of suffering is a core value in clinical practice, which is shared by surgery, palliative care, chaplaincy, and other spiritual care professionals.[57] Spiritual/existential suffering involves a loss of certainty and a fear of the unknown, and is expressed, albeit differently, in every major religious tradition (**Box 2**).[58–61] Søren Kierkegaard[62] explained that, etymologically, existence is to "stand out of being." The psychological manifestation of existence is dread, and the fundamental mysteries (sin, faith, incarnation, and so forth) then become obstacles to well-being. All sentient beings tragically

Table 1
Responding to emotions using the NURSE mnemonic

Name it (tone down the emotion: ie, fear becomes concern)	"That must be frustrating." "I can see how upsetting this is." "Was that difficult to hear?" "What is your greatest concern … about the future?" "What are you most afraid of?" "What are you hoping for?"
Understanding (you do not!)	"I can't image what it must be like to hear this." "I cannot imagine being in your shoes." "Anyone confronting these issues would feel scared." "These discussions are not easy. Are you okay with continuing?"
Respect (and commend)	"I am very impressed by how you have been taking care of your mother through all of this." "I want to commend you on your unswerving commitment to …" "I can see that you really care about …"
Support	"How can I help you?" "I will do my best to honor your values and goals/support you." "I am in your court. We will not abandon you; I will be with you every step of the way."
Explore	"Could you explain that to me?" "What are you willing to go through in order to try to get you over this crisis?" "What do you mean by … ?" "Tell me more."
Example of addressing anger with NURSE	Avoid fight/flight or freeze. Defensiveness and avoidance are counterproductive. Anger displayed to a surgeon is a sign of vulnerability and respect. An underlying fear is there somewhere. Naming/understanding/respecting/supporting/exploring is a particularly efficacious response to anger Say: "Mr Smith, I can see you're frustrated/upset. These are very difficult conversations … and I can't imagine being in your shoes. What did I say that bothered you the most?" Support is implicit in the continued engagement. "Yes sir … please let me clarify what I meant. I want to assure you that I, too, am hoping for the best, … and [avoid but] I also think we need to prepare for the worst. How can I help you explore how we might do that … together?"

NURSE mnemonic Fischer G, Tulsky J, Arnold R: Communicating a poor prognosis, in Portenoy R, Bruera E (eds): Topics in Palliative Care. New York, NY, Oxford University Press, 2000. *Data from* Refs.[37,44–48]

ex-ist, and suffer angst in that we can all imagine our nonbeing, and we therefore imaginatively strive for more being (eternal ist-ness).[62] Pain and suffering can be a diagnostic tool for thinking about relationships to the Divine, others, or the community, but pain and suffering can also cause people to question their image of Reality/God/cosmic justice.[63] Nazi death camp survivor and psychiatrist Viktor Frankl[64] maintained that meaning can be found in any situation, including great suffering, and that meaning-making in gravely difficult situations affords people the will to continue living even in the worst of circumstances.

Religious traditions are resources that patients both lean on and reevaluate when faced with existential threats, such as the possibility of death. Most surgical patients are staring loss and uncertainty directly in the face, sometimes after prolonged periods

Box 1
Spirituality – 3 definitions

"Spirituality is a dynamic, life-long process, described with common themes of meaning and purpose in life, self-transcendence, transcendence with a higher being, feelings of communion and mutuality, ... and hope."[49]

"Spirituality is a dynamic and intrinsic aspect of humanity through which persons seek ultimate meaning, purpose, and transcendence, and experience relationship to self, family, others, community, society, nature, and the significant or sacred. Spirituality is expressed through beliefs, values, traditions, and practices."[50]

The three vital themes of spirituality are meaning, purpose, and connectedness/relationality. Although many imagine/feel/believe that connectedness, purpose and meaning must be associated with an extrinsic transcendent force, eg, God; that is not necessary. To be spiritual is to be human.[51]

in which they subconsciously spend a lot of time in "safety." This is not denial. Few people can dwell in spiritual suffering, or live with their finitude/mortality all the time. Emanuel and colleagues[65] claim that, in order for humans to process external realities, "we oscillate between comfort and horror, contentment and anxiety, togetherness and isolation, synthesis and fragmentation, feeling replete and longing, and being at ease and aggressively activated." Adapting their model, we also oscillate from touching on overt mortal fear back to the relative safety of future hopes, whether they are reasonable hopes or unrealistic wishes/fantasies, as we cope with suffering and trauma (**Fig. 1**).[66,67] When faced with the prospect of loss of limb and life, patients in crisis tend to oscillate very quickly past realistic hope because realistic hope resides in the chaotic, highly energized, liminal and transcendent center of the "stream." Furthermore, the angle of the trajectory across the river of hope and the unknown is influenced by fear itself.[68] People are much more comfortable living in fear, whether it is conscious or subconscious, than they are in embracing the transcendent hope that is found in chaos.

Box 2
Selected religious views of suffering

Islam: pain and suffering are viewed as a means for the expiation of moral evil and sins (although excruciating pain may inhibit a Muslim's worship and memory of God).[58]

Hindu faith traditions: in one of the earliest Hindu scriptures, dukkha (suffering, sorrow, distress) awaits all who have not come to fully know ātman, or self (*Bṛhadāraṇyaka Upaniṣad* 4.4.14),[59] as unified with Brahman, or Ultimate Reality.

Buddhist traditions: the Buddha taught that dukkha (suffering, distress, despair, pain, unsatisfactoriness) "is holy only if we embrace it and look deeply into it," and dukkha arises as people crave and cling to permanence and (egoic) self, or remain in ignorance, anger, or arrogance.[60]

Christianity: the Apostle Paul boasted/gloried in his suffering, because he knew "that suffering produces endurance, and endurance produces character, and character produces hope, and hope does not disappoint us, because God's love has been poured into our hearts through the Holy Spirit that has been given to us" (Romans 5:3b-5, New Revised Standard Version).

Judaism: suffering is a problem to be addressed, and is rarely construed positively. According to Rabbi Abraham Joshua Heschel, absurdity is the greatest challenge to existence, and the deepest passion in any real human person is a craving for meaning in existence.[61]

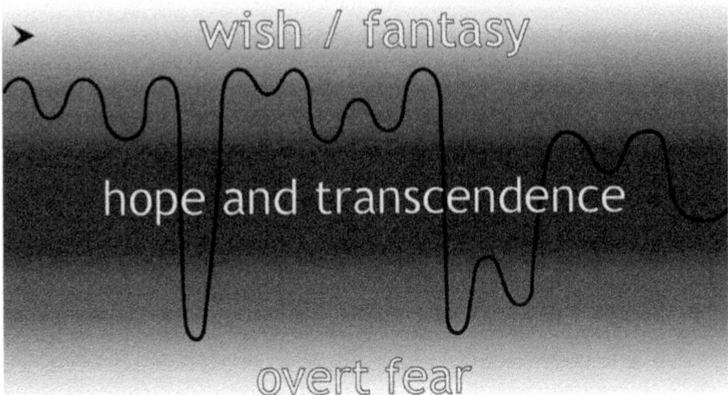

Fig. 1. Fear-hope oscillations. As people in spiritual crisis look to the future, they typically hug one of the clearer fear "shores" (either overt death anxiety or wishes/fantasies) and only rapidly oscillate across the unclear waters of hope and transcendence in the liminal center of the river of life and certain death. Eventually, some reach a degree of transcendent hopeful acceptance with the murky unknown.

Patients and families in spiritual crisis typically hug one of the clearer fear "shores" of **Fig. 1** and only rapidly oscillate across the dark and uncertain waters of hope and transcendence in the center of the river of life and certain death.[69] Eventually, by navigating through a tumultuous emotional and spiritual process, some people do reach a degree of transcendent hopeful acceptance with the murky unknown.[70] When they do, they usually express this as an uncanny sense of calm or peace.[63] Surgeons nobly embrace nonabandonment, and readily lean into physical uncertainty and size up material risk mathematically, make decisions under pressure, and perform bailout plans when necessary, and yet they must learn to lean into their own emotions and fear in order to effectively help patients navigate the river of hope and mitigate their suffering.

The Third Step: Leaning into Our Own Fear

Surgeons pride themselves on staying busy. Most surgeons are very uncomfortable with stillness. Could surgeons be suffering from unconscious spiritual pain, which simultaneously places them in the position of not being able to slow down, reflect on and lean in to suffering, and begin to heal, for the good of their own and their patients' well-being?[71] Do surgeons insidiously project overconfident positivity onto high-risk patients and assume that their patients have bought into their personal strength, which comes complete with prolonged heroic postoperative care in an unspoken covenant,[72–77] as they push toward their own purposes and value of self-efficacy, all the while staying busy to avoid their own spiritual suffering? Do surgeons stay busy out of the weakness of spiritual insecurity, as a diversion toward what they know how to do well, and away from the mysteries of the unknown? Why do many surgeons avoid holding silent space for patients to express feelings of deep regret, existential questions, and nonphysical pain? Because it is too risky? Surgeons are fixers, and these pain-inducing conundrums and fear-filled questions do not have easy answers or solutions. Even basic spiritual screening and care takes self-awareness and emotional sensitivity, or "heart." In addition, many surgeons' hearts, lamentably, are grossly underdeveloped, not because they do not have them, but because they are covered by layers and layers of ego (which, frankly, were needed and successfully embraced in the pursuit to become excellent surgeons).

To be experts at their craft, surgeons rightly use a scientific, linear, cause-and-effect epistemology, and yet this empirical way of knowing allows the surgical "vessel" to take on water,[78,79] particularly when interfacing with patients who use a romantic or religious epistemology.[80] Knowledge is multifaceted, and anyone who applies a single narrow view does so foolishly. As Buddhist Nun Pema Chödrön[81] says, "[T]he only way to ease our pain is to experience it fully. [We must] learn to stay with uneasiness." Stereotypical surgeons need to slow their rolls, practice quieting their minds, rest in awareness, and embrace the alien territory of existential questions and personal fear, in order to better support their patients' suffering.

Critically ill surgical patients with grave diagnoses are, almost universally, experiencing some degree of spiritual suffering.[82–87] Whether surgeons listen and attend to their suffering is crucial to their well-being. When existential angst is ignored or dismissed by the medical team, then patients feel disaffirmed at a core level of personal identity and meaning. Rapport and trust bridges break down.[88] There are, however, some tools that every clinician can use to help identify patients' spiritual needs, as well as basic strategies for addressing spiritual distress.

PRACTICAL SPIRITUAL TOOLS AND RESOURCES IN THE CLINIC AND HOSPITAL

Chaplains are religion and spirituality professionals. They have master's degrees, are eligible for board certification, and are endorsed by their governing religious bodies to do the work of addressing patients' spiritual needs. Particularly if the patient's spiritual distress is significant, consult a chaplain. Surgeons' recommendations should be supported by demonstrating how they are the patient's advocate, and how the chaplain's input will align with the patient's whole-person needs. Chaplains are experts who glean in-depth spiritual assessments[89] and provide in-depth and effective spiritual care to patients of all faith traditions and none.[90–93] They intend to connect the patient, family, and medical staff to each person's own spiritual frame of reference and inner strong spirits, not superimposing or proselytizing any specific religious or spiritual tradition. They meet each person where they are; address purpose, meaning, and loss; and provide specially skilled spiritual care interventions, such as empathic listening, life review and dignity therapy,[36,87,94,95] prayer, religious rituals, and sacred scripture reading. They provide spiritual care not only for patients and families but also to health care workers (including surgeons).[21,54,82,87,96–98]

Although chaplain availability is highly variable in hospitals across the country,[99] by law, hospitals are required to provide spiritual care and assessment, and, ideally, acute and specialized spiritual/religious work is done by chaplains. Although all health care professionals are called to provide basic spiritual care, there are many barriers that prevent this ideal.[29,32,100–104] Although patients uncommonly expect to receive in-depth, specialized spiritual care from their physicians, they do express a strong preference for some basic spiritual inquiry and care,[105] including active listening, presence, and empathy. Chaplains excel at navigating amid fear, hope, and coping with spiritual suffering, particularly near the end of life.[91,106] Spiritual care is the shared work of chaplains and other health care professionals,[12,54,82,87,96,107–109] including surgeons. All doctors can take a spiritual history.

Taking a Spiritual History

Spirituality is a private and sensitive matter. People's relationship to the sacred is, well, sacred. Spiritual histories must be taken with the utmost tact and compassion,[110] and without judgment.[17,111] Spirituality assessors must simultaneously be in tune with their patients' emotions and spirituality as well as their own. An openness to others' spirituality deeply affirms human dignity and allows the other to exercise agency/self-efficacy/personal control, particularly during chaotic health crises. Sacred discussions are highly powerful, with both negative and positive potential. Surgeons who accomplish them build trust and rapport with patients and families with extreme effectiveness[88,112]; those who do not, may not.

Taking a spiritual history requires emotional intelligence as well as some specific skills (See **Table 3**).[54,82,107,113–118] The American Cancer Society (ACS) 2016 Commission on Cancer has mandated that every patient receiving treatment of cancer be screened for psychosocial distress "at a pivotal medical visit."[119] Every health care provider should be able to perform spiritual screening.[108,109] Spiritual screening lends an opportunity for doctors to lean into their own discomfort of spiritual history taking, as a first step toward deeper inquiry. Single-question screens for religious/spiritual distress are inadequate; combining one question of meaning/joy and another of self-described spiritual struggle is better.[120]

Spiritual histories are more detailed than screening,[121] but they still have less depth than the spiritual assessment that a chaplain undertakes. Just gleaning a basic understanding of the patient's values and spiritual disposition with empathy can buoy the inner human spirit, which is a strong source of healing.[122–126] Importantly, during the course of a spiritual history or follow-up inquiries, the patient may reveal a deeper level of distress.

Diagnosing Spiritual and Existential Pain Crises

The best way to discern significant spiritual distress is through active listening. Questions such as "What's the point?" or "Why is this happening to me?" signal potential meaninglessness and hopelessness.[127] Similarly, the question, "What can I hope for?" is not a request for information; it is a request for inspiration.[128] Most doctors think that questions are posed in search of answers. Within the surgeon's "wheelhouse" of expertise (pathophysiology, anatomy, and treatment principles) answers are frequently helpful.

Questions like the ones presented above are not questions that have easy answers, however; they are expressions of fear and spiritual/existential pain. If clinicians offer information in response to them, they will only make the situation worse. Clergy and other well-meaning caregivers who offer pat answers to these deep spiritual questions concretize the mysterious and, in doing so, cause spiritual harm.[122,129] Rather than answer, maintain reverence for mystery,[130] ascertain where the patient is and try to keep the patient between the shores of the oscillating fear-hope river (see **Fig. 1**) by saying, "I don't know; what do you think?" Such statements affirm the patient's self-efficacy, which is critical to hope and spiritual growth.[63,131] They also open the patient's imagination, with which hope cooperates.[132,133] In order to recognize questions that point to spiritual pain, refer to **Box 3**.[63,134–137] If a patient is thought to be in significant spiritual suffering, consider a chaplaincy/spiritual expert consult.[54,96,138,139] Some language cues in **Box 3** include mention of a Divine figure (eg, God), but not all do. Just offering a safe empathic space with deep listening allows many patients in existential pain to engage their own inner human spirit and do the work; others need expert guidance and support.[43,65,114,130,140,141]

REFRAMING AND MAINTAINING HOPE: ALL THE WAY TO THE END

How should surgeons engender hope in their patients, and what kinds of hope is it responsible to facilitate for them? Both hopes and fears are future-oriented and dynamic, complementary, and interconnected in the face of the unknown[1] (see **Fig. 1**).

Box 3
Diagnosing spiritual and existential pain crises

Significant spiritual/existential distress requires a spiritual professional (eg, Chaplain) consult. Many clinicians will recognize spiritual distress when they see it. If they are not asked, (with a spiritual history; see **Table 3**), many patients do not tell. Other patients give cues that are adeptly avoided by physicians.

Typically, in spiritual suffering, 1 or more of the vital 3 elements of spirituality (meaning, purpose, connectedness/relational) is fractured or suffering in some way. For theists, shattered images of God and broken faith relationships frequently accompany existential distress. Many theists are frightened by expressing anger at God, and do not mention it, but their feelings are causing them tremendous distress.

The authors offer the following overlapping categories, which contextualize some typical patient and family comments and questions that may be an expression of existential or spiritual pain crises:

Existential/meaninglessness: "Why is this happening to me? Why is this happening now? What will happen to me after I die? Is this all there is?"

Hopelessness/ purposelessness/despair: "What's the point? Why should I go on? There's nothing left for me to live for. So there's no hope then. I feel useless."

Unworthiness/shame: "I don't want to be a burden. My life doesn't matter. I hate myself. I'm a bad person."

Abandonment/ isolation/vulnerability: "I feel all alone. No one understands me. No one visits me anymore. God [or my family] doesn't care about me. I'd just like to be able to tell my kids how much I love them/that I'm sorry."

Guilt/ shame/punishment : "I've made some really bad choices in my life. I'm a horrible person. I'm beginning to think that God hates me. I don't deserve to die pain-free."

Shattered relationship with/image of God: "I am angry at God. I have tried my whole life to do what is right, and pray and trust in God ... and now look! I'm not sure God even exists anymore..."

Powerlessness: "I can't believe I'm facing this; I can't deal with it. So what you're saying is ... that I have no hope of ever getting over this."

Intense fear of dying: "What if God doesn't think I should get into heaven? I'm really scared."

Some "hopes" are really unrealistic wishes,[142] which are expressions of subconscious fear, based on one's lack of confidence in their agency to bring about their goal.[132] Realistic hope is defined here as having 3 major components: feasible goals, pathways to achieve those goals, and agency or self-efficacy to navigate those paths.[143,144]

All 3 components apply to aggressive surgical care, even in apparently hopeless clinical situations. The problems that arise in futile or near-futile cases are mainly 2: the feasibility of the goal; and that the agency and the pathways to meet those goals are heavily technologically based and entirely within the purview of the surgeon. Surgeons, and the technologies that they wield, are the agents and the pathways. Surgical moral distress ensues when the surgeon seriously doubts their ability to effect the patient's goals, at least in a way that does not dramatically increase suffering. Even in technically feasible cases, escalating to a more aggressive treatment does not always mesh with the patient's values in a goal-concordant fashion,[145] particularly once the patient's hopes and fears and how much suffering they are willing to endure are considered. It is easy to become complacent with the original plan, while allowing slippage into areas that patients never dreamed of, even in their worst nightmares. For instance, the best way to slow the momentum of the surgical/trauma intensive care unit (SICU/TICU) and/or surgical oncology ship toward inordinate burden with miniscule benefit[101,146] is to revisit (the surgeon's and the patient's) hopes and fears regularly.

Hope has been described as a human life-force.[128] Hope has clearly been shown to be associated with reduced physical symptoms and psychological distress, for both patients and their caregivers.[147–149] Hope prevents and/or decreases psychological distress (depression),[149] and it helps people to adjust to and cope with challenges, be they physical, psychological, social, and/or spiritual. Hope has been shown to lead to a faster rate of recovery and improved quality of life at 6 months following coronary artery bypass surgery.[150] Anecdotally, many surgeons have noticed the association of a patient's hope with better outcomes on multiple levels. How can surgeons convey an accurate and honest prognosis, which is what patients need to continue on their meaning-making spiritual journey[151], when the realistic hopeful outcome is highly discordant with their wishes?

Erich Fromm[152] wrote that active hope empowers people "to think the unthinkable, yet to act within the limits of the realistic possible." Even when people undertake fanciful wishes about the future–which are not mentally contrasted with present reality (as in realistic hope)–their fantasies can still help them endure suffering in a goal-directed manner.[153] Hope is spiritual. Meaning-making, purpose, and self-efficacy are key aspects to hope.[154] Self-efficacy is the power of "believing you can,"[155] but what if a patient's body is failing, dying, and they cannot? Hope becomes more complex when medical-surgical treatments and/or critical organ systems are failing. Core human values, the 3 key elements of spirituality, may persist when someone is dying, but hope's agency must change to include others and inner spiritual strength must supplant bodily self-efficacy when it becomes limited.

When patients are struggling with core values and beliefs (for instance, with their image of God),[71,156–161] often they hope for miraculous divine intervention even though it has not been forthcoming.[15,38,41,53] Is that based on fear? It depends. Some miracle wishes are just wishes that illuminate love and well-being on another person; other miracle wishes are an expression of spiritual suffering[38,40] and covert fear. Responsible hope seeks goals that are realistic possibilities[162]; fantasies portend unrealistic outcomes. Either way, clinicians who discount the grounding and significance of wishes for a miracle do so at the risk of losing all trust and rapport with their patients.[88] This is sure to cause the surgical ship to take on water.

Although (unrealistic) hope for a miracle is not justification to continue aggressive treatment near the end of life, clinicians should never (further) fracture their patients' theological views unless invited, willing, and trained to help them rebuild. That is clearly outside the wheelhouse of surgeons (see **Table 2** for dealing with miracle wishes). Religious patients, in particular, have relied on a belief and practice system that has been supported by ancient and modern stories within their faith traditions and worship communities for most of their lives, and it has served them well. Now, however, in the face of death, their beliefs and images of God (which can be cognitively dissonant in anyone) may be shattered.[63] The surgeon walks into a spiritual crisis and is asked to provide hope.

Is this something surgeons can do? Should do?[6,9,14,16] Surgeons are typically pragmatic realists, but they are also experts at mental preparation, and their mental readiness planning processes include the processes of visualization and creative imagining.[163,164] Surgeons are also typically positive, instilling hope in their patients routinely. Surgeons can chip away at a densely scarred vascular anastomosis with exceedingly fine strokes of the scalpel primarily because they imagine where the vessels might be before encountering their borders, all the time picking up on clues such as old suture lines and other geometric hints. The anatomy progressively unfolds in their minds before it is realized in the flesh. Surgeons also mentally and inventively

Table 2
Family meeting pearls

Premeeting		Each interdisciplinary representative updates others. Establish a leader. Communicate preference for intermingled seating
Who?		Involve patients as dictated by their ability, decision-making capacity, energy, and interest. It can help to involve weak or incapacitated patients at the end
Where/how?		Private, comfortable space. Sit down. Avoid us-vs-them seating arrangements; intermingle health care providers and family
Introductions		Write down preferred names and refer to each by name
Assess and update: Ask-empathize-tell-empathize-ask	Ask	"Tell me what you know about your condition." "How do you feel he's doing today? What do you think about … ?"
	Tell	"Here's what the tests show: …" "Since we last met, his [breathing, blood pressure, kidney function, and so forth] has …"
	Empath	Make eye contact. Allow silence for emotional processing. Use NURSE (see **Table 1**). Use appropriate physical touch, tissues
	Ask	Involve quiet, despondent participants: "Where are you right now, Ms. Jones? I want to check in with you." Inquire for cognitive understanding: "Does that make sense?"
Elicit stories, values, goals, un/acceptable outcomes; diagnose spiritual suffering		Reflect, paraphrase and echo (use their words) to understand their values, hopes, fears, and what are they willing to lose or how much suffering they are willing to endure to achieve their goals. Diagnose spiritual and existential distress (see **Box 2**)
Dealing with miracle wishes and the do-everything request		Expressions of miracle wishes come from a deeply private spiritual place. Dishonor them at the peril of major distrust. Affirm their strong sense of divine sovereignty/providence: "God is ultimately in charge. Only God knows." Respectfully ask: "How can I know when a miracle has happened? How might we know when it is your time?" Explore what they mean by "do everything" (do not assume that they are requesting more technological intervention). There is usually an underlying fear to this request. Ask: "What is worrying you the most? What are you most afraid of … going forward? What is the hardest part of this for you? Tell me more about what you mean by 'everything'."
Ask permission and align your recommendations with their values and goals		"Would it be alright if I made some recommendations, … based on what's important to her?" Make recommendations that are aligned with the patient's values, addressing fears gently, even, and particularly, when they differ from your plan Do-everything requests and miracle wishes are perfect opportunities for a time-limited trial. Help them weigh burden vs benefit with: "How much suffering is he willing to endure to achieve his goals?" And come back another day
Debrief with team		Coordinate tasks. Because everyone is learning, ask: "What went well? Where were the challenges?" The ideal positive affirmation to constructive criticism ratio for learners is >3:1

Data from Refs.[24,37–42]

practice imaginative clinical scripts to help themselves develop skills in diagnosis, problem solving, judgment, and visualization.[165–167]

Supporting Realistic Hope is Compassionate Care

No one can fix another's spiritual pain. As fixers, most surgeons feel like a fish out of water when dealing with this. One of the greatest powers clinicians can wield in this situation is to guide their patients back to a realistic positive future and help them find hope once again. This guidance is done, in part, by reawakening their imaginations.[133] Although hopelessness in the face of shattered belief systems seems devastating, it rarely persists. Most people, even when faced with extreme loss and trauma, have the inner strength to rebound and find a glimpse of hope as they rebuild their images of God/Reality.

These difficult conversations can typically take place as a gradual process over time.[66] Particularly in the surgical oncology population, there is plenty of time to have multiple conversations.[168] Prognostic (time and/or functionality) awareness within the context of uncertainty can be promoted,[66] and burden versus benefit can be revisited with regoaling conversations and appropriate shifts to comfort care. Patients and families want accurate and honest information[132,169]; they need it to sustain hope.[151]

Balancing truth telling with nurturing hope when the prognosis/future looks grim can be tricky. Expert surgeons, however, know but transcend logical algorithms (with hope) and solve complex clinical problems creatively by using pattern recognition repeatedly so that they can develop a sharp edge to their surgical intuition.[163] Surgeons bring an essential mixture of realism, pragmatism, creativity, imagination, and hope to the problem of promoting hope to their palliative surgical patients. Fears cannot be conquered, but they can be handled creatively, with imagination. Imagination helps all of us reframe hope.

Reframing Hope: from Cure to Comfort

Hope protects against despair, restores meaning, and helps people realize purpose.[170] It is critical to spiritual peace and coping when faced with a grave diagnosis. Family members and patients may or may not be tacking back and forth between various forms of fear, scooting past hope quickly (see **Fig. 1**), and thinking that surgery or more aggressive postoperative treatments may still offer a curative option for their problems.[145] Avoid the temptation to offer a treatment option that cannot be provided with reasonable certainty (eg, in an patient with incurable cancer in the last few months of life, saying: "If 'things' improve with the total parenteral nutrition,[171–176] we might consider more surgery"). Engaging in such fantasies is a pathologic form of subconscious psychological projective identification of the surgeon's own death anxiety and/or fears of powerlessness onto the patient. Instead, refocus the patient's hopes away from outcomes and onto meanings and connectedness, gently exposing fears, and addressing them with open, courageous discussion.

Hope is entrenched in meaning,[13,154] and meanings are socially constructed. Determining what is most important to the patient (**Table 3**) is key to helping a person reframe hope.[177] Connectedness (relationships with loved ones and/or the Divine) top the list for most people.[134] As the focus of hope shifts from cure to comfort, allow the patient's wishes for a (miraculous) cure to persist. Many surgeons have an admirable helper/rescuer mentality, but no one can rescue another from death; there is no fix. Beginning each encounter by asking, rather than telling, and listening to wishes for cure in a nonjudgmental fashion empowers the patient/family (see **Table 2**). After asking about fears and hopes, it is important to pay attention to how people respond.

Table 3
Spiritual history taking

	Techniques and Sample Questions
Spiritual Screening	"Are you a spiritual person? Tell me more about that." "Do you struggle with meaning and joy in your life?" "Do you have any religious or spiritual struggles? Tell me more."
Discerning spirituality implicitly	Requires an open interview, with an open-ended starter question, facilitated with periods of silence, and further exploration of some storylines. Acknowledge and normalize the patient's concerns. Initially, after introductions, inquire about what the patient knows about their condition, and then switch subjects (away from the clinical) with a leading question; eg, "Tell me a little about yourself, as a person." Then listen to the story. While listening for symptoms, also: Listen intently for values, what is most important, meaning, and purpose Listen specifically for hopes, fears, and un/supportive relationships Take note of other losses and sources of suffering; eg, uncertainty, grief, regret, guilt, anger, abandonment, rejection, unreconciled/hurtful relationships Frequently, people mention their principal spiritual values (perhaps with anxiety of loss or change) first. Spirituality is about meaning, purpose (hopes, fears, goals), and connection. Many patients, but not all, mention their loved ones, and/or faith tradition/beliefs (eg, in God, church/temple attendance/participation, or not). Fewer mention practices Listen for supportive resources, coping strategies, spiritual/faith communities, spiritual/religious pain, as well as areas that they are uncomfortable pursuing Reflect: use their language to echo/paraphrase: "So what I hear you saying is ..." Inquire about any key elements you think they may have left out Gently question apparent inconsistencies for better understanding: "Help me to understand..." Respect: "How can I make sure I honor your spirituality in your care plan?" Whenever you get stuck, say: "Tell me more." Resist answering spiritual questions; maintain reverence for mystery
Taking an explicit spiritual history without a tool	After introductions, inquire about what they know about their condition, and then switch subjects away from the clinical and establish some rapport and trust by getting to know the patient as a person. Alternately, when you have finished asking about symptoms, transition into open-ended spiritual questions: Ask about (1) hopes, (2) fears, (3) meaning, and (4) the big 3 types of relationships (intrapersonal [with self]; interpersonal [with others]; transpersonal [with the transcendent/sacred]) and support. Helpful questions include: 1. What is your goal? What are your hopes?" 2. What is your greatest concern? What else are you concerned about?" 3. How have you made sense of why this is happening to you?" 4. Who or what has helped you cope with stressful, difficult times in the past?"

(*continued on next page*)

Table 3
(*continued*)

	Techniques and Sample Questions
	If the patient does not offer the following, ask: "What is your faith tradition? Which spiritual practices [eg, meditation, prayer, reading sacred texts, music, exercise, communing with nature]) do you find helpful? Have you experienced significant negative religious or spiritual events?" Many theists fear expressing anger at God, and will not bring it up. If you suspect this, generate a safe environment/ normalize this first, watching the patient's reaction, and then ask: "Sometimes people are afraid to talk about being angry with God. If you are, that's perfectly okay. Have you been angry with God?" In addition, ask: "How can I make sure I honor your spirituality in your care plan?" Whenever you get stuck, say: "Tell me more." Resist answering spiritual questions; maintain reverence for mystery
Spiritual history taking tools	These tools are less likely to uncover spiritual pain or religion-associated suffering/regrets, because they are all positively oriented. A common shortcoming is that no tool addresses fear, which is ubiquitous in surgical patients: FICA[115] HOPE[116] iCARING [117] SPIRIT[118]

When dying patients use the word hope as a noun, it invariably relates to the absolute medically-mediated black-and-white possibilities of cure versus no cure, and expresses powerlessness, which typically takes a negative form (ie, there is no hope). However, patients who use hope as a verb emphasize their active engagement in life, and the strengthening of connectedness.[169] Hope seeks the "beyond," and patients who have a realistic understanding of their approaching death integrate transcendent sources of inner strength with positive reappraisal as they reframe the verb form of hope.[162]

Focusing on the values and meanings that the patient has articulated rather than biological outcomes helps to facilitate a shift toward hope for comfort rather than cure. If a patient has prognostic awareness, then there are only 3 other things that the surgeon needs to know to recommend a new plan in a shared decision-making model: (1) the patient's goals, (2) the patient's fears, and (3) how much suffering the patient is willing to endure for the *possibility* of achieving their goals. The conversation should not be about test results, ventilators, or the addition of another technology, which is likely to fail.[178,179] Once the patient's hopes, fears, and acceptable trade-offs have been accurately determined, the medical-surgical details of the new plan will just fall into place.[180] Then the surgeon's goal-concordant plan can be recommended,[45,181] and can be backed up by returning to and echoing meanings and acceptable trade-offs.[182]

Remember that curiosity is the first problem-solving component to the Zen mind (and listening is the second).[183] Inquire further about unachievable long-term event-based goals and plans (wishes) and facilitate the patient's distillation of the meaning and value beneath them. As Dunn and colleagues[55] say, "One may be honest with patients and still maintain hope through a change in focus, away from hopes that are long-term, to hopes that are short-term [and] spiritual."

Most patients and families still want realism, both in the disclosure of their prognosis and when discussing attainable hopes.[132,151,169] Honest assessments can be communicated effectively without numbers, percentages, or medical jargon that only widens the patient-surgeon power gap. Although that information is critical to the surgeon's thought processes, it is unhelpful to the patient's. When reframing hope from cure to comfort, a good way to respond to unrealistic wishes, particularly in the context of family demands for aggressive treatment in the context of a poor prognosis, is with an I-wish statement,[184] or a wish-worry statement (**Box 4**).[37,177,184] Using these communication techniques is not easy, and yet effort and practice is the only way to sharpen these skills.[185]

A common trap for surgeons arises when their patients' surrogates request more heroic and aggressive treatments in situations that they have deemed goal-discordant and burdensome. This request places the surgeon and their agency in the center of the maelstrom. Surgeons experience their own moral distress because they have already done the benefit-versus-burden calculations in their heads, and may be simultaneously sickened by being dehumanized/instrumentalized[186] by fantastical demands.[187] Surgeons themselves may begin to wonder what the point is even as they grapple with their personally-defined ideals as healers, not torturers.[188] Serious surgical moral distress has the potential to capsize the ship. To keep the ship afloat, rather than assume that the family wants the surgeon to fix it, paradoxically step away from the helm when families ask that everything be done, and consider that this request originates from their fear. Rather than assume that they are requesting more technical heroism, ask what they mean (see **Box 4** and **Table 2**). "Do-everything" requests are an opening to discuss hopes, fears, and how much suffering they are willing to watch their loved one endure to achieve the possibility of reaching their goals.

Box 4
Examples of statements/questions to facilitate realistic hope

Delivering bad news: "I wish I had better news for you."

For addressing unrealistic wishes: "I wish the very best for you; I'm concerned that..."

When waiting on a miracle: "How might we know when God thinks it is her time?"

To address demands for continued aggressive treatment in (relatively) futile cases: "It must be very difficult to see so little change in [their loved one's name]. I wish we had the power to change things around. I'm concerned too. Unfortunately, we don't have any more treatments that won't just prolong his suffering. He's not getting better like we have all hoped."

"I'm concerned that you're/he's dying. And all we're doing here is increasing your/his suffering. How much more suffering do you think you're/he's willing to endure? What are you hoping we might accomplish with continuing his life support?"

When asked to do everything to keep a loved one alive: "What are you most afraid of? What are you hoping for? What impact do you think these treatments might have? How much suffering do you think she's willing to endure?"

To reframe hope for unrealizable events: "I hear your concern about not being able to attend your granddaughter's wedding. I can't imagine being in your shoes. What does [use the granddaughter's name] mean to you? What do you think you mean to your granddaughter? Is there something you could do for her in lieu of attending her wedding to show her that?"

Data from Refs.[37,177,184]

Hope is the positive expectation of meanings,[13,154] not specific future events or outcomes. Imaginatively rediscovering new meanings beneath the fear allows both surgeons and their patients to gain a sense of control in otherwise immensely challenging circumstances.

Maintaining Hope: from Comfort to a Peaceful Dying Process

The second major shift for patients, families, and surgeons is from hope for comfort to hope for a peaceful dying process. Can a dying patient still have responsible hope? Charles Corr[142] thinks so: "dying persons ... can, in fact, be hopeful—full of hope—in ways that are often a source of awe to those around them." People who are dying have tangible and meaningful needs. As they more closely approach death, there is a right-shift in the focus of the 4 elements of their humanity: from the biological, psychological, and social, toward the spiritual.[140,189] Spiritually, they seek to identify, develop, or reaffirm meaningful relationship to transcendent energy.[142] Christina Puchalski[63] writes, "[T]here are no easy answers or concrete solutions to the process of dying.... The mystery surrounding life and death can frighten us, and clinging to certitude is woefully inadequate." As people die, the psychosociologic tools that they have developed for coping throughout their lives lose their potency, even as they begin to face the awe and chaos in the liminal center of the stream of life and death (see **Fig. 1**) with more urgency.

When patients begin to confront this unique phase of life, including those who have no religious affiliation, the quest for meaning and peace typically intensifies.[63] Most patients want to be told that they are dying,[55,177] and many patients need to be told by an expert who cares in order to take the first step onto this very difficult pathway. Euphemisms are unhelpful for facilitating hope.[132] Many patients are in touch with their bodies and spirits and already know–at least on a deep, if enigmatic, level–what is happening. Powerfully, an expert who says the words, "I'm concerned that you're dying" can encourage their patient to further face this hard reality and prepare. The necessary pathway[143,144] involved in hope for a peaceful dying process typically becomes more transcendent.[49,113,124,147,190,191] Can a surgeon help with this, and, if so, how?[14,16]

Dying is hard work. Emanuel and colleagues[65] write: "[E]xistential maturity is an achievement beyond [all] other major developmental achievements" and "[P]resence, understanding, listening, and appreciating ... provide the most powerful psychological milieu for developing ... what it takes to face mortality."[65] Kathleen Dowling Singh[131] describes the spiritual transformation process of dying as one of moving from chaos toward surrender to transcendence. This process requires compassionate presence from those attending to the patient.[130] Unfolding compassionate action is the third and final problem-solving component to the Zen mind.[183] In *On Death and Dying*, Elisabeth Kübler-Ross[192] writes: "It is the one who is beyond medical help who needs as much if not more care than the one who can look forward to another discharge." If clinicians offer presence and deep listening, patients and families "will keep [their] glimpse of hope and continue to regard [their] physician as a friend who will stick it out to the end."[192]

Compassionate presence opens the door to hope as the transcending possibilities of finding spiritual meaning and purpose unfold.[65,130] Offering presence is inherently healing.[114,141,193–195] Although listening to stories takes time that most surgeons do not have, even listening to a little bit each day can be therapeutic[14] (this is an excellent opportunity for expert chaplaincy care[89,91,92,106]). Surgeons can act as catalysts, and even guides, in this process,[55] if they are so privileged and willing to try.

A common task that dying people confront is the need to make amends with estranged/strained friends and family members.[63,84,196] Memories of deep harm and feelings of regret spur the dying to reconsider dis/connectedness in new meaning-making ventures as they approach the ends of their lives. Ira Byock[197–199] offers 11 words that can be said to help repair fractured relationships and strengthen once-cherished bonds near the end of life. For the intimate (whether estranged/strained or not, because no human relationship is flawless) who are willing to courageously exercise love by saying these simple phrases to their dying beloved, a powerful opportunity to aid a peaceful dying process can be seized. Surgeons who gently suggest these 4 phrases to loved ones can wield simple but powerful spiritual care. The phrases are: "Please forgive me," "I forgive you," "I love you," and "Thank you." In addition, for all caregivers, surgeons included, there is: "Goodbye."

SUMMARY

Caring for the dying, staying present, and facilitating new meaning-making during another's suffering is emotionally trying and spiritually challenging, and yet this work offers spiritual and professional growth opportunities,[200–202] and deep personal rewards.[203] The gratitude expressed by families and patients is profound and priceless. As Susan Block[113] says: "The intimacy of the experience offers deeper understanding about the nature of life, an appreciation of the gift of being alive, and constantly renewed inspiration and hopefulness about human resilience."

Being the captain of the surgical ship for palliative patients involves rethinking long-held skills and cultivating a few new ones. One of the most challenging skills for surgeons is to slow down and hold the silence and the tension without trying to fix it. Surgeons are, by definition, fixers, but, as surgeons better understand that they cannot fix spiritual suffering, they will notice that most patients fix it themselves. Or they do not. Patients and surgeons alike have deep spiritual resources. In the face of suffering, any clinician can guide their patients/families to imagine hope, even as they revise their own faith and images of God/Reality. The most vulnerable things a person can share with another are their hopes, dreams, and fears. Attentively listening is how clinicians best honor those vulnerabilities, but holding the space for that is not easy.

Staying afloat with excellent process–in the present moment–requires that we all attend to our own emotions and nurture spiritual resources that we already have available deep within ourselves, and resonating with them. Chödrön[204] writes that, "[T]he spiritual journey involves going beyond hope and fear, stepping into unknown territory, continually moving forward. The most important aspect of being on the spiritual path may be to just keep moving." Nobel Laureate Rabindranath Tagore[205] said, "You can't cross the sea merely by standing and staring at the water." So let's put a spiritual hand on the wheel.

REFERENCES

1. Descartes R. The Passions of the Soul. An English Translation of Legras H. Les Passions de l'âme, 1649. Translated and Annotated by Stephen Voss. Indianapolis: Hackett Publishing Company; 1989.
2. McDonald J, Orlick T. Excellence in surgery: psychological considerations. 2005. Available at: http://www.zoneofexcellence.ca/free/surgery.html.
3. Moulton C-AE, Regehr G, Mylopoulos M, et al. Slowing down when you should: a new model of expert judgment. Acad Med 2007;82(10 Suppl):S109–16.
4. Flin R, Youngson GG, Yule S, editors. Enhancing surgical performance: a primer in non-technical skills. Boca Raton (FL): CRC Press; 2015.
5. Csikszentmihalyi M, Figurski TJ. Self-awareness and aversive experience in everyday life. Journal of Personality 1982;50(1):15–28.

6. Krizek TJ. Spiritual dimensions of surgical palliative care. Surg Oncol Clin N Am 2001;10(1):39–55.
7. Hollis RH, Theiss LM, Gullick AA, et al. Emotional intelligence in surgery is associated with resident job satisfaction. J Surg Res 2017;209:178–83.
8. Cassel EJ. The nature of suffering and the goals of medicine. N Engl J Med 1982;306(11):639–45.
9. Ravenscroft P, Ravenscroft E. Spirituality and surgery. In: Dunn GP, Johnson AG, editors. Surgical palliative care. Oxford (United Kingdom): Oxford University Press; 2004. p. 65–84.
10. de Leval MR, Carthey J, Wright DJ, et al. Human factors and cardiac surgery: a multicenter study. J Thorac Cardiovasc Surg 2000;119(4):661–72.
11. Gawande AA, Zinner MJ, Studdert DM, et al. Analysis of errors reported by surgeons at three teaching hospitals. Surgery 2003;133(6):614–21.
12. Handzo G, Koenig HG. Spiritual care: whose job is it anyway? South Med J 2004;97(12):1242–4.
13. Moadel A, Morgana C, Fatone A, et al. Seeking meaning and hope: self-reported spiritual and existential needs among an ethnically-diverse cancer patient population. Psychooncology 1999;8(5):378–85.
14. Turcotte JG. Invited commentary on “The spiritual needs of the dying patient.” J Am Coll Surg 2002;195(4):568–9.
15. Cassell J. Expected miracles: surgeons at work. Philadelphia: Temple University Press; 1991.
16. Hinshaw DB. The spiritual needs of the dying patient. J Am Coll Surg 2002; 195(4):565–8.
17. Smyre CL, Yoon JD, Rasinski KA, et al. Limits and responsibilities of physicians addressing spiritual suffering in terminally ill patients. J Pain Symptom Manage 2015;49(3):562–9.
18. Kruizinga R, Scherer-Rath M, Schilderman HJBAM, et al. Toward a fully fledged integration of spiritual care and medical care. J Pain Symptom Manage 2018; 55(3):1035–40.
19. El Nawawi NM, Balboni MJ, Balboni TA. Palliative care and spiritual care: the crucial role of spiritual care in the care of patients with advanced illness. Curr Opin Support Palliat Care 2012;6(2):269–74.
20. Rivet E. Palliative care ‘in my hands’. ACS Surgery News 2017. Available at: https://www.mdedge.com/acssurgerynews/article/132324/hospice-palliative-medicine/palliative-care-my-hands. Accessed August 12, 2018.
21. Schmidt R. The role of chaplaincy in caring for the seriously ill: Fast Fact #347. In: Fast facts. Milwaukee (WI): Palliative Care Network of Wisconsin; 2017. Available at: https://www.mypcnow.org/fast-fact-347. Accessed April 5, 2018.
22. Joseph-Williams N, Elwyn G, Edwards A. Knowledge is not power for patients: a systematic review and thematic synthesis of patient-reported barriers and facilitators to shared decision making. Patient Educ Couns 2014;94(3):291–309.
23. Sharot T. The influential mind: what the brain reveals about our power to change others. New York: Henry Holt and Company; 2017.
24. Hurd C, Gibbon L, Back A. Harnessing emotions in decision making. graduate certificate in palliative care. 2016. Available at: http://apps.nursing.uw.edu/grants/palliative-care/emotions/index.html. Accessed October 17, 2018.
25. Ecker B, Ticic R, Hulley L. Unlocking the emotional brain: eliminating symptoms at their roots using memory reconsolidation. London: Routledge; 2012.
26. LeDoux JE. Emotions: a view through the brain. In: Russell RJ, Murphy N, Meyering TC, et al, editors. Neuroscience and the Person: Scientific

perspectives on Divine action. A series on "Scientific Perspectives on Divine Action." Città del Vaticano, vol. 4. Berkeley (CA): University of Notre Dame Press; 2002. p. 101–17.

27. Back A, Arnold R, Tulsky J. Mastering communication with seriously ill patients: balancing honesty with empathy and hope. New York: Cambridge University Press; 2009.
28. Task force on surgical palliative care and the committee on ethics. Statement of principles of palliative care. Bull Am Coll Surg 2005;90(8):34–5.
29. Orgel E, McCarter R, Jacobs S. A failing medical educational model: a self-assessment by physicians at all levels of training of ability and comfort to deliver bad news. J Palliat Med 2010;13(6):677–83.
30. Cooper Z, Meyers M, Keating NL, et al. Resident education and management of end-of-life care: the resident's perspective. J Surg Educ 2010;67(2):79–84.
31. Wancata LM, Hinshaw DB, Suwanabol PA. Palliative care and surgical training: are we being trained to be unprepared? Ann Surg 2017;265(1):32–3.
32. Suwanabol PA, Reichstein AC, Suzer-Gurtekin ZT, et al. Surgeons' perceived barriers to palliative and end-of-life care: a mixed methods study of a surgical society. J Palliat Med 2018. https://doi.org/10.1089/jpm.2017.0470.
33. Levinson W, Hudak P, Tricco AC. A systematic review of surgeon–patient communication: strengths and opportunities for improvement. Patient Educ Couns 2013;93(1):3–17.
34. Soto-Rubio A, Sinclair S. In defense of sympathy, in consideration of empathy, and in praise of compassion: a history of the present. J Pain Symptom Manage 2018;55(5):1428–34.
35. Rogers CR. Empathic: an unappreciated way of being. Couns Psychol 1975; 5(2):2–10.
36. Chochinov HM. Dignity and the essence of medicine: The A, B, C, and D of dignity conserving care. BMJ 2007;335(7612):184–7.
37. Quill TE, Arnold R, Back AL. Discussing treatment preferences with patients who want "everything." Ann Intern Med 2009;151(5):345–9.
38. Shinall MC, Stahl D, Bibler TM. Addressing a patient's hope for a miracle. J Pain Symptom Manage 2018;55(2):535–9.
39. Back A, Arnold R, Edwards K, et al. Family conference. VitalTalk. 2018. Available at: https://www.vitaltalk.org/guides/family-conference/. Accessed January 27, 2019.
40. Bibler TM, Shinall MC Jr, Stahl D. Responding to those who hope for a miracle: practices for clinical bioethicists. Am J Bioeth 2018;18(5):40–51.
41. Widera EW, Rosenfeld KE, Fromme EK, et al. Approaching patients and family members who hope for a miracle. J Pain Symptom Manage 2011;42(1):119–25.
42. Quill TE, Holloway R. Time-limited trials near the end of life. JAMA 2011;306(13): 1483–4.
43. Thoele SP. Inspiring people. Living life fully. Available at: http://www.livinglifefully.com/people/suepattonthoele.htm. Accessed February 2, 2019.
44. Back A, Arnold R, Edwards K, et al. Responding to emotion: respecting. VitalTalk. 2018. Available at: https://www.vitaltalk.org/guides/responding-to-emotion-respecting/. Accessed January 27, 2019.
45. Cooper Z, Koritsanszky LA, Cauley CE, et al. Recommendations for best communication practices to facilitate goal-concordant care for seriously ill older patients with emergency surgical conditions. Ann Surg 2016;263(1):1–6.
46. Groves JE. Taking care of the hateful patient. N Engl J Med 1978;298(16):883–7.

47. Gerhart JI, Varela VS, Burns JW. Brief training on patient anger increases oncology providers' self-efficacy in communicating with angry patients. J Pain Symptom Manage 2017;54(3):355–60.e2.
48. Kitzinger C, Kitzinger J. Grief, anger and despair in relatives of severely brain injured patients: responding without pathologising. Clin Rehabil 2014;28(7): 627–31.
49. Vachon M, Fillion L, Achille M. A conceptual analysis of spirituality at the end of life. J Palliat Med 2009;12(1):53–9.
50. Puchalski CM, Vitillo R, Hull SK, et al. Improving the spiritual dimension of whole person care: reaching national and international consensus. J Palliat Med 2014; 17(6):642–56.
51. Handzo G, Meyerson EM. What are sources of spiritual and existential suffering for patients with advanced disease?. In: Goldstein NE, Morrison RS, editors. Evidence-based practice of palliative medicine: expert consult. Philadelphia: Saunders; 2013. p. 480–3.
52. Jacobs C. Reflection on the role of the spirit in finding meaning and healing as clinicians. J Pain Symptom Manage 2018;55(1):151–4.
53. Sulmasy DP. Spiritual issues in the care of dying patients: " . . . It's okay between me and God." JAMA 2006;296(11):1385–92.
54. Puchalski C, Ferrell B, Virani R, et al. Improving the quality of spiritual care as a dimension of palliative care: the report of the consensus conference. J Palliat Med 2009;12(10):885–904.
55. Discussing spiritual issues— maintaining hope. In: Dunn GP, Martensen R, Weissman D, editors. Surgical palliative care: a resident's guide. Chicago: American College of Surgeons; 2009. p. 241–50.
56. Schultz M, Meged-Book T, Mashiach T, et al. Distinguishing between spiritual distress, general distress, spiritual well-being, and spiritual pain among cancer patients during oncology treatment. J Pain Symptom Manage 2017;54(1):66–73.
57. Cassell EJ. The nature of suffering and the goals of medicine. 2nd edition. New York: Oxford University Press; 2004.
58. Choong KA. Islam and palliative care. Glob Bioeth 2015;26(1):28–42.
59. Upaniṣads. Oxford (United Kingdom): Oxford University Press; 1996.
60. Hanh TN. The heart of the Buddha's teaching: transforming suffering into peace, joy, and liberation. New York: Broadway Books; 1999.
61. Freire E. A conversation with Abraham Joshua Heschel - 1972. Burbank (CA): NBC Studios; 2015. Available at: https://www.youtube.com/watch?v=FEXK9xcRCho. Accessed April 8, 2018.
62. Kierkegaard S. Concluding unscientific postscript. Paperback Edition. Princeton (NJ): Princeton University Press; 1968.
63. Puchalski CM. Spiritual stages of dying. In: Puchalski CM, editor. A time for listening and caring: spirituality and the care of the chronically ill and dying. Oxford (United Kingdom), New York: Oxford University Press; 2006. p. 55–81.
64. Frankl VE. Man's search for meaning. 2006 Paperback Edition. Boston: Beacon Press; 1959.
65. Emanuel LL, Reddy N, Hauser J, et al. "And yet it was a blessing": the case for existential maturity. J Palliat Med 2017;20(4):318–27.
66. Jackson VA, Jacobsen J, Greer JA, et al. The cultivation of prognostic awareness through the provision of early palliative care in the ambulatory setting: a communication guide. J Palliat Med 2013;16(8):894–900.

67. Jacobsen J, Kvale E, Rabow M, et al. Helping patients with serious illness live well through the promotion of adaptive coping: a report from the Improving Outpatient Palliative Care (IPAL-OP) Initiative. J Palliat Med 2014;17(4):463–8.
68. Stefanucci JK, Proffitt DR, Clore GL, et al. Skating down a steeper slope: fear influences the perception of geographical slant. Perception 2008;37(2):321–3.
69. Masel EK, Schur S, Watzke HH. Life is uncertain. Death is certain. Buddhism and palliative care. J Pain Symptom Manage 2012;44(2):307–12.
70. Singh KD. The grace in dying: how we are transformed spiritually as we die. San Francisco (CA): HarperSanFrancisco; 2000.
71. Kézdy A, Martos T, Robu M. God image and attachment to God in work addiction risk. Studia Psychologica 2013;55(3):209–14.
72. Cassell J, Buchman TG, Streat S, et al. Surgeons, intensivists, and the covenant of care: administrative models and values affecting care at the end of life-updated. Crit Care Med 2003;31(5):1551–9.
73. Cooper Z, Courtwright A, Karlage A, et al. Pitfalls in communication that lead to nonbeneficial emergency surgery in elderly patients with serious illness: description of the problem and elements of a solution. Ann Surg 2014;260(6): 949–57.
74. Nabozny MJ, Kruser JM, Steffens NM, et al. Patient-reported limitations to surgical buy-in: a qualitative study of patients facing high-risk surgery. Ann Surg 2017;265(1):97–102.
75. Pecanac KE, Kehler JM, Brasel KJ, et al. It's big surgery: preoperative expressions of risk, responsibility, and commitment to treatment after high-risk operations. Ann Surg 2014;259(3):458–63.
76. Schwarze ML, Redmann AJ, Alexander GC, et al. Surgeons expect patients to buy-in to postoperative life support preoperatively: results of a national survey. Crit Care Med 2013;41(1):1–8.
77. Schwarze ML, Bradley CT, Brasel KJ. Surgical "Buy-In": The contractual relationship between surgeons and patients that influences decisions regarding life-supporting therapy. Crit Care Med 2010;38(3):843–8.
78. Swinton J. Healthcare spirituality: a question of knowledge. In: Cobb M, Puchlaski CM, Rumbold B, editors. Oxford textbook of spirituality in healthcare. Oxford (United Kingdom): Oxford University Press; 2012. p. 99–104.
79. Whipp M. Spirituality and the scientific mind: a dilemma for doctors. In: Cobb M, Robshaw V, editors. The spiritual challenge of health care. Edinburgh (Scotland): Churchill Livingstone; 1998. p. 137–50. New York.
80. Farley E. The fragility of knowledge: hermeneutic paradigms in the enlightenment tradition. In: Fragility of knowledge: theological education in the church and the university. Philadelphia: Fortress Press; 1988. p. 3–16.
81. Chödrön P. Taking the leap: freeing ourselves from old habits and fears. Boston: Shambhala; 2009. London.
82. Puchalski CM, Ferrell B. Making health care whole: integrating spirituality into patient care. West Conshohocken (PA): Templeton Press; 2010.
83. Mako C, Galek K, Poppito SR. Spiritual pain among patients with advanced cancer in palliative care. J Palliat Med 2006;9(5):1106–13.
84. McNichols KZ, Feldman DB. Spirituality at the end of life: issues and guidelines for care. In: Plante TG, Thoresen CE, editors. Spirit, science, and health: how the spiritual mind fuels physical wellness. Westport (CT): Praeger Publishers; 2007. p. 191–203.
85. Balboni TA, Balboni MJ. The spiritual event of serious illness. J Pain Symptom Manage 2018;56(5):816–22.

86. Balboni TA, Balboni MJ. Religion and spirituality in palliative medicine. In: Balboni MJ, Peteet JR, editors. Spirituality and religion within the culture of medicine: from evidence to practice. New York: Oxford University Press; 2017. p. 147–64.
87. Puchalski CM, editor. A time for listening and caring: spirituality and the care of the chronically ill and dying. Oxford (United Kingdom), New York: Oxford University Press; 2006.
88. Pellegrini CA. Trust: the keystone of the patient-physician relationship. J Am Coll Surg 2017;224(2):95–102.
89. Cooper RS. The palliative care chaplain as story catcher. J Pain Symptom Manage 2018;55(1):155–8.
90. Kestenbaum A, Shields M, James J, et al. What impact do chaplains have? A pilot study of spiritual AIM for advanced cancer patients in outpatient palliative care. J Pain Symptom Manage 2017;54(5):707–14.
91. Bay PS, Beckman D, Trippi J, et al. The effect of pastoral care services on anxiety, depression, hope, religious coping, and religious problem solving styles: a randomized controlled study. J Relig Health 2008;47(1):57–69.
92. Piderman KM, Breitkopf CR, Jenkins SM, et al. The impact of a spiritual legacy intervention in patients with brain cancers and other neurologic illnesses and their support persons. Psychooncology 2017;26(3):346–53.
93. Flannelly KJ, Emanuel LL, Handzo GF, et al. A national study of chaplaincy services and end-of-life outcomes. BMC Palliat Care 2012;11(1):10.
94. Vuksanovic D, Green HJ, Dyck M, et al. Dignity therapy and life review for palliative care patients: a randomized controlled trial. J Pain Symptom Manage 2017;53(2):162–70.e1.
95. Kissane DW, Treece C, Breithart W, et al. Dignity, meaning, and demoralization: emerging paradigms in end-of-life care. In: Chochinov HM, Breitbart W, editors. Handbook of psychiatry in palliative medicine. Second Edition. Oxford (United Kingdom): Oxford University Press; 2009. p. 324–40.
96. Hall EJ, Hughes BP, Handzo GH. Spiritual care: what it means, why it matters in health care 2016. Available at: https://www.healthcarechaplaincy.org/docs/about/spirituality.pdf. Accessed August 15, 2018.
97. Millspaugh D. Assessment and response to spiritual pain: part I. J Palliat Med 2005;8(5):919–23.
98. Millspaugh D. Assessment and response to spiritual pain: part II. J Palliat Med 2005;8(6):1110–7.
99. Cadge W, Freese J, Christakis NA. The provision of hospital chaplaincy in the United States: a national overview. South Med J 2008;101(6):626–30.
100. Balboni MJ, Sullivan A, Enzinger AC, et al. Nurse and physician barriers to spiritual care provision at the end of life. J Pain Symptom Manage 2014;48(3):400–10.
101. Berlin A, Kunac A, Mosenthal AC. Perioperative goal-setting consultations by surgical colleagues: a new model for supporting patients, families, and surgeons in shared decision making. Ann Palliat Med 2017;6(2):178–82.
102. Edwards A, Pang N, Shiu V, et al. The understanding of spirituality and the potential role of spiritual care in end-of-life and palliative care: a meta-study of qualitative research. Palliat Med 2010;24(8):753–70.
103. Karlekar M, Collier B, Parish A, et al. Utilization and determinants of palliative care in the trauma intensive care unit: results of a national survey. Palliat Med 2014;28(8):1062–8.

104. Taylor LJ, Johnson SK, Nabozny MJ, et al. Barriers to goal-concordant care for older patients with acute surgical illness: communication patterns extrinsic to decision aids. Ann Surg 2017. https://doi.org/10.1097/SLA.0000000000002282.
105. Roze des Ordons AL, Sinuff T, Stelfox HT, et al. Spiritual distress within inpatient settings—a scoping review of patients' and families' experiences. J Pain Symptom Manage 2018;56(1):122–45.
106. Nolan S. Spiritual care at the end of life: the chaplain as a 'hopeful presence'. London: Jessica Kingsley Publishers; 2011. Philadelphia.
107. Balboni TA, Fitchett G, Handzo GF, et al. State of the science of spirituality and palliative care research part II: screening, assessment, and interventions. J Pain Symptom Manage 2017;54(3):441–53.
108. Ahluwalia SC, Chen C, Raaen L, et al. A systematic review in support of the national consensus project clinical practice guidelines for quality palliative care, fourth edition. J Pain Symptom Manage 2018;56(6):831–70.
109. National coalition for hospice and palliative care. Clinical practice guidelines for quality palliative care. 4th edition. Available at: https://www.nationalcoalitionhpc.org/ncp. Accessed January 13, 2019.
110. Morse DS, Edwardsen EA, Gordon HS. Missed opportunities for interval empathy in lung cancer communication. Arch Intern Med 2008;168(17):1853–8.
111. Smyre CL, Tak HJ, Dang AP, et al. Physicians' opinions on engaging patients' religious and spiritual concerns: a national survey. J Pain Symptom Manage 2018;55(3):897–905.
112. Bayer–Fetzer conference on physician–patient communication in medical education participants, May 1999. Essential elements of communication in medical encounters: the Kalamazoo consensus statement. Acad Med 2001;76(4):390–3.
113. Block SD. Psychological considerations, growth, and transcendence at the end of life: the art of the possible. JAMA 2001;285(22):2898–905.
114. Sulmasy DP. Ethos, mythos, and thanatos: spirituality and ethics at the end of life. J Pain Symptom Manage 2013;46(3):447–51.
115. Puchalski C, Romer AL. Taking a spiritual history allows clinicians to understand patients more fully. J Palliat Med 2000;3(1):129–37.
116. Anandarajah G, Hight E. Spirituality and medical practice: using the HOPE questions as a practical tool for spiritual assessment. Am Fam Physician 2001;63(1):81–8.
117. Hodge DR. Spiritual assessment in social work and mental health practice. New York: Columbia University Press; 2015.
118. Maugans TA. The SPIRITual history. Arch Fam Med 1996;5(1):11–6.
119. Commission on cancer. Cancer program standards: ensuring patient-centered care 2016. Available at: https://www.facs.org/quality-programs/cancer/coc/standards. Accessed February 10, 2019.
120. King SDW, Fitchett G, Murphy PE, et al. Determining best methods to screen for religious/spiritual distress. Support Care Cancer 2017;25(2):471–9.
121. Lo B, Ruston D, Kates LW, et al. Discussing religious and spiritual issues at the end of life: a practical guide for physicians. JAMA 2002;287(6):749–54.
122. Pargament KI. The psychology of religion and coping: theory, research, practice. New York: The Guilford Press; 1997.
123. Ano GG, Vasconcelles EB. Religious coping and psychological adjustment to stress: a meta-analysis. J Clin Psychol 2005;61(4):461–80.
124. López-Sierra HE, Rodríguez-Sánchez J. The supportive roles of religion and spirituality in end-of-life and palliative care of patients with cancer in a culturally

diverse context: a literature review. Curr Opin Support Palliat Care 2015;9(1): 87–95.

125. Vallurupalli M, Lauderdale K, Balboni MJ, et al. The role of spirituality and religious coping in the quality of life of patients with advanced cancer receiving palliative radiation therapy. J Support Oncol 2012;10(2):81–7.
126. Woll ML, Hinshaw DB, Pawlik TM. Spirituality and religion in the care of surgical oncology patients with life-threatening or advanced illnesses. Ann Surg Oncol 2008;15(11):3048–57.
127. Farran CJ, Herth KA, Popovich JM. Hope and hopelessness: critical clinical constructs. Thousand Oaks (CA): SAGE Publications; 1995.
128. Leget C. Art of living, art of dying: spiritual care for a good death. London: Jessica Kingsley Publishers; 2017. Philadelphia.
129. Pargament KI, Smith BW, Koenig HG, et al. Patterns of positive and negative religious coping with major life stressors. Journal for the Scientific Study of Religion 1998;37(4):710–24.
130. Puchalski CM. Spiritual care: compassionate service to others. In: Puchalski CM, editor. A time for listening and caring: spirituality and the care of the chronically ill and dying. Oxford (United Kingdom), New York: Oxford University Press; 2006. p. 39–51.
131. Singh KD. The psychospiritual stages of dying. In: The grace in dying: how we are transformed spiritually as we die. San Francisco (CA): HarperSanFrancisco; 2000. p. 167–214.
132. Hagerty RG, Butow PN, Ellis PM, et al. Communicating with realism and hope: incurable cancer patients' views on the disclosure of prognosis. J Clin Oncol 2005;23(6):1278–88.
133. Whittaker R, Bansal P. On hopelessness and hope: a conversation with deep psychologist Michael Penn. Parabola: The Search for Meaning 2018;43(4): 88–94.
134. Maiko S, Johns SA, Helft PR, et al. Spiritual experiences of adults with advanced cancer in outpatient clinical settings. J Pain Symptom Manage 2019;57(3): 576–86.e1.
135. Grech A, Marks A. Existential suffering part 1: definition and diagnosis #319. J Palliat Med 2016;20(1):93–4.
136. Grech A, Marks A. Existential suffering part 2: clinical response and management #320. J Palliat Med 2016;20(1):95–6.
137. Saunders CM. Spiritual pain. J Palliat Care 1988;4(3):29–32.
138. Back AL, Anderson WG, Bunch L, et al. Communication about cancer near the end of life. Cancer 2008;113(7 Suppl):1897–910.
139. Peteet JR, Balboni MJ, D'Ambra MN. Approaching spirituality in clinical practice. In: Peteet JR, D'Ambra MN, editors. The soul of medicine: spiritual perspectives and clinical practice. Baltimore (MD): Johns Hopkins University Press; 2011. p. 23–44.
140. Anandarajah G. The 3 H and BMSEST models for spirituality in multicultural whole-person medicine. Ann Fam Med 2008;6(5):448–58.
141. Engel JD, Pethtel L, Zarconi J. Caring for patients at the end of life: honoring the patient's story. In: Puchalski CM, editor. A time for listening and caring: spirituality and the care of the chronically ill and dying. Oxford (United Kingdom), New York: Oxford University Press; 2006. p. 253–68.
142. Corr CA. A task-based approach to coping with dying. OMEGA - Journal of Death and Dying 1992;24(2):81–94.

143. Snyder CR, Rand KL, Sigmon DR. Hope theory: a member of the positive psychology family. In: Gallagher MW, Lopez SJ, editors. The Oxford handbook of hope. New York: Oxford Library of Psychology; 2018. p. 27–43. Oxford University Press.
144. Rand KL, Cheavens JS. Hope theory. In: Lopez SJ, Snyder CR, editors. The Oxford handbook of positive psychology. 2nd Edition. Oxford: Oxford University Press; 2009. p. 323–33. New York.
145. Kruser JM, Cox CE, Schwarze ML. Clinical momentum in the intensive care unit. A latent contributor to unwanted care. Ann Am Thorac Soc 2017;14(3):426–31.
146. Berlin A. Goals of care and end of life in the ICU. Surg Clin North Am 2017;97(6): 1275–90.
147. Duggleby WD, Williams AM. Living with hope: developing a psychosocial supportive program for rural women caregivers of persons with advanced cancer. BMC Palliat Care 2010;9(1):3.
148. Utne I, Miaskowski C, Bjordal K, et al. The relationship between hope and pain in a sample of hospitalized oncology patients. Palliat Support Care 2008;6(4): 327–34.
149. Berendes D, Keefe FJ, Somers TJ, et al. Hope in the context of lung cancer: relationships of hope to symptoms and psychological distress. J Pain Symptom Manage 2010;40(2):174–82.
150. Scheier MF, Matthews KA, Owens JF, et al. Dispositional optimism and recovery from coronary artery bypass surgery: the beneficial effects on physical and psychological well-being. J Pers Soc Psychol 1989;57(6):1024–40.
151. Clayton JM, Hancock K, Parker S, et al. Sustaining hope when communicating with terminally ill patients and their families: a systematic review. Psycho-Oncology 2008;17(7):641–59.
152. Fromm E. The revolution of hope: toward a humanized technology. New York: Harper & Row; 1968.
153. Oettingen G, Chromik MP. How Hope influences goal-directed behavior. In: Gallagher MW, Lopez SJ, editors. The Oxford handbook of hope. New York: Oxford Library of Psychology. Oxford University Press; 2018. p. 69–79.
154. Feldman DB, Snyder CR. Hope and the meaningful life: theoretical and empirical associations between goal-directed thinking and life meaning. J Social Clin Psychol 2005;24(3):401–21.
155. Maddux JE. Self-efficacy: the power of believing you can. In: Lopez SJ, Snyder CR, editors. The Oxford handbook of positive psychology. 2nd Edition. Oxford (United Kingdom): Oxford University Press; 2009. p. 335–43.
156. Bradshaw M, Ellison CG, Marcum JP. Attachment to God, images of God, and psychological distress in a nationwide sample of Presbyterians. Int J Psychol Religion 2010;20(2):130–47.
157. Davis EB, Moriarty GL, Mauch JC. God images and God concepts: definitions, development, and dynamics. Psychology of Religion and Spirituality 2013;5(1): 51–60.
158. Hoffman L. Cultural constructs of the God image and God concept: implications for culture, psychology, and religion. Presented at the Annual Meeting of the Society for the Scientific Study of Religion. Kansas City, MO, October 2005. https://doi.org/10.13140/RG.2.1.2498.2480.
159. van Laarhoven HWM, Schilderman J, Vissers KC, et al. Images of God in relation to coping strategies of palliative cancer patients. J Pain Symptom Manage 2010;40(4):495–501.
160. Moriarty GL, Hoffman L, Grimes C. Understanding the God image through attachment theory. J Spiritual Ment Health 2006;9(2):43–56.

161. Rizzuto A-M. Object relations and the formation of the image of God. Br J Med Psychol 1974;47(1):83–99.
162. Duggleby W, Hicks D, Nekolaichuk C, et al. Hope, older adults, and chronic illness: a metasynthesis of qualitative research. J Adv Nurs 2012;68(6):1211–23.
163. Abernathy CM, Hamm RM. Surgical intuition: what it is and how to get it. Philadelphia: Hanley & Belfus; 1995.
164. Korn ER, Johnson K. The uses of imagery in surgery and with surgical patients. In: Visualization: the uses of imagery in the health professions. Goshen (VA): Transpersonal Publishing; 2005. p. 185–96.
165. McDonald J, Orlick T, Letts M. Mental readiness in surgeons and its links to performance excellence in surgery. J Pediatr Orthop 1995;15(5):691–7.
166. Csikszentmihalyi M. Creativity: flow and the psychology of discovery and invention. New York: HarperCollins Publishers; 1996.
167. Wiley J. Expertise as mental set: the effects of domain knowledge in creative problem solving. Mem Cognit 1998;26(4):716–30.
168. Schulman-Green D, Smith CB, Lin JJ, et al. Oncologists' and patients' perceptions of initial, intermediate, and final goals of care conversations. J Pain Symptom Manage 2018;55(3):890–6.
169. Eliott JA, Olver IN. Hope and hoping in the talk of dying cancer patients. Soc Sci Med 2007;64(1):138–49.
170. Dufault K, Martocchio BC. Symposium on compassionate care and the dying experience. Hope: its spheres and dimensions. Nurs Clin North Am 1985; 20(2):379–91.
171. Mirhosseini M, Fainsinger R. Parenteral nutrition in patients with advanced cancer #190. J Palliat Med 2009;12(3):260–1.
172. Cass-Garcia M, Hodul PJ, Almhanna K. Use of total parenteral nutrition (TPN) in terminally ill gastrointestinal (GI) cancer patients (pts) compared to other malignancies (OM): a single-institution experience. JCO 2013;31(4 suppl):309.
173. Mitchell J, Jatoi A. Parenteral nutrition in patients with advanced cancer: merging perspectives from the patient and healthcare provider. Semin Oncol 2011; 38(3):439–42.
174. Virizuela JA, Camblor-Álvarez M, Luengo-Pérez LM, et al. Nutritional support and parenteral nutrition in cancer patients: an expert consensus report. Clin Transl Oncol 2018;20(5):619–29.
175. Cotogni P. Enteral versus parenteral nutrition in cancer patients: evidences and controversies. Ann Palliat Med 2016;5(1):42–9.
176. Pernar LIM, Peyre SE, Smink DS, et al. Feasibility and impact of a case-based palliative care workshop for general surgery residents. J Am Coll Surg 2012; 214(2):231–6.
177. Parker-Oliver D. Redefining hope for the terminally ill. Am J Hosp Palliat Care 2002;19(2):115–20.
178. Schwartz B. The paradox of choice. In: Joseph S, editor. Positive psychology in practice: promoting human flourishing in work, health, education, and everyday life. 2nd edition. Hoboken (NJ): Wiley; 2015. p. 121–38.
179. Speerstra K, Anderson H. Decisions, decisions, decisions. In: The Divine art of dying: how to live well while dying. 1st edition. Studio City (CA): Divine Arts; 2014. p. 29–40.
180. How to talk end-of-life care with a dying patient - Atul Gawande. New York: FORA.tv; 2010. Available at: https://www.youtube.com/watch?v=45b2QZxDd_o. Accessed January 29, 2019.

181. Jacobsen J, Blinderman C, Cole CA, Jackson V. "I'd recommend ..." how to incorporate your recommendation into shared decision making for patients with serious illness. J Pain Symptom Manage 2018;55(4):1224–30.
182. Roeland E, Cain J, Onderdonk C, et al. When open-ended questions don't work: the role of palliative paternalism in difficult medical decisions. J Palliat Med 2014;17(4):415–20.
183. Halifax J. Being with dying: cultivating compassion and fearlessness in the presence of death. Boston: Shambhala; 2009.
184. Quill TE, Arnold RM, Platt F. "I wish things were different": expressing wishes in response to loss, futility, and unrealistic hopes. Ann Intern Med 2001;135(7): 551–5.
185. Miner TJ. Communication skills in palliative surgery: skill and effort are key. Surg Clin North Am 2011;91(2):355–66. Dunn GP, ed. Update on surgical palliative care.
186. Schroeder J, Fishbach A. The 'empty vessel' physician: physicians' instrumentality makes them seem personally empty. Soc Psychol Personal Sci 2015;6(8): 940–9.
187. Halifax J. Falling over the edge of integrity: moral suffering. In: Standing at the edge: finding freedom where fear and courage meet. New York: Flatiron Books; 2018. p. 101–17.
188. Nuland SB. A Surgeon's reflections on the care of the dying. Surg Oncol Clin N Am 2001;10(1):1–5.
189. Sulmasy DP. A biopsychosocial-spiritual model for the care of patients at the end of life. Gerontologist 2002;42(Special III):24–33.
190. Patton JF. Jungian spirituality: a developmental context for late-life growth. Am J Hosp Palliat Care 2006;23(4):304–8.
191. Delgado-Guay MO. Spirituality and religiosity in supportive and palliative care. Curr Opin Support Palliat Care 2014;8(3):308–13.
192. Kübler-Ross E. On death and dying. Paperback. New York: MacMillan Publishing Co; 1969.
193. Charon R. Narrative medicine: a model for empathy, reflection, profession, and trust. JAMA 2001;286(15):1897–902.
194. Charon R. Narrative medicine: honoring the stories of illness. Oxford: Oxford University Press; 2006. New York.
195. Teske JA. Knowing ourselves by telling stories to ourselves. Zygon 2017;52(3): 880–902.
196. Irwin SA, Fairman N, Montross L. Alleviating psychological and spiritual pain. 4th Edition. Glenview (IL): American Academy of Hospice and Palliative Medicine; 2013.
197. Byock IR. The nature of suffering and the nature of opportunity at the end of life. Clin Geriatr Med 1996;12(2):237–52.
198. Byock I. Dying well: peace and possibilities at the end of life. New York: Riverhead Books; 1998.
199. Canadian Virtual Hospice. The 4 things that matter most. Canada; Available at: https://www.youtube.com/watch?v=vcMmx-6RIUY. Accessed January 1, 2019.
200. Carlin N, Cole T, Strobel H. Guidance from the humanities for professional formation. In: Cobb M, Puchlaski CM, Rumbold B, editors. Oxford textbook of spirituality in healthcare. Oxford (United Kingdom): Oxford University Press; 2012. p. 443–9.

201. Gardner F. Training and formation: a case study. In: Cobb M, Puchlaski CM, Rumbold B, editors. Oxford textbook of spirituality in healthcare. Oxford (United Kingdom): Oxford University Press; 2012. p. 451–7.
202. Puchalski CM, Guenther M. Restoration and Re-creation: spirituality in the lives of healthcare professionals. Curr Opin Support Palliat Care 2012;6(2):254–8.
203. Byock I. The meaning and value of death. J Palliat Med 2002;5(2):279–88.
204. Chödrön P. When things fall apart: heart advice for difficult times. 20th Anniversary Edition. Boulder (CO): Shambhala; 2016.
205. Tagore R. The king of the dark chamber. New York: Drama League of America; MacMillan Company; 1914.

Transitioning to Comfort-Focused Care at the End of Life

Christine C. Toevs, MD, MA (Bioethics)[a,b,*]

KEYWORDS

- Surgical buy-in • Goals of care • Advanced directives • Advance care planning
- Surrogate decision makers • Comfort measures • Symptom management
- End-of-life decision making

KEY POINTS

- Basic end-of life care is within the scope of surgical practice.
- Framework for goals of care should be presented preoperatively with best-case/worst-case discussions, especially in the context of emergency surgery or high-risk elective surgical cases.
- Do not resuscitate does not mean do not treat. Palliation and comfort-focused care are valuable and necessary forms of treatment of patients with serious life-limiting illness and at the end of life.
- Symptom management is a critical component of end-of life care.

INTRODUCTION

Surgeons spend their careers taking care of complex surgical problems with high risk that have the potential to improve patient quality of life. Regrettably, patients do not always do well and the goal of improved quality of life through surgical palliation is not always achieved. Sometimes surgical complications arise, and patients fail to recover, or their disease progresses and the reality of cure changes, necessitating transparent communication. Ideally, surgeons address end-of-life issues as potentialities over the continuum of care within the framework of the surgeon-patient relationship, rather than during a crisis when all treatment options have been exhausted. This article helps surgeons with the components of transitioning to comfort-focused care at the end of life, beginning with preoperative preparation and by encouraging ongoing goals of care discussions thereafter.

Disclosures: None.
[a] Terre Haute Regional Hospital, 3901 South 7th Street, Terre Haute, IN 47802, USA; [b] Indiana University School of Medicine, Terre Haute, IN, USA
* Terre Haute Regional Hospital, 3901 South 7th Street, Terre Haute, IN 47802.
E-mail address: ctoevs@pghphysician.com

Surg Clin N Am 99 (2019) 1019–1027
https://doi.org/10.1016/j.suc.2019.06.014

BEFORE THE OPERATION

Surgical decision making involves recognizing a surgical problem, determining the indicated surgical treatment, and planning for surgical intervention. Whether this process is completed over time in a controlled elective outpatient setting or in the chaos of an acute hospitalization, the steps are the same. Surgeons tend to focus on the technical aspects of surgery rather than on the complexity of the perioperative period for patients and their loved ones. Patients are often ill-informed about the time and effort involved to achieve optimal recovery from their surgical procedures. The literature discusses this process as surgical buy-in. Patients need to be educated and understand what it means to have a surgical intervention in the context of their current condition and desired quality of life; being informed about the operative risks, benefits, and alternatives is not enough for informed decision making. For some patients, preoperative preparation and postoperative recovery may be extensive and more than the patient is willing to endure. For example, the postoperative recovery period may require an intensive care unit (ICU) stay, prolonged mechanical ventilation, education and teaching about how to care for a stoma, renal replacement therapy, or recovery away from home in a rehabilitation center or skilled nursing facility.[1,2] All of these challenges, when disclosed, might change a patient's desire to embark on the intended procedure. Discussions that address perioperative expectations before surgical intervention can help prevent the crisis that occurs when a family requests withdrawal of life-sustaining medical therapy, because they did not realize their loved one would require a ventilator postoperatively.[3]

ADVANCED DIRECTIVES AND GOALS OF CARE

In an ideal world, patients would be clear about their goals of care; have advance directives completed; and share their preferences, goals, and values with their surrogate decision makers. This clarity would help facilitate patient-concordant care when decisions need to be made during an acute change in a patient's clinical condition or at the end of life. It often takes the prompting of the surgeon and treatment team during perioperative planning for patients to express their wishes. Many surgical procedures, from elective to emergent, would benefit from the best-case/worst-case framework for discussion.[4,5] The goal being to decrease "unwanted burdensome treatments near the end of life," and to "create boundaries around what is possible."[5] In the best-case scenario, discussions about the surgical procedure, postoperative course, expectations for functional recovery, discharge destination, and common complications would all occur before surgery, rather than at the time of a crisis. Surgeons have a professional responsibility to inform patients and their families about reasonable expectations for recovery and expected outcomes, especially because popular media sources tend to distort the successes of medical intervention (ie, 66% short-term survival and 87% long-term survival with in-hospital cardiopulmonary resuscitation on television).[6] In a culture that glorifies autonomy and patient preferences, clinicians tend to defer all decision making to the patients. However, patient autonomy is not irrefutable, because surgeons also have autonomy.[7–9] Surgeons have a professional responsibility to help guide patients through shared decision making, including making patient-centric recommendations.[7–9]

THE DECISION TO FORGO FURTHER TREATMENTS

The decision to forgo further treatments and interventions can take many forms, from no chemotherapy or dialysis to withdrawal of mechanical ventilation. Critically ill patients may refuse life-extending surgery, resulting in a transition to end-of-life care, the implementation of which is usually not managed by surgeons. Postoperative patients may refuse further surgery or interventions, especially if they have a complication (failure to rescue).[10,11] For some patients, the limitation of further intervention may be in changing their code status to a do-not-attempt-resuscitation (DNR) order, which can be misunderstood as a do-not-treat order.[12] From a medical, legal, and ethical standpoint, the decision to withhold treatment is the same as the decision to withdraw treatment, although withholding is perceived as easier than withdrawing therapy once it has begun.[13] The decision not to intervene further, whether through refusal of interventions or by withdrawal of care that could be curative, can be distressing for a surgeons.[14]

WITHDRAWAL OF LIFE-SUSTAINING MEDICAL TREATMENT IN THE INTENSIVE CARE UNIT

Once the patient/family has decided to transition to comfort-focused care, the goal of treatment should be focused on patient comfort and family support through the patient's dying process. All nonbeneficial treatment that does not confer comfort should be discontinued. The patient may have a faith-based or spiritual tradition, which should provoke the support of spiritual services. Most deaths in the ICU are preceded by either deescalating care or deciding not to escalate care, as in initiating a DNR order.[15,16] Administering opioids is often indicated at the end of life for treatment of pain and dyspnea. When death is imminent from the patient's medical condition, administering opioids for symptom management should not be construed as the cause of death.[17] If the care plan becomes a compassionate extubation, it is likely that the hospital already has a protocol in place; if not, there are many available online.[18] If the patient is on paralytics, those should be discontinued before withdrawing ventilatory support, metabolically clearing the patient, and a train-of-four with recovery of 4 twitches or clinical assessment of extremity movement confirmed before proceeding. Opioids and sedatives are often administered following serial assessments based on need, and route, frequency, and doses are variable and titrated to meet the individual needs of each patient. In general, the mantra used for the administration of opioids is to start low and go slow; however, as is the case with many hospitalized patients, they are not opioid naive and already have been exposed to opioids and some sedatives. Escalation of pharmaceuticals occurs if a patient's symptoms no longer respond appropriately to existing doses. Sometimes frequent intermittent doses are changed to continuous infusions to ensure patient comfort during the compassionate extubation process. Continuous opioid and/or sedative infusions may be appropriate to continue if that is where the patient is starting out and seems comfortable or the patient's symptoms do not respond to frequent intermittent doses. Using opioid/sedative infusions should not be predicated on time to death but on optimal symptom management. If the patient does not die shortly after withdrawal of life-sustaining medical treatment (LSMT), transfer to the medical/surgical ward, dedicated palliative unit, or affiliated general inpatient hospice unit (GIP) for ongoing comfort-focused care may be preferable. Patient visitation is often restricted in hospital ICUs, whereas it is not in most hospice units; this is an important consideration because greater family time with larger families may be a priority for some dying patients. Intubated patients can also be transferred to the associated GIP for compassionate extubation if this is desired by the decision maker and there is bed availability. Besides more liberal visitation parameters before compassionate extubation, the GIP staff are specifically trained and practice under the expectations of helping people die peacefully, which is a practice divergence for ICU nurses who more commonly are trained to assist in life prolongation. These practice competency differences can affect the end-of-life care delivered in the ICU versus the GIP setting. For ICU nurses who have been caring for the surgical patient for a prolonged period of time and who may have bonded with the patient and the family, consider informing them of the planned withdrawal of LSMT and inviting them to be present, especially when requested by the patient and/or family. Debriefing with all the members of the treatment team after a compassionate extubation may be helpful to guard against moral distress or any residual conflicts that may be present among the treatment team members.[19,20]

COMFORT MEASURES OUTSIDE OF THE INTENSIVE CARE UNIT

If the patient is on the medical/surgical ward and the plan of care has changed from restoration of health to comfort-focused care, there are steps to be taken. Often these decisions happen within the broader context of goals-of-care discussions, but the patient may decide on no further surgery/interventions. Should the patient decide on no further surgery when it could potentially be lifesaving, some understanding of prognosis helps guide the discussion and logistics of end-of-life care. Prognostic tools such as the Palliative Performance Scale, Palliative Prognostic Score, and Palliative Prognostic Index are designed for use in patients with cancer, but can be applied to other clinical conditions. As a general rule, physicians tend to overestimate survival and functional outcomes of patients, giving patients and families little time to prepare for and address pressing matters before death.[21]

Too often, end-of-life care is presented as a menu for patients to choose each and every intervention (eg, intubation, chest compressions, tube feedings, antibiotics). Patients and families may find themselves presented with decisions when realistically they are not choices; for example, a discussion of code status and chest compressions in a patient with uncontrolled hemorrhage.[22–24] Instead, a goals-of-care discussion about the patient's understanding of the disease, prognosis, how the patient wants to spend the remaining time, and what the patient is willing to undergo for more time (eg, intubation, prolonged ICU time, procedures, surgeries) is critical for shared decision making to occur.[25] Surgeons should give patients recommendations about options that align with the patient's stated goals and preferences.[22] Again, too often clinicians present all options as equivalent when in reality they are not, and some options do not support patient-concordant care. Surgeon autonomy also plays a role in these discussions.[7–9] Surgeons should determine whether a surgical intervention is indicated in the context of the patient's preferred care plan, as well as assessing technical feasibility and whether the benefit outweighs the harm. Surgeons determine the availability of resources. The surgeon in discussion with the patient through shared decision making determines whether the desired outcome by the patient is even a possibility.[9]

WHEN TO CALL PALLIATIVE MEDICINE

Patients and physicians still confuse palliative medicine with hospice. The goal of palliative medicine is to support patients and their families during serious life-limiting illness. Palliative medicine can be concurrent with disease-directed therapy to optimize symptom management and adhere to a plan of care that remains patient-concordant. Palliative medicine providers often discuss goals of care, including preferences for care at the end of life, to enhance patient understanding of options, elicit patient engagement, and promote multidisciplinary care coordination while optimizing symptom management. The palliative care team often consists of a physician, nurse practitioner and/or physician assistant (advance practice provider), social worker, and chaplain who provide interdisciplinary comprehensive whole-person care. Surgeons should have basic palliative care skills, including the ability to lead a goals-of-care discussion, and provide basic symptom management, and surgeons should integrate these skills into everyday practice.[26] Palliative medicine can help with more complex decision making, conflict among decision makers, uncontrolled refractory symptoms, and ongoing needs in an inpatient and outpatient setting.

Hospice is a Medicare benefit that is designed to support patients and their loved ones with a life expectancy of 6 months or less. Hospice care is provided by an interdisciplinary team composed of a physician, nurse practitioner, nurse, social worker, and chaplain. One way to determine whether a patient is eligible for hospice care is by asking the so-called surprise question: "Would you be surprised if this patient was alive in 6 months?"[27] If the answer is yes, then it is appropriate to discuss the benefits of hospice care with patients and their loved ones. Hospice can be provided in a patient's home or another residential community setting with the frequency of provider visits tailored to the individual needs of the patient. Patients and families often think that home hospice will provide 24/7 nursing care, which should be clarified in hospice discussions to set accurate expectations of the hospice benefit. Admission criteria for GIP include refractory symptoms, complex hospital discharges when a patient is transitioning to hospice care, and respite when a patient lives at home and the caregiver needs a break.

SYMPTOM MANAGEMENT

Patients often have many symptoms at the end of life that need therapeutic intervention. If surgeons are to provide basic palliative care for their patients, an understanding of treatment options is important. An evidence-based multimodal approach to pain management should be considered that includes both nonpharmacologic and pharmacologic therapies. For considering initiation of pharmacotherapy, the World Health Organization (WHO) pain relief ladder for analgesia is an accepted standard to follow. Dosing and route of administration are dictated by patient metabolic limitations, capability, and access. Routes of administration include sublingual, oral dissolving tablet, rectal, subcutaneous, transdermal, and intravenous. In certain cases, consulting anesthesia pain specialists or interventional radiologists for nerve blocks, epidural, and intrathecal catheters may be the best way to palliate a patient's pain.[26]

All patients receiving opioids should receive preventive treatment to reduce the risk of opioid-induced constipation (OIC).[26] Constipation can be distressing and painful for patients and their caregivers. With every opioid prescription/order there should be a concurrent bowel program recommended commensurate with the patient's needs and ability to comply. As patients become less mobile and take in less oral hydration and nutrition, OIC becomes a significant problem. Therefore, an aggressive bowel regimen is critical to the care of palliative or hospice patients on opioids.

Dyspnea can occur during compassionate extubations or in any patient at the end of life regardless of primary or secondary pulmonary disease. Protocols for compassionate extubations include premedication and ongoing treatment with opioids and sedatives. Nonpharmacologic therapy using an electric fan has proved beneficial and, for some patients with dyspnea, oxygen is also therapeutic. Opioids are an evidence-based standard for the treatment of dyspnea with the goal of decreasing air hunger and increasing comfort and function without hastening death.[26]

ARTIFICIAL NUTRITION AND HYDRATION

Artificial nutrition and hydration are considered medical therapies and can be refused or withdrawn. Anorexia, fatigue, and weight loss are common during the terminal phase of disease. For awake and interested patients at the end of life, the best option for nutrition and hydrations is pleasure drinking and eating. In patients who cannot hold a drink or feed themselves, hand feeding and assistance with liquids are encouraged via sipping, sucking, or with sponges to keep the mouth moist. Families appreciate participating in providing hydration and nourishment for their loved ones. The experience can be pleasurable for all involved. Families may be reluctant to stop artificial hydration and nutrition because of concerns for dehydration and starvation. However, at the end of life, the body usually shuts down and cannot reasonably negotiate oral intake, tube feeding, or intravenous infusions. Patients become bloated, constipated, edematous, dyspneic, and have increased oropharyngeal secretions, increasing their discomfort.[28] Refocusing the family's attention to comfort at the end of life is a critical component of the ongoing end-of-life discussion.

MALIGNANT BOWEL OBSTRUCTION

High-grade malignant bowel obstruction is a common consult for surgeons, and a poor prognostic indicator for patients. Although about half the time patients have potentially treatable adhesions, rather than cancer causing the obstruction, these patients do very poorly with surgical intervention and often spend the rest of their lives recovering from surgery in the hospital, skilled nursing facility, or nursing home with or without significant postoperative complications.[29] Rather than offering major intestinal surgery, a variety of medical interventions have been shown to improve symptoms and allow patients to enjoy some limited amount of oral intake (glucocorticoids, antiemetic agents, analgesics, and antisecretory agents, including anticholinergic drugs, somatostatin analogues, and proton-pump inhibitors.)[30] If pharmacotherapy is not effective in palliating obstructive symptoms, inserting a venting gastrostomy for decompression instead of maintaining a nasogastric tube (NGT) is an indicated palliative intervention that can often be achieved endoscopically or with image guidance. It rare for patients' quality of life not to be impaired by living with an NGT. Surgically placed gastrostomies should be avoided at the end of life. Percutaneous transesophageal gastrotubing is another option at some centers when traditional endoscopic or interventional approaches are technically unsafe.

DEACTIVATION OF CARDIAC DEVICES

Because more and more patients are living longer with cardiac disease, the use of implantable cardiac devices has increased. These devices include implantable cardioverter-defibrillators (ICDs), pacemakers, and left ventricular assist devices (LVADs). Ideally, deactivation of these devices is discussed at time of implantation. Patients have the option of requesting deactivation of their ICDs at the end of life, to prevent unwanted electrical shocks. LVADs are perceived as ethically more difficult to deactivate because this usually results in imminent death. In these situations, a cardiologist can facilitate the deactivation[31,32] and palliative medicine should be comanaging to ensure symptoms are managed before circulatory failure ensues. It is important to recognize that, once the LVAD is deactivated, subsequently infused medications may not be circulated effectively and therefore may fail to achieve the desired therapeutic benefit.[31,32]

RECOGNIZING IMPENDING DEATH

Patients who are dying within days to weeks start sleeping more, and there is less interaction with family and friends. They slowly decrease their oral intake until they stop eating and drinking completely. Death can usually be anticipated within days to a couple of weeks after cessation of all oral intake. However, this trajectory is variable depending on the patients age, general condition, terminal diagnosis, and baseline reserve. As oral intake decreases, so does bowel and bladder elimination. Activity significantly decreases as fatigue increases and metabolism slows down, often rendering patients bedridden. Confusion is common and hallucinations can occur.[33] Skin may feel cool to the touch, and then become mottled in appearance. Agonal respirations are present in the last days to hours before death. Physicians often recognize imminent death but are reluctant to discuss it. Recognizing and relaying that death is imminent can help patients and their loved ones prepare for the end of life by saying their goodbyes and being intentional about meaning making and the patient's legacy. Communication with the patients and their families during this phase of care is crucial[34]

SUMMARY

"To cut is to cure" is the surgeon's mantra. However, sometimes surgeons do not cure and the patients do not recover as they had hoped when they performed surgery. End-of-life care in some surgical patient populations is a common occurrence. Applying primary palliative care principles and integrating primary palliative care skills should be within the scope of practice of every surgeon.[35] Goals-of-care discussions, education, addressing advanced directives, managing symptoms, and helping patients and their families make these challenging decisions should be integrated into the practice of all surgeons. The purpose is to help the patients seek the treatment that best aligns with their goals and values and, when appropriate, make a smooth transition to comfort-focused care at the end of life, promoting a natural death rather than a death encumbered by unwanted aggressive life-prolonging measures.

REFERENCES

1. Schwarze ML, Bradley CT, Brasel KJ. Surgical "buy-in": the contractual relationship between surgeons and patients that influences decisions regarding life-supporting therapy. Crit Care Med 2010;38:843–8.
2. Schwarze ML, Redmann AJ, Alexander GC. Surgeons expect patients to buy-in to postoperative life support preoperatively: results of a national survey. Crit Care Med 2013;41:1–8.
3. Pecana KE, Kehler JM, Brasel KL, et al. It's big surgery: preoperative expressions of risk, responsibility, and commitment to treatment after high-risk operations. Ann Surg 2014;259:458–63.
4. Kruser JM, Nabozny MJ, Steffens NM, et al. "Best case/worst case": qualitative evaluation of a novel communication tool for difficult-in-the-moment surgical decisions. J Am Geriatr Soc 2015;63:1805–11.
5. Kruser JM, Taylor LJ, Campbell TC, et al. "Best case/worst case": training surgeons to use a novel communication tool for high0risk acute surgical problems. J Pain Symptom Manage 2017;53:711–9.
6. Monahan K, Ducach G, Olympia RP. Cardiopulmonary resuscitation survival rates depicted in emergency department-associated medical television shows. Resuscitation 2019. https://doi.org/10.1016/j.resuscitation.2018.12.017.

7. Pellegrino ED. Patient and physician autonomy: conflicting rights and obligations in the physician-patient relationship. J Contemp Health Law Policy 1994;10: 47–68.
8. Wright MS. End of life and autonomy: the case for relational nudges in end-of-life decision-making law and policy. Md Law Rev 2018;44:1062–141.
9. Wancata LM, Hinshaw DB. Rethinking autonomy: decision making between patient and surgeon in advanced illness. Ann Transl Med 2016;4:77.
10. Khan M, Jehan F, Zeeshan M, et al. Failure to rescue after emergency general surgery in geriatric patients: does frailty matter? J Surg Res 2019;233:397–402.
11. Sharoky CE, Martin ND, Smith BP, et al. The location and timing of failure-to-rescue events across a statewide trauma system. J Surg Res 2019;235:529–35.
12. Patel K, Sinvani L, Patel V, et al. Do-not-resuscitate orders in older adults during hospitalization: a propensity score-matched analysis. J Am Geriatr Soc 2018;66: 924–9.
13. Welie JVM, ten Have HAMJ. The ethics of forgoing life-sustaining treatment: theoretical considerations and clinical decision making. Multidiscip Respir Med 2014; 9:14.
14. Murphy J, Fayanju O, Brown D, et al. Withdrawal of care in a potentially curable patient. Surgery 2010;147:441–5.
15. Bacchetta MD, Eachempati SR, Fins JJ, et al. Factors influencing DNR decision-making in a surgical ICU. J AM Coll Surg 2006;202:995–1000.
16. Murthi SB, Scalea TM. Defining the space between life and death: fatal critical illness. J Trauma Acute Care Surg 2015;79:493–4.
17. Papadimos TJ, Maldonado Y, Tripathi RS, et al. An overview of end-of-life issues in the intensive care unit. Int J Crit Illn Inj Sci 2011;1:138–46.
18. Massachusetts General Hospital. Ventilator withdrawal guidelines. Available at: https://www.massgeneral.org/palliativecare/assets/WithdrawalProtocol.pdf. Accessed February 02, 2019.
19. Smith L, Hough CL. Using death rounds to improve end-of-life education for internal medicine residents. J Palliat Med 2011;14:55–8.
20. Browning ED, Cruz JS. Reflective debriefing: a social work intervention addressing moral distress among ICU nurses. J Soc Work End Life Palliat Care 2018;14: 44–72.
21. Campbell ML. How to withdraw mechanical ventilation: a systematic review of the literature. AACN Adv Crit Care 2007;18:397–403.
22. Soliman IW, Cremer OL, DeLange DW, et al. The ability of intensive care unit physicians to estimate long-term prognosis in survivors of critical illness. J Crit Care 2018;43:148–55.
23. Nabozny MJ, Steffens NM, Schwarze ML. When do not resuscitate is a nonchoice choice: a teachable moment. JAMA Intern Med 2015;175:1444–5.
24. Anesi GL, Halpern SD. Choice architecture in code status discussion with terminally ill patients and their families. Intensive Care Med 2016;42:1065–7.
25. Bernacki RE, Block SD. Communication about serious illness care goals: a review and synthesis of best practice. JAMA Intern Med 2014;174:1994–2003.
26. Dunn GP, Milch RA, Mosenthal AC, et al. Palliative care by the surgeon: how to do it. J Am Coll Surg 2002;194:509–37.
27. White N, Kupell N, Vicerstaff V, et al. How accurate is the "Surprise Question" at identifying patients at the end of life? A systematic review and meta-analysis. BMC Med 2017;15:139.
28. Druml C, Ballmer PE, Druml W, et al. ESPEN guideline on the ethical aspects of artificial nutrition and hydration. Clin Nutr 2016;35:545–56.

29. Olson TJP, Pinkerton C, Brasel K, et al. Palliative surgery for malignant bowel obstruction from carcinomatosis: a systematic review. JAMA Surg 2014;149: 383–92.
30. Laval G, Marcelin-Benazech B, Guirimand F, et al. Recommendations for bowel obstruction with peritoneal carcinomatosis. J Pain Symptom Manage 2014;48: 75–91.
31. Nakagawa S, Garan AR, Takayama H, et al. End of life with left ventricular assist device in both bridge to transplant and destination therapy. J Palliat Med 2018; 21:1284–9.
32. Warraich HJ, Hernandez AF, Allen LA. How medicine has changed the end of life for patients with cardiovascular disease. J Am Coll Cardiol 2017;70:1276–89.
33. Matsunami K, Tomita K, Touge H, et al. Physical signs and clinical findings before death in ill elderly patients. Am J Hosp Palliat Care 2018;35:712–7.
34. Houttekier D, Witkamp FE, van Zuylen L, et al. Is physician awareness of impending death in hospital related to better communication and medical care? J Palliat Med 2014;17:1238–43.
35. American College of Surgeons. Statement on principles of palliative care. Available at: https://www.facs.org/about-acs/statements/50-palliative-care. Accessed February 02, 2019.

Mitigating Burnout

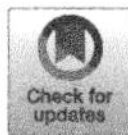

Timothy R. Siegel, MD[a,b,*], Andrea K. Nagengast, MD[c]

KEYWORDS

- Burnout • Compassion fatigue • Self-care • Resilience • Self-awareness
- Job satisfaction • Compassion satisfaction

KEY POINTS

- Burnout and compassion fatigue have far-reaching effects on nearly all members of the health care system, including surgeons, and significant focus on physician well-being has helped identify factors that both influence and mitigate burnout.
- Commitment to self-care and self-awareness help improve job satisfaction, job engagement, and compassion satisfaction.
- The combination of support within health care organizations and personal commitment to self-care creates the optimal framework for mitigating burnout.

INTRODUCTION

Burnout is ubiquitous when considering the topic of physician well-being in modern medical and surgical practice. As focus on physician wellness and self-care has gained significant momentum, considerable credence has been given to the effects of burnout on all members of the health care team. This explores strategies for mitigating burnout among physicians.

BURNOUT

Burnout is characterized by emotional exhaustion, depersonalization, and a reduced sense of personal accomplishment.[1] Feelings associated with each of these characteristics are outlined[3] in **Table 1**. Depression, anxiety, hypochondria, irritability, combativeness, lack of control, and inability to concentrate are features associated with burnout.[2,3]

Disclosure: No disclosures for either author.

[a] Department of Surgery, Oregon Health and Sciences University, 3181 Southwest Sam Jackson Park Road, Mail Code: UHS-3, Portland, OR 97239, USA; [b] Department of Medicine, Oregon Health and Sciences University, 3181 Southwest Sam Jackson Park Road, Mail Code: UHS-3, Portland, OR 97239, USA; [c] Trauma, Critical Care and Acute Care Surgery, Department of Surgery, Oregon Health and Sciences University, 3181 Southwest Sam Jackson Park Road, Mail Code: L611, Portland, OR 97239, USA

* Corresponding author. 3181 Southwest Sam Jackson Park Road, Mail Code: UHS-3, Portland, OR 97239.

E-mail address: siegelti@ohsu.edu

Surg Clin N Am 99 (2019) 1029–1035
https://doi.org/10.1016/j.suc.2019.06.015 surgical.theclinics.com

Table 1
Characteristics of burnout with associated feelings

Characteristic	Associated Feelings
Emotional exhaustion	Overextended; "stretched too thin"
Depersonalization	Impersonal response to people; unfeeling
Decreased sense of personal accomplishment	Decreased competence and achievement at work

A myriad of implications for both physicians and patients exist as a result of the effects of burnout. For physicians, burnout causes decreased empathy, decreased communication skills, and decreased clinical performance. The additive effect of these deficiencies leads to increased medical errors, increased adverse events, and a significantly compromised quality of patient care.[4,5] Ultimately, the snowball effect of burnout leads to poorer patient outcomes.

Additional physician consequences include decreased job satisfaction, increased job turnover, and poor health.[6] Self-medication with alcohol, prescription medications, or illicit substances, and ultimately suicide,[7] are sequelae of burnout.

COMPASSION FATIGUE

Compassion fatigue occurs in people who are emotionally affected by another's trauma. Despite sharing certain features of burnout, it is more like posttraumatic stress disorder. Characteristic feelings of emptiness and depletion, lack of energy, and questioning of professional purpose define compassion fatigue. Physicians who have compassion fatigue maintain the ability to engage in patient care, albeit to a lesser extent than normal, whereas burnout may ultimately result in affected physicians who are unable to care for patients or connect with colleagues, friends, and family.[2,3]

RISK FACTORS

All physicians face the potential for burnout. Surgeons of any type have a high incidence of developing burnout, with several studies citing rates up to 40%.[8] This particularly high incidence is attributed to the demanding nature of surgical residency and practice, all within the scope of the rigorous medical training required to earn a medical degree in the first place.[9–12]

Most medical school applicants cite an altruistic commitment to helping others and a desire to alleviate suffering in their personal statements.[13] As the didactic medical school years segue into the clinical arena, the focus shifts from rote memorization of new medical language and disease processes to developing clinical skills at patients' bedsides in the hospital or clinic. Sometimes the ideal does not match the reality, and the attributes that led students to the practice of medicine are muted early in those clinical years and continue to diminish further during postgraduate training. Facing the computer screen instead of the patient, navigating an electronic medical record system, and learning the necessary documentation to achieve the highest billable patient encounter begin to take precedence over honing the personal side of patient interactions and understanding patients in the context of disorders that were studied in medical texts. For surgical trainees and practitioners, the dedication, time commitment, and personal sacrifice (all widely acknowledged as inherent in achieving a successful career as a surgeon) manifest as attitudes that precipitate a higher rate of burnout compared with their medical specialist counterparts.[10–13]

Although risk factors for physician burnout include a previous personal or family history of psychiatric illness; a personal history of childhood illness, death, or emotional neglect; lack of social support; and certain personality traits,[14,15] these are not the only relevant risk factors for those who have chosen a surgical career.

Surgeons routinely care for critically ill patients, some of whom have experienced clinical complications born out of their own surgical technique. Surgical oncologists may care for patients for an extended period and, when no further medical or surgical options remain, they must guide end-of-life and goals-of-care discussions. Trauma surgeons often care for patients who have endured particularly disturbing injuries, some of which prove rapidly fatal either in the operating room or in the trauma surgical intensive care unit. No matter the surgical specialty and regardless of the acute or chronic nature of the patient's illness or death, repeated exposure to patient (and caregiver) fatigue, grief, suffering, and death increases the susceptibility to physician burnout.

Burnout is rarely, if ever, attributable to 1 isolated antecedent factor, but is the additive effect of many factors that influence overall physician wellness. A major precipitant of burnout is job stress. Job stress is multifactorial and often exacerbated by both organization-specific issues and discordant workplace relationships. Clinical overload, lack of resources, mismanagement, and conflicts with administration or staff are potential contributors. If personal stress is present outside of work, it may also serve as an agitator to job-related stress and dissatisfaction.[16]

MITIGATING BURNOUT

The best strategies for mitigating burnout mimic a modern approach to medicine: the development of preventive practices to protect, promote, and maintain health and well-being. However, just as it is impossible to prevent every case of colon, breast, or lung cancer despite the use of thoughtful and well-defined screening practices, it is impossible to prevent all cases of physician burnout. Typically, physicians develop burnout over a protracted time course with acute, chronic, situational, and systemic factors playing different, but important, roles. The same strategies that help prevent burnout may also be used to assist in recovery from it.

Job Satisfaction and Job Engagement

Both job satisfaction and job engagement protect from burnout and are realized by healthy relationships with patients, their caregivers, and workplace colleagues at all levels.[16]

Using key elements that define burnout (see **Table 1**), one strategy for mitigating burnout may be created by contrasting those very characteristics and feelings that define it. Job satisfaction results in greater enjoyment with work and a sense of both control and competence. Job engagement creates sustained energy, involvement, and efficacy in the workplace. Ultimately, a fair, just, and supportive work environment that provides appropriate recognition and reward, a sustainable workload, and belief in the meaning and value of work results in high levels of satisfaction.[16]

Compassion Satisfaction

Compassion satisfaction is the sense of achievement that is derived from helping others and is a powerful contributor to protecting against burnout.[2] By recalling the humanistic attributes that often lead students to medicine, it is clear that the dampening of these critical attributes factor into burnout. The loss of the tangible desire to help others happens to most physicians at differing time points in their careers.

Recognizing this is of the utmost importance because compassion satisfaction is often the easiest strategy to use. To surgeons who show signs of burnout as a result of a serious patient complication or who endure repeated exposures to patient fatigue, grief, suffering, and death, a quick and simple reminder that their efforts have profound effects on patients and their families provides tremendous support.[17] To have the self-awareness to remind themselves shows both strength and forgiveness.

Resilience and Self-awareness

Resilience is a multifaceted concept that enables a healthy and adaptive response to stress. It is the ability to "bounce back" quickly after facing challenging situations, growing stronger in the process. Resilience is thought to be both innate and teachable, allowing deeper insight into personal coping skills and improved sense of self-awareness.[18,19]

Self-awareness is a major component of self-care that can lead to increased resilience. It combines the concepts of self-knowledge and dual awareness, which is the ability to attend to and monitor the needs of patients, work environments, and personal objective experiences. This concept is realized as an ability to both provide and experience increased empathy, or to experience the mutual healing connections formed between physician and patients and use that as a means to derive and promote compassion satisfaction. Improved job engagement also results because physicians perceive less stress in the work environment with better ability to be emotionally available in stressful workplace situations. With the improved coping skills and resilience enabled by a strong sense of self-awareness, job dissatisfaction is overcome by the belief that work can be regenerative and fulfilling.[20,21]

Self-care

Self-care is the foundation for physician well-being. It is a dynamic concept that requires a commitment to nurturing and protecting personal and professional wellness. Attention to physical, emotional, psychological, and spiritual dimensions is necessary.[22–24] The new age of medical and surgical training underscores the practice of self-care as a way for clinicians to provide compassionate patient care, enjoy job satisfaction and engagement, and facilitate compassion satisfaction in themselves and others.

Cognitive behavioral interventions, self-reflection, practicing active and passive coping skills, and an active spiritual life are all individual stress-reduction strategies. Spirituality is what gives meaning and purpose to an individual's life and comes in multiple forms. Organized religion, meditation, athletics, exercise, and nature are examples of spirituality. Engaging in any form of spirituality improves wellness, reduces stress, and protects from burnout.[25]

Given the high incidence of surgeon burnout,[8] it is imperative that surgeons incorporate self-care into their lives. Surgeons are prone to overwork not just because of a desire to do the best for their patients but also because of the normalization of extreme work hours during residency and the examples set forth by unhealthy role models. Survival mode, an existence with which most surgeons are overly familiar, does not align with a fulfilled life.

Surgeons are motivated, intelligent, and driven individuals whose tremendous personal and emotional sacrifice affords the privilege to care for some of the sickest patients.[9] These patients are often in their most vulnerable state, exposed on a cold and sterile operating room table, and not only rely on the superior technical skills of the surgeons but also believe that the surgeons have compassion. When a surgeon experiences dissatisfaction, cynicism, and moral distress, ultimately leading to burnout, compassion is lost and all patients, especially the most vulnerable, suffer the consequences.

Filling the Toolbox

Time and commitment are necessary to cultivate the multimodal toolbox that helps protect from burnout. Exercising, learning and practicing relaxation techniques such as mindfulness meditation, developing boundaries at work, sleeping regularly, relaxing, and spending time with friends and family are but a few examples of self-care. **Box 1** provides more examples of self-care techniques.

Factors that help promote wellness include focusing on work-life balance, personal relationships, spiritual practice, and finding value and meaning in work. For surgeons, participating in research and educational activities outside of work, connecting with colleagues, nurturing hobbies outside of work, and identifying personal support systems are important to promoting wellness.[26,27] Maintaining good physical health is a necessity that goes beyond the sense of well-being that a nonsedentary lifestyle provides. Surgeons have a physically demanding job, both in and out of the operating room. Intense operations that last several hours, sometimes requiring heavy lifting and retracting, suboptimal body positioning for sustained amounts of time, and long stretches of being on call with little sleep are all potential risk factors for developing physical disability. For surgeons, the benefits of maintaining good physical health are 2-fold because of the effects on both daily job satisfaction and overall self-care.

Health Care Organizations: a Group Effort

The greatest chance that physicians have to refine these habits is the combination of personal commitment to self-care and support at an institutional level. Frameworks within health care organizations have become increasingly robust with the overall increased focus on self-care. Incentive programs that help cultivate healthy habits vary across health care organizations of all locations, sizes, and types. Other important elements that lead to a healthy workplace environment and help combat burnout focus on issues other than physical health.

Once it is understood, compassion satisfaction is more readily available as a tool to help mitigate burnout, but improving job satisfaction and engagement often requires infrastructural changes that take time and commitment. Health care organizations can show physicians their commitment to improving job satisfaction and engagement by holding town hall meetings and small work unit meetings. Transparently examining workload and efficiency, allowing flexibility within work hours, and supporting work-life balance are other ways to facilitate a healthier work environment. Team training focused on improving communication skills, management techniques, and team

Box 1
Self-care techniques

Mindfulness meditation

Narrative competence
- Close reading of literature
- Reflective writing

Centering before each new patient encounter

Taking time to eat with colleagues at work

Listening to music on the commute home

work dynamics are integral to the development of coping skills that protect from burnout.[28,29]

Physician leaders are critical to the success of institutions' ability to affect change and help shape workplace culture. Surgeons are often called on to fill this role by the nature of their inherent ability as leaders within their specialties. Physician leaders must be exceptional listeners who can engage, develop, and motivate their colleagues. They must also be able to distill the concerns and suggestions of their groups into practical solutions that can be effectively communicated to their organizational administration. Physician leaders can be powerful tools in promoting change, improving job satisfaction and engagement, and thereby helping to mitigate burnout.[28]

SUMMARY

The effects of burnout are far reaching, with professional and personal consequences that ultimately lead to poorer patient outcomes. Mitigating burnout requires buy-in from all stakeholders in the health care system, at both individual and institutional levels. Embracing a multimodal approach ensures the best chance at mitigation and recovery from burnout. Focusing on self-care enables increased job satisfaction, job engagement, and compassion satisfaction, and a commitment to this is integral to overcoming the personal and professional burden of burnout.

REFERENCES

1. Sanchez-Reilly S, Morrison LJ, Carey E, et al. Caring for oneself to care for others: physicians and their self-care. J Support Oncol 2013;11(2):75–81.
2. Slocum-Gori S, Hemsworth D, Chan WW, et al. Understanding compassion satisfaction, compassion fatigue and burnout: a survey of the hospice palliative care workforce. Palliat Med 2013;27(2):172–8.
3. Wright B. Compassion fatigue: how to avoid it. Palliat Med 2004;18(1):3–4.
4. West CP, Tan AD, Habermann TM, et al. Association of resident fatigue and distress with perceived medical errors. JAMA 2009;302(12):1294–300.
5. Dewa CS, Loong D, Bonato S, et al. How does burnout affect physician productivity? A systematic literature review. BMC Health Serv Res 2014;14:325.
6. Kuerer HM, Eberlein TJ, Pollock RE, et al. Career satisfaction, practice patterns and burnout among surgical oncologists: report on the quality of life of members of the Society of Surgical Oncology. Ann Surg Oncol 2007;14(11):3043–53.
7. Gold KJ, Sen A, Schwenk TL. Details on suicide among US physicians: data from the National violent death reporting system. Gen Hosp Psychiatry 2013;35(1):45–9.
8. Balch CM, Shanafelt T. Combating stress and burnout in surgical practice: a review. Adv Surg 2010;44(1):29–47.
9. Oskrochi Y, Maruthappu M, Henriksson M, et al. Beyond the body: a systematic review of the nonphysical effects of a surgical career. Surgery 2016;159(2):650–64.
10. Dimou FM, Eckelbarger D, Riall TS. Surgeon burnout: a systematic review. J Am Coll Surg 2016;222(6):1230–9.
11. Dyrbye LN, Shanafelt TD, Balch CM, et al. Relationship between work-home conflicts and burnout among American surgeons: a comparison by sex. Arch Surg 2011;146(2):211–7.
12. Pulcrano M, Evans SR, Sosin M. Quality of life and burnout rates across surgical specialties: a systematic review. JAMA Surg 2016;151(10):970–8.

13. Jager AJ, Tutty MA, Kao AC. Association between physician burnout and identification with medicine as a calling. Mayo Clin Proc 2017;92(3):415–22.
14. Amoafo E, Hanbali N, Patel A, et al. What are the significant factors associated with burnout in doctors? Occup Med (Lond) 2015;65(2):117–21.
15. Gundersen L. Physician burnout. Ann Intern Med 2001;135(2):145–8.
16. Siegel T. Self care and the surgeon. In: Mosenthal A, Dunn G, editors. Palliative surgery. New York: Oxford University Press; 2018.
17. Kuerer HM, Breslin T, Shanafelt TD, et al. Road map for maintaining career satisfaction and balance in surgical oncology. J Am Coll Surg 2008;207(3):435–42.
18. Epstein RM, Krasner MS. Physician resilience: what it means, why it matters, and how to promote it. Acad Med 2013;88(3):301–3.
19. Zwack J, Schweitzer J. If every fifth physician is affected by burnout, what about the other four? Resilience strategies of experienced physicians. Acad Med 2013;88(3):382–9.
20. Makowski SK, Epstein RM. Turning toward dissonance: lessons from art, music, and literature. J Pain Symptom Manage 2012;43(2):293–8.
21. Meier DE, Back AL, Morrison RS. The inner life of physicians and care of the seriously ill. JAMA 2001;286(23):3007–14.
22. Brandt ML. Sustaining a career in surgery. Am J Surg 2017;214(4):707–14.
23. Page DW. Are surgeons capable of introspection? Surg Clin North Am 2011;91(2):293–304, vii.
24. West CP, Dyrbye LN, Erwin PJ, et al. Interventions to prevent and reduce physician burnout: a systematic review and meta-analysis. Lancet 2016;388(10057):2272–81.
25. Doolittle BR, Windish DM, Seelig CB. Burnout, coping, and spirituality among internal medicine resident physicians. J Grad Med Educ 2013;5(2):257–61.
26. Balch CM, Freischlag JA, Shanafelt TD. Stress and burnout among surgeons: understanding and managing the syndrome and avoiding the adverse consequences. Arch Surg 2009;144(4):371–6.
27. Kearney MK, Weininger RB, Vachon ML, et al. Self-care of physicians caring for patients at the end of life: "Being connected... a key to my survival". JAMA 2009;301(11):1155–64. E1.
28. Shanafelt TD, Noseworthy JH. Executive leadership and physician well-being: nine organizational strategies to promote engagement and reduce burnout. Mayo Clin Proc 2017;92(1):129–46.
29. Bertges Yost W, Eshelman A, Raoufi M, et al. A national study of burnout among American transplant surgeons. Transplant Proc 2005;37(2):1399–401.

Surgical Palliative Care Education

Jessica H. Ballou, MD, MPH*, Karen J. Brasel, MD, MPH

KEYWORDS

• Palliative care • Medical student education • Surgical resident education
• Continuing medical education • End-of-life care

KEY POINTS

- Without palliative care training, surgeons often miss empathic moments with patients, and surgical patients are less likely to receive palliative care services than medicine patients.
- Palliative care is increasingly recognized as an essential component to undergraduate and graduate surgical training. Opportunities for formal education decrease as trainees enter practice.
- Most research on palliative care education consists of surveys from single academic centers with limited longitudinal data.
- Of the studies available, witnessed interactions with feedback have been shown to be the most consistent in showing improvements in provider comfort and skill.
- Most educational initiatives and requirements focus on end-of-life care, although providing comprehensive palliative care requires intervention at all stages of disease.

INTRODUCTION

Palliative care and the relief of suffering have always been at the heart of surgical practice. Many of the most well-known operations, ranging from the Billroth and Whipple procedures to the Halsted radical mastectomy and coronary artery bypass, initially served palliative rather than curative purposes.[1–5] Despite the long-standing role that surgery has played in the provision of de facto palliative care, teachings on the principles of palliative and end-of-life care have not traditionally been a part of the surgical education curriculum. As a result, surgeons at all levels of training, from medical school to advanced practice, struggle with communicating and implementing palliative care.

Disclosure: The authors have no disclosures.
Division of Trauma, Acute Care, and Emergency General Surgery, Department of Surgery, Oregon Health and Science University, L223, 3181 Southwest Sam Jackson Park Road, Portland, OR, USA
* Corresponding author.
E-mail address: ballouj@ohsu.edu

Surg Clin N Am 99 (2019) 1037–1049
https://doi.org/10.1016/j.suc.2019.06.016
surgical.theclinics.com

The US population is aging: by the year 2030, 1 in 5 adults in the United States will be more than 65 years old and the number of persons more than 85 years old will have doubled to nearly 12 million.[6] Epidemiologic studies reveal that nearly one-third of elderly Medicare beneficiaries have surgery in the final year of life.[7] The growing elderly and surgical population makes integration of palliative care into surgical education necessary. In recognition of the surgeon's role in eliciting patients' needs and assessing treatment options, palliative and end-of-life care have also been adopted as core competencies by numerous professional societies, including the American College of Surgeons, National Comprehensive Cancer Network, the American Society of Clinical Oncology, and the Institute of Medicine.[8–11] Moreover, although the past three decades have seen an exponential increase in the number of medical schools, residency, and fellowship level programs incorporating palliative care into their programs, the degree and manner of implementation vary dramatically by institution.[12]

SURGICAL EXPERIENCE IS NOT A SURROGATE FOR DELIVERING QUALITY PALLIATIVE CARE

Until the 1970s, patients with advanced cancer were unlikely to be told of their diagnoses.[13] A 1961 study at a Chicago hospital found that nearly 90% of physicians and surgeons did not regularly disclose a cancer diagnosis and none had a policy of informing every patient.[14] As a profession, the focus of the patient-physician interaction has shifted from one of paternalism to that of a shared decision making and open communication. However, the vestiges of the days when physicians withheld end-of-life discussions for fear that it would cause "disturbing psychological effects"[14] remain in the modern era as a generalized discomfort with palliative and end-of-life discussions.

Although surgeon experience may be associated with increased comfort with end-of-life conversations and fewer nontherapeutic interventions, multiple studies report discomfort with difficult conversations, particularly about prognosis and goals of care, among surgical trainees and staff.[15,16] In 1997, Wilson and colleagues[17] surveyed 230 seriously ill hospitalized adults on their desires for cardiopulmonary resuscitation, their quality of life, and their attitudes toward 6 other common adverse outcomes. They then asked the same questions of the intern and attending providers. Neither medical interns nor the attending physicians were consistently accurate in assessing patients' preferences.

The Wilson study is only 1 example of how experience alone is an unreliable surrogate for comfort and competency applying palliative care principles. Although surgeons play a central role in palliative care delivery, surgical patients are less likely to receive palliative care services than their medicine counterparts.[18] For all the progress in recognizing patient autonomy and improving patient-centered communication, without training in palliative and end-of-life care and communication, physicians at all stages of their careers have been shown to lack confidence in their communication skills and miss opportunities for empathetic communication in patient encounters.[16,19]

CURRENT STATE OF UNDERGRADUATE MEDICAL EDUCATION IN PALLIATIVE CARE

In 1997, Billings and Block[20] published their report in the *Journal of the American Medical Association* on palliative care education in US medical schools. Their principal findings were as follows:

- Although nearly all medical schools offer some formal teaching about end-of-life care, there is considerable evidence that current training is inadequate, most strikingly in the clinical years.

- Teaching about palliative care is received favorably by students, positively influences student attitudes, and enhances communication skills.
- Curricular offerings are not well integrated: the dominant teaching format is the lecture; formal teaching is predominantly preclinical; clinical experiences are mostly elective; and there is little attention to home care, hospice, and nursing home care.
- Role models are few and students are not encouraged to examine their reactions to these clinical experiences.[20]

The investigators called on medical schools to address their "responsibility to prepare students to provide skilled, compassionate end-of-life care"[20] in a comprehensive manner that reflects the student's level of training. In 2000, the Liaison Committee on Medical Education (LCME) made it a formal requirement that all medical schools provide experiential training in end-of-life care.[21] By 2011, all accredited medical schools in the United States and Canada had some form of teaching on death and dying within their medical curricula.[22]

The LCME mandate makes no further requirements on how to implement such training, nor does it touch on the components of palliative care beyond end-of-life needs. In a recent editorial in the *Journal of Palliative Medicine*, Dr. Weissman[23] laments: "the unfortunate linkage of palliative care with end-of-life care is a major deterrent to widespread adoption of core palliative care educational domains." Beyond hospice and end-of-life care, essential palliative domains that are amenable to medical student teaching include, but are not limited to, discussions of code status, dyspnea management, informed consent, treatment goals and prognosis, and management of the family meeting.[24]

The Formal, Informal, and Hidden Curricula

There are 3 principal modalities by which palliative and end-of-life care teaching take place within medical schools: formal teaching (either lecture based or simulation), informal clinical experience, and the so-called hidden curriculum.[25]

Formal palliative care curricula range dramatically within undergraduate medical education. Surveys reveal that training can span from a couple of hours in a classroom to weeks of palliative care training or hospice-based clinical rotations.[26,27] There is also little consensus on when these courses should be incorporated into the curriculum.[28] Multiple studies support combining palliative care classroom teachings with clinical experience because medical student attitudes toward palliative care are more strongly affected by personal experience than by previous education in the subject.[29]

The informal curriculum refers to the unstructured lessons that take place outside of a palliative care–focused learning session. It can include discussions on clinical rounds or otherwise unstructured learning environments. However, without awareness of the learning opportunities and an active role on the part of the instructor, these opportunities can be missed and ineffective. In one study of junior residents, one-third (35%) noted that they had not observed a patient being told about a terminal prognosis during medical school and only 5% of residents report a faculty member being present during their first experience delivering bad news.[25]

When the formal and informal curricula do not provide students with the lessons that they need, students must resort to eliciting cues from the hidden curriculum.[30] The hidden curriculum consists of student-identified role models, rules and regulations, medical ethics, medical lingo and jargon, the embodiment of professionalism, and the power hierarchy in medicine.[30] When the content of the hidden curriculum conflicts with formal classroom teachings, students must internally reconcile any conflicts between their ideal image and character of a physician with what they witness in reality.

Recognizing the struggle that students experience early in their clinical years between the ideal and the perceived clinical experience provides the opportunity for discussion and character development. Although the traditional formal medical curriculum offers little opportunity to discuss the emotional experiences of students, self-reflection through small group discussions and mentorship within the formal and informal learning experiences can identify and solidify productive, positive themes within the hidden curriculum.[30]

A Focus on Empathy

The primary danger of not addressing the negative aspects of the hidden curriculum is the loss of empathy. Studies have found that surgeons at all levels of training often miss empathic opportunities in patient interviews.[31] Although there is little consensus on the definition of empathy, the Jefferson Scale of Physician Empathy defines it as "a cognitive attribute that involves an ability to understand the patient's pain, suffering, and perspective combined with a capability to communicate this understanding and an intention to help."[32,33] Studies have shown that the negative impressions within the hidden curriculum, unstable learning environments, loss of idealism, and the perceived need for detachment can lead to a decrease in empathy (as measured by standardized scales) as students advance through their training.[34,35] These findings have widespread ramifications because empathy is central to practicing quality palliative care, and addressing these issues should be central to teaching palliative care. In addition, physician empathy has been shown to have a positive impact on patient satisfaction, greater adherence to therapy, better clinical outcomes, and lower malpractice liability.[34]

There is evidence that empathy can be taught and maintained, although the studies are often limited to single sites with small sample sizes. Regardless, examples of these positive interventions include reflective writing, didactics, early clinical exposure to hospice and palliative care, and apprenticeships with empathetic faculty or advisors.[29,36,37]

CURRENT STATE OF GRADUATE MEDICAL EDUCATION IN PALLIATIVE CARE

Although medical schools are progressively incorporating more palliative care education into their curricula, training for surgical residents and fellows lags despite requirements from the American Board of Surgery, the American College of Graduate Medical Education (ACGME) Residency Review Committee, and various fellowships. Most general surgery residencies lack formal palliative care training because many programs struggle to meet the clinical and professional demands imposed on them by the various accrediting agencies.[38]

Palliative care skills are both desired and needed in surgical residency and fellowship.[39,40] In a 2015 study of New England surgical residents, Cooper and colleagues[41] found that although 90% of residents were expected to discuss end-of-life issues with patients and surrogates, only 59% were comfortable managing such discussions. Multiple survey studies find residents are often not present at pivotal moments, such as during the decision to withdraw life-sustaining treatments, or they are alone in these conversations without faculty observation and feedback.[41,42] Fellows similarly lack opportunities for both role models and feedback: a recent survey of hepatobiliary fellows found that most observed faculty discussing surgical complications, but only

54% had witnessed faculty discussing end-of-life goals,[43] with fewer receiving feedback on their palliative skills.[44] Further, even when trainees do have integrated palliative care teaching in their curricula, care must be given to the content and clinical application of the material because the teachings may be perceived as inappropriate for the resident's level of training.[40]

The most commonly cited barrier to teaching palliative care skills is time.[44] Because residents must meet all clinical, operative, and didactic milestones within the 80-hour work week restrictions, it has become essential for residency programs to develop flexible, adult-learning methods to meet the trainees' learning needs.

Formal Didactic Training in Palliative Care for Surgical Trainees

First developed in 2006 to establish a foundation for didactic training among US surgical residents, the Surgical Council on Resident Education (SCORE) is a nonprofit consortium consisting of the American Board of Surgery, the American College of Surgeons, the American Surgical Association, the Association of Program Directors in Surgery, the Association for Surgical Education, the Review Committee for Surgery of the ACGME, and the Society of American Gastrointestinal and Endoscopic Surgeons.[45] The topics within the SCORE curriculum represent the potentially testable material that general surgery residents need to learn in order to pass their board examinations. With regard to palliative care, SCORE includes in its curriculum modules on advance directives:

1. Do-not-resuscitate orders and power of attorney
2. Frailty
3. Goal setting with elderly patients and families
4. Palliative and hospice care
5. Perioperative management of geriatric patients

Each of these modules consists of selected readings and questions meant to provide a broad overview of the topic. The method in which each training institution chooses to incorporate or implement the SCORE curriculum into their didactics varies between sites. The list highlights the unfortunate linkage of palliative care and end-of-life care described by Dr Weissman,[23] showing that even those leading educational efforts in surgery need further education in palliative care.

Clinical Applications for Residents and Fellows

All surgical residents must show a certain level of competency with procedures or tasks as defined by the ACGME to graduate. Although the ACGME dictates how many mastectomies or thoracotomies are needed or how many times the resident leads a resuscitation, there is no requirement for palliative procedures or palliative conversations. Structured palliative care curricula have been shown to improve knowledge, but only integration with clinical experiences increased confidence in managing pain, breaking bad news, or addressing ethical issues.[46] These efforts include written assignments, interactive lectures, case-based discussions and presentations, problem-based learning sessions, skills laboratories, and simulator laboratories.[46–48]

In 2009, the American College of Surgery Committee on Surgical Palliative Care published its *Resident's Guide to Palliative Care* as a comprehensive educational tool for applying palliative care knowledge and skills to clinical situations. Specifically, the text "provides a basic knowledge of palliative care. [Residents] will learn how to be clear with patients, their families, colleagues and [themselves] about the realities of the patient's disease picture and what [the resident's] judgment and skill in the art of surgery can provide for their comfort, function, and longevity."[49]

The text, which is available free through the American College of Surgeons, offers guidance on discrete topics ranging from managing constipation to discussing spiritual issues and maintaining hope. It represents a substantial milestone in the practical application of palliative care principles to surgical practice, but it is unclear how training programs incorporate this text into their program and practice.

CONTINUING SURGICAL PALLIATIVE CARE EDUCATION

On graduation, the opportunities for structured palliative care education dwindle for surgeons. The most common method of educational development posttraining for surgeons in practice is through continuing medical education (CME) courses and credits. At present, most state medical boards require that providers participate in CME courses.[50] Colorado, South Dakota, and Montana have no CME requirements for practicing physicians. States with CME requirements range from 2 hours on opioid prescribing every 2 years (Indiana) to 100 hours every 2 years (California). Except for California, there is no requirement that the CME be related to palliative care. California certification requires that "all physicians (except pathologists and radiologists) are required to take, as a one-time requirement, twelve units on pain management and the appropriate care and treatment of the terminally ill."[50] The onus is therefore on providers to seek out opportunities to advance their skill sets in palliative care principles and communication within the confines of a demanding clinical and academic schedule.

There is little consensus on the optimal method for teaching palliative care principles and communication to providers in practice. In a single-site study of academic surgeons, Hutul and colleagues[44] (2006) found that faculty preferred to use structured forms when evaluating students (93%), online teaching resources (82%), and workshops (63%) to improve their communication skills. However, these preferences reflect a tiny sample of attending physicians at an academic center. It may not be fair to assume that surgeons practicing at community or nonteaching hospitals have the same preferences or have the same incentives or barriers to implementing physician development initiatives related to palliative care.

Teaching Specific Skills: Communication Initiatives

For providers and students who wish to improve their palliative care skills, obtaining information and developing skills efficiently and effectively is a priority. Much of the educational focus in palliative care is on teaching providers to be more effective communicators, particularly as it relates to delivering bad news or discussing end-of-life care. Unlike the standardized history-taking communication skill that medical students are taught early in their training, learning how to communicate information on symptom management or end-of-life issues is more nuanced and has a greater emotional component.[19] Although learning to deliver bad news alone does not equate to delivering competent palliative care, there is good reason to place an emphasis on provider-patient communication: inadequate discussions have been shown to result in more aggressive, unwanted management as well as increased psychological and existential distress for patients and their loved ones.[19,51,52] Surveys show that it is common for surgeons to report feeling unprepared and ill-equipped to handle the emotional and logistical challenges that these conversations entail.[53] Improving confidence, knowledge, comfort, and self-efficacy in palliative and end-of-life communication has been shown to be a teachable skill, although the data are weak and studies are often limited to surveys and single sites.[54]

Formal communication training sessions include in-person or Web-based classroom lessons, interactive workshops, role playing, or an objective structured clinical examination (OSCE) with performance feedback by standardized patients and faculty.[53,55] These curriculum-based teachings vary widely, ranging from 20 minutes to multiple days depending on the extent of the curriculum.[53] However, there are limited data on whether classroom or lecture-based sessions result in improved patient-provider interactions.[56,57] If anything, didactic sessions have been shown to improve specific task-oriented communication initiatives such as discussing informed consent or documenting goals of care.[16] Similarly, in-person or Web-based workshops, although more effective than standard lecture-based didactics, show no consistent relationship between the length of training and efficacy.[54,58,59] To be effective, online curricula must include face-to-face interactions with feedback and discussion.[60]

Although the best data for improving provider practice, comfort, and confidence in communication are obtained through witnessed interactions with feedback,[54] communication tools have been developed to assist with specific interactions or situations. Among the most prevalent are mnemonics (eg, SPIKES and NURSE [discussed later), the ask-tell-ask style of provider communication, and the best-case-worst-case method for providing a framework for discussing high-risk operations.

The mnemonics SPIKES and NURSE were developed by oncologists to assist providers in delivering bad news (often about a new cancer diagnosis) as well as how to respond to patient emotions with empathy.[19,61] SPIKES refers to a 6-step protocol for delivering bad news[61]:

1. Setting up the interview,
2. Assessing the patient's perception
3. Obtaining the patient's invitation
4. Giving knowledge and information to the patient
5. Addressing the patient's emotions with an empathic response
6. Strategy and summary

NURSE refers to a method of responding to emotions: naming, understanding, respecting, supporting, and exploring.[19] Similarly the oncology literature supports the ask-tell-ask method for communicating information. It consists of (1) asking the patients to describe their understanding of the issue, (2) telling the patients in straightforward language what needs to be communicated, and (3) asking the patients about their understanding of what was discussed.[19] Although these methods are easy to incorporate into practice, the data are mixed on their effectiveness in improving patient-provider interactions.[54,62,63]

Although these tools may be adapted to surgical scenarios, few interventions specifically target surgical populations. However, the best-case-worst-case method was developed specifically as a communication tool and decision aid for patients undergoing high-risk surgical procedures.[64,65] In this model, the surgeon identifies the best, most likely, and worst case scenarios to compare and contrast the likely outcomes of undergoing certain procedures.[65] This model can be adapted to consider the individual patients' current fitness levels, the complexity of the proposed procedures, as well as their values and goals. Studies of the method have found that although surgeons can quickly and effectively adopt the model into their practices, the outcomes presented are subject to each surgeon's biases and could potentially conflict with patient autonomy.[64] A summary of the various teaching modalities is listed in **Table 1**.

Efforts have been made to develop quality indicators for communication between patients and physicians as it pertains to palliative care. Sinuff and colleagues[52] (2015) proposed a comprehensive list of quality indicators within the domains of

Table 1
Examples of teaching modalities for improving provider-patient communication

Communication Teaching Methods	Examples	Pros	Cons	Evidence of Effectiveness
Didactics	Classroom teachings, SCORE curriculum, CME	Requirement in many programs	Variability in use and implementation. Most effective when it incorporates face-to-face interactions with feedback	Useful for specific tasks (eg, informed consent)
Role playing/witnessed interaction with feedback	OSCE, interactive workshops	Simulates clinical experience	Requires trained participant to critique roles; time intensive	"Most consistently demonstrated significant improvements in reported outcomes amongst the healthcare professional interventions"[54]
Communication tools	Ask-tell-ask Best case/worst case Mnemonics	Easy to learn, implement	Limited in scope	Limited data on effectiveness[62]
Role modeling	Clinical rounds, witnessing faculty/mentor lead palliative conversation	Demonstrates clinical application	Highly dependent on mentor	Limited because of mentor variability

advance care planning, goals-of-care discussions, documentation, and organization/system. The principal indicators included (1) discussions of the use of life-sustaining therapies before hospitalization; (2) whether a member of the health care team has talked to the patient or surrogate about a poor prognosis or indicated in some way that the patient has a limited time left to live; (3) documentation of goals of care present in the medical record; and (4) ensuring that a mechanism is in place to enable access to the most current advance care planning documents in other settings within the health care system.[52]

Ultimately, the goal of patient-provider communication in the context of palliative care is to ensure that patient goals and values are understood in a way that allows the provider to address the patient's physical and psychological needs.

LIMITATIONS AND FUTURE DIRECTIONS

There are 2 significant shortcomings in palliative care education research and initiatives. First, there is a lack of rigorous scientific data on educational interventions and outcomes. Second, there is a shortage of palliative care experts relative to the need.

Many of the published studies regarding palliative care interventions and educational models consist of a single academic site with a small sample size and lack the long-term follow-up data to describe how these efforts affect clinical practice in surgical patients.[16,34,53,56,66] Community providers and trainees are often left out of these surveys and, as such, more information is required to identify the needs and barriers that community surgeons face in delivering quality palliative care.

Much of what is known about palliative care education has its origins in oncology. Although the oncology literature provides a substantial foundation for developing palliative care educational tools for surgeons, palliative principles in surgery extend beyond oncology. In surgical critical care, for example, a substantial proportion of patients are unable to communicate, and making decisions via a surrogate presents unique challenges.[67] Similarly, providers with pediatric or adolescent patients cannot be assumed to have the same palliative care challenges as those who manage adults or the elderly.[68,69] Going forward, both qualitative and quantitative studies are needed to assess the impact of specific interventions and educational models within different populations.

Addressing the needs of a growing and diverse population takes a strong workforce that is well versed in palliative care principles. With an estimated 6000 palliative care specialists in practice and fewer than 250 fellowship-trained physicians entering the workforce annually, there is a substantial shortage of specialty-trained palliative care providers.[70] Moreover, an aging population places demands on the few palliative providers and leaves limited availability for teaching. With a subject as complex and personal as palliative care, the fate of the curriculum often rests on the shoulders of palliative care "champions" who are single-handedly responsible for maintaining the courses.[23]

SUMMARY

Palliative care is increasingly recognized as central to surgical practice, but incorporating palliative care education into surgical training remains in its infancy. There are ample data on the discomfort that surgeons at all stages of practice feel with regard to delivering palliative care, but there is a dearth of data on the impact of educational modalities and interventions. Although efforts have been made by accrediting agencies and centers of higher learning to develop palliative care skills and principles early in training, the proposed curricula are too often lecture based and solely focused on end-of-life care. Such practices limit the acquisition of skills and narrow the scope of palliative care for future generations of physicians and surgeons.

In practice, palliative care is a multidisciplinary field designed to improve the quality of life for patients and their loved ones. Meeting the palliative care needs of an expanding, aging population requires participation from a variety of clinicians, including, but not limited to, those in nursing, social work, mental health, pastoral care, and pharmacy, as well as a variety of therapists depending on the circumstances. Harnessing the interdisciplinary nature of the field could help stem the burden of the limited palliative care educators and serve as a model for interdisciplinary collaboration.[66]

REFERENCES

1. Dunn GP, Milch RA. Introduction and historical background of palliative care: where does the surgeon fit in? J Am Coll Surg 2001;193(3):325–8.
2. Yuan SM, Jing H. Palliative procedures for congenital heart defects. Arch Cardiovasc Dis 2009;102(6–7):549–57.
3. Mueller RL, Rosengart TK, Isom OW. The history of surgery for ischemic heart disease. Ann Thorac Surg 1997;63(3):869–78.
4. Miner TJ. Communication as a core skill of palliative surgical care. Anesthesiol Clin 2012;30(1):47–58.
5. Hanna NN, Bellavance E, Keay T. Palliative surgical oncology. Surg Clin North Am 2011;91(2):343–53, viii.
6. Vespa J, Armstrong DM, Medina L. Demographic turning points for the United States: population projections for 2020 to 2060. Washington, DC: U.S. Census Bureau; 2018. p. P25–1144.
7. Kwok AC, Semel ME, Lipsitz SR, et al. The intensity and variation of surgical care at the end of life: a retrospective cohort study. Lancet 2011;378(9800):1408–13.
8. American College of Surgeons. Statement of principles of palliative care bulletin of the American College of Surgeons, vol. 2017. Chicago: American College of Surgeons Task Force on Surgical Palliative Care and the Committee on Ethics; 2005.
9. Dans M, Smith T, Back A, et al. NCCN guidelines insights: palliative care, version 2.2017. J Natl Compr Canc Netw 2017;15(8):989–97.
10. Ferris FD, Bruera E, Cherny N, et al. Palliative cancer care a decade later: accomplishments, the need, next steps – from the American Society of Clinical Oncology. J Clin Oncol 2009;27(18):3052–8.
11. Committee on approaching death: addressing key end of life issues; Institute of Medicine. Dying in America: improving quality and honoring individual preferences near the end of life. Washington, DC: National Academies Press (US); 2015.
12. Walker S, Gibbins J, Barclay S, et al. Progress and divergence in palliative care education for medical students: a comparative survey of UK course structure, content, delivery, contact with patients and assessment of learning. Palliat Med 2016;30(9):834–42.
13. Sisk B, Frankel R, Kodish E, et al. The truth about truth-telling in american medicine: a brief history. Perm J 2016;20(3):74–7.
14. Oken D. What to tell cancer patients. A study of medical attitudes. JAMA 1961;175:1120–8.
15. Suwanabol PA, Kanters AE, Reichstein AC, et al. Characterizing the role of U.S. surgeons in the provision of palliative care: a systematic review and mixed-methods meta-synthesis. J Pain Symptom Manage 2018;55(4):1196–215.e5.

16. Bakke KE, Miranda SP, Castillo-Angeles M, et al. Training surgeons and anesthesiologists to facilitate end-of-life conversations with patients and families: a systematic review of existing educational models. J Surg Educ 2018;75(3):702–21.
17. Wilson IB, Green ML, Goldman L, et al. Is experience a good teacher? How interns and attending physicians understand patients' choices for end-of-life care. SUPPORT Investigators. Study to understand prognoses and preferences for outcomes and risks of treatments. Med Decis Making 1997;17(2):217–27.
18. Olmsted CL, Johnson AM, Kaboli P, et al. Use of palliative care and hospice among surgical and medical specialties in the Veterans Health Administration. JAMA Surg 2014;149(11):1169–75.
19. Back AL, Arnold RM, Baile WF, et al. Approaching difficult communication tasks in oncology. CA Cancer J Clin 2005;55(3):164–77.
20. Billings JA, Block S. Palliative care in undergraduate medical education. Status report and future directions. JAMA 1997;278(9):733–8.
21. International Association of Medical Colleges. LCME accreditation standards. 2004. Available at: http://www.iaomc.org/lcme.htm. Accessed January 22, 2019.
22. Dickinson GE. Thirty-five years of end-of-life issues in US medical schools. Am J Hosp Palliat Care 2011;28(6):412–7.
23. Weissman DE. Technology and the future of palliative care education. J Palliat Med 2016;19(1):2–3.
24. Tchorz KM, Binder SB, White MT, et al. Palliative and end-of-life care training during the surgical clerkship. J Surg Res 2013;185(1):97–101.
25. Billings ME, Engelberg R, Curtis JR, et al. Determinants of medical students' perceived preparation to perform end-of-life care, quality of end-of-life care education, and attitudes toward end-of-life care. J Palliat Med 2010;13(3):319–26.
26. Horowitz R, Gramling R, Quill T. Palliative care education in U.S. medical schools. Med Educ 2014;48(1):59–66.
27. von Gunten CF, Mullan P, Nelesen RA, et al. Development and evaluation of a palliative medicine curriculum for third-year medical students. J Palliat Med 2012;15(11):1198–217.
28. Lloyd-Williams M, MacLeod RD. A systematic review of teaching and learning in palliative care within the medical undergraduate curriculum. Med Teach 2004; 26(8):683–90.
29. Wechter E, O'Gorman DC, Singh MK, et al. The effects of an early observational experience on medical students' attitudes toward end-of-life care. Am J Hosp Palliat Care 2015;32(1):52–60.
30. Bandini J, Mitchell C, Epstein-Peterson ZD, et al. Student and faculty reflections of the hidden curriculum. Am J Hosp Palliat Care 2017;34(1):57–63.
31. Easter DW, Beach W. Competent patient care is dependent upon attending to empathic opportunities presented during interview sessions. Curr Surg 2004; 61(3):313–8.
32. Sulzer SH, Feinstein NW, Wendland CL. Assessing empathy development in medical education: a systematic review. Med Educ 2016;50(3):300–10.
33. Hojat M, Gonnella JS, Nasca TJ, et al. The Jefferson scale of physician empathy: further psychometric data and differences by gender and specialty at item level. Acad Med 2002;77(10 Suppl):S58–60.
34. Batt-Rawden SA, Chisolm MS, Anton B, et al. Teaching empathy to medical students: an updated, systematic review. Acad Med 2013;88(8):1171–7.
35. Rosenthal S, Howard B, Schlussel YR, et al. Humanism at heart: preserving empathy in third-year medical students. Acad Med 2011;86(3):350–8.

36. Han JL, Pappas TN. A review of empathy, its importance, and its teaching in surgical training. J Surg Educ 2018;75(1):88–94.
37. Parikh PP, White MT, Buckingham L, et al. Evaluation of palliative care training and skills retention by medical students. J Surg Res 2017;211:172–7.
38. Klaristenfeld DD, Harrington DT, Miner TJ. Teaching palliative care and end-of-life issues: a core curriculum for surgical residents. Ann Surg Oncol 2007;14(6): 1801–6.
39. Gorman TE, Ahern SP, Wiseman J, et al. Residents' end-of-life decision making with adult hospitalized patients: a review of the literature. Acad Med 2005; 80(7):622–33.
40. Bonanno AM, Kiraly LN, Siegel TR, et al. Surgical palliative care training in general surgery residency: an educational needs assessment. Am J Surg 2019; 217(5):928–31.
41. Cooper Z, Meyers M, Keating NL, et al. Resident education and management of end-of-life care: the resident's perspective. J Surg Educ 2010;67(2):79–84.
42. Falcone JL, Claxton RN, Marshall GT. Communication skills training in surgical residency: a needs assessment and metacognition analysis of a difficult conversation objective structured clinical examination. J Surg Educ 2014;71(3):309–15.
43. Amini A, Miura JT, Larrieux G, et al. Palliative care training in surgical oncology and hepatobiliary fellowships: a national survey of the fellows. Ann Surg Oncol 2015;22(6):1761–7.
44. Hutul OA, Carpenter RO, Tarpley JL, et al. Missed opportunities: a descriptive assessment of teaching and attitudes regarding communication skills in a surgical residency. Curr Surg 2006;63(6):401–9.
45. American Board of Surgery. SCORE - surgical council on resident education. Available at: http://www.absurgery.org/default.jsp?aboutscre. Accessed January 25, 2019.
46. Bradley CT, Webb TP, Schmitz CC, et al. Structured teaching versus experiential learning of palliative care for surgical residents. Am J Surg 2010;200(4):542–7.
47. Webb TP, Weigelt JA, Redlich PN, et al. Protected block curriculum enhances learning during general surgery residency training. Arch Surg 2009;144(2): 160–6.
48. Pernar LI, Peyre SE, Smink DS, et al. Feasibility and impact of a case-based palliative care workshop for general surgery residents. J Am Coll Surg 2012;214(2): 231–6.
49. Dunn GP, Martensen R, Weissman DE. Surgical palliative care: a resident's guide. Chicago: American College of Surgeons; 2009.
50. Federation of State Medical Boards. Continuing medical education: boardby-board overview. Available at: http://www.fsmb.org/siteassets/advocacy/keyissues/continuing-medical-education-by-state.pdf. Accessed January 25, 2019.
51. Heyland DK, Barwich D, Pichora D, et al. Failure to engage hospitalized elderly patients and their families in advance care planning. JAMA Intern Med 2013; 173(9):778–87.
52. Sinuff T, Dodek P, You JJ, et al. Improving end-of-life communication and decision making: the development of a conceptual framework and quality indicators. J Pain Symptom Manage 2015;49(6):1070–80.
53. Lamba S, Tyrie LS, Bryczkowski S, et al. Teaching surgery residents the skills to communicate difficult news to patient and family members: a literature review. J Palliat Med 2016;19(1):101–7.

54. Walczak A, Butow PN, Bu S, et al. A systematic review of evidence for end-of-life communication interventions: who do they target, how are they structured and do they work? Patient Educ Couns 2016;99(1):3–16.
55. Alexander SC, Keitz SA, Sloane R, et al. A controlled trial of a short course to improve residents' communication with patients at the end of life. Acad Med 2006;81(11):1008–12.
56. Oczkowski SJ, Chung HO, Hanvey L, et al. Communication tools for end-of-life decision-making in the intensive care unit: a systematic review and meta-analysis. Crit Care 2016;20:97.
57. Davis D, O'Brien MA, Freemantle N, et al. Impact of formal continuing medical education: do conferences, workshops, rounds, and other traditional continuing education activities change physician behavior or health care outcomes? JAMA 1999;282(9):867–74.
58. Forsetlund L, Bjorndal A, Rashidian A, et al. Continuing education meetings and workshops: effects on professional practice and health care outcomes. Cochrane Database Syst Rev 2009;(2):CD003030.
59. Clayton JM, Adler JL, O'Callaghan A, et al. Intensive communication skills teaching for specialist training in palliative medicine: development and evaluation of an experiential workshop. J Palliat Med 2012;15(5):585–91.
60. Schmitz CC, Braman JP, Turner N, et al. Learning by (video) example: a randomized study of communication skills training for end-of-life and error disclosure family care conferences. Am J Surg 2016;212(5):996–1004.
61. Baile WF, Buckman R, Lenzi R, et al. SPIKES-a six-step protocol for delivering bad news: application to the patient with cancer. Oncologist 2000;5(4):302–11.
62. Berlin A. Goals of care and end of life in the ICU. Surg Clin North Am 2017;97(6): 1275–90.
63. Dean A, Willis S. The use of protocol in breaking bad news: evidence and ethos. Int J Palliat Nurs 2016;22(6):265–71.
64. Kruser JM, Nabozny MJ, Steffens NM, et al. "Best case/worst case": qualitative evaluation of a novel communication tool for difficult in-the-moment surgical decisions. J Am Geriatr Soc 2015;63(9):1805–11.
65. Schwarze ML, Kehler JM, Campbell TC. Navigating high risk procedures with more than just a street map. J Palliat Med 2013;16(10):1169–71.
66. DeCoste-Lopez J, Madhok J, Harman S. Curricular innovations for medical students in palliative and end-of-life care: a systematic review and assessment of study quality. J Palliat Med 2015;18(4):338–49.
67. Hsieh HF, Shannon SE, Curtis JR. Contradictions and communication strategies during end-of-life decision making in the intensive care unit. J Crit Care 2006; 21(4):294–304.
68. Wiener L, Weaver MS, Bell CJ, et al. Threading the cloak: palliative care education for care providers of adolescents and young adults with cancer. Clin Oncol Adolesc Young Adults 2015;5:1–18.
69. Section on Hospice and Palliative Medicine and Committee on Hospital Care. Pediatric palliative care and hospice care commitments, guidelines, and recommendations. Pediatrics 2013;132(5):966–72.
70. Kamal AH, Bull JH, Swetz KM, et al. Future of the palliative care workforce: preview to an impending crisis. Am J Med 2017;130(2):113–4.

UNITED STATES POSTAL SERVICE®

Statement of Ownership, Management, and Circulation (All Periodicals Publications Except Requester Publications)

1. Publication Title	2. Publication Number	3. Filing Date
SURGICAL CLINICS OF NORTH AMERICA	529 – 800	9/18/2019
4. Issue Frequency	5. Number of Issues Published Annually	6. Annual Subscription Price
FEB, APR, JUN, AUG, OCT, DEC	6	$417.00

7. Complete Mailing Address of Known Office of Publication (*Not printer*) (*Street, city, county, state, and ZIP+4®*)
ELSEVIER INC.
230 Park Avenue, Suite 800
New York, NY 10169

Contact Person
STEPHEN R. BUSHING
Telephone (*Include area code*)
215-239-3688

8. Complete Mailing Address of Headquarters or General Business Office of Publisher (*Not printer*)
ELSEVIER INC.
230 Park Avenue, Suite 800
New York, NY 10169

9. Full Names and Complete Mailing Addresses of Publisher, Editor, and Managing Editor (*Do not leave blank*)

Publisher (*Name and complete mailing address*)
TAYLOR BALL, ELSEVIER INC.
1600 JOHN F KENNEDY BLVD. SUITE 1800
PHILADELPHIA, PA 19103-2899

Editor (*Name and complete mailing address*)
JOHN VASSALLO, ELSEVIER INC.
1600 JOHN F KENNEDY BLVD. SUITE 1800
PHILADELPHIA, PA 19103-2899

Managing Editor (*Name and complete mailing address*)
PATRICK MANLEY, ELSEVIER INC.
1600 JOHN F KENNEDY BLVD. SUITE 1800
PHILADELPHIA, PA 19103-2899

10. Owner (*Do not leave blank. If the publication is owned by a corporation, give the name and address of the corporation immediately followed by the names and addresses of all stockholders owning or holding 1 percent or more of the total amount of stock. If not owned by a corporation, give the names and addresses of the individual owners. If owned by a partnership or other unincorporated firm, give its name and address as well as those of each individual owner. If the publication is published by a nonprofit organization, give its name and address.*)

Full Name	Complete Mailing Address
WHOLLY OWNED SUBSIDIARY OF REED/ELSEVIER, US HOLDINGS	1600 JOHN F KENNEDY BLVD. SUITE 1800 PHILADELPHIA, PA 19103-2899

11. Known Bondholders, Mortgagees, and Other Security Holders Owning or Holding 1 Percent or More of Total Amount of Bonds, Mortgages, or Other Securities. If none, check box → ☐ None

Full Name	Complete Mailing Address
N/A	

12. Tax Status (*For completion by nonprofit organizations authorized to mail at nonprofit rates*) (*Check one*)
The purpose, function, and nonprofit status of this organization and the exempt status for federal income tax purposes:
☒ Has Not Changed During Preceding 12 Months
☐ Has Changed During Preceding 12 Months (*Publisher must submit explanation of change with this statement*)

13. Publication Title: SURGICAL CLINICS OF NORTH AMERICA

14. Issue Date for Circulation Data Below: AUGUST 2019

15. Extent and Nature of Circulation			Average No. Copies Each Issue During Preceding 12 Months	No. Copies of Single Issue Published Nearest to Filing Date
a. Total Number of Copies (*Net press run*)			410	462
b. Paid Circulation (*By Mail and Outside the Mail*)	(1)	Mailed Outside-County Paid Subscriptions Stated on PS Form 3541 (Include paid distribution above nominal rate, advertiser's proof copies, and exchange copies)	172	197
	(2)	Mailed In-County Paid Subscriptions Stated on PS Form 3541 (*Include paid distribution above nominal rate, advertiser's proof copies, and exchange copies*)	0	0
	(3)	Paid Distribution Outside the Mails Including Sales Through Dealers and Carriers, Street Vendors, Counter Sales, and Other Paid Distribution Outside USPS®	165	219
	(4)	Paid Distribution by Other Classes of Mail Through the USPS (e.g., First-Class Mail®)	0	0
c. Total Paid Distribution [*Sum of 15b (1), (2), (3), and (4)*] ▶			337	416
d. Free or Nominal Rate Distribution (*By Mail and Outside the Mail*)	(1)	Free or Nominal Rate Outside-County Copies included on PS Form 3541	60	28
	(2)	Free or Nominal Rate In-County Copies Included on PS Form 3541	0	0
	(3)	Free or Nominal Rate Copies Mailed at Other Classes Through the USPS (e.g., First-Class Mail)	0	0
	(4)	Free or Nominal Rate Distribution Outside the Mail (*Carriers or other means*)	0	0
e. Total Free or Nominal Rate Distribution (*Sum of 15d (1), (2), (3) and (4)*)			60	28
f. Total Distribution (*Sum of 15c and 15e*) ▶			397	444
g. Copies not Distributed (*See Instructions to Publishers #4 (page #3)*) ▶			13	18
h. Total (*Sum of 15f and g*)			410	462
i. Percent Paid (*15c divided by 15f times 100*) ▶			84.89%	93.69%

* If you are claiming electronic copies, go to line 16 on page 3. If you are not claiming electronic copies, skip to line 17 on page 3.

16. Electronic Copy Circulation	Average No. Copies Each Issue During Preceding 12 Months	No. Copies of Single Issue Published Nearest to Filing Date
a. Paid Electronic Copies ▶		
b. Total Paid Print Copies (Line 15c) + Paid Electronic Copies (Line 16a) ▶		
c. Total Print Distribution (Line 15f) + Paid Electronic Copies (Line 16a) ▶		
d. Percent Paid (Both Print & Electronic Copies) (16b divided by 16c × 100) ▶		

☒ **I certify that 50% of all my distributed copies (electronic and print) are paid above a nominal price.**

17. Publication of Statement of Ownership
☒ If the publication is a general publication, publication of this statement is required. Will be printed in the OCTOBER 2019 issue of this publication. ☐ Publication not required.

18. Signature and Title of Editor, Publisher, Business Manager, or Owner
Stephen R. Bushing
STEPHEN R. BUSHING - INVENTORY DISTRIBUTION CONTROL MANAGER
Date: 9/18/2019

I certify that all information furnished on this form is true and complete. I understand that anyone who furnishes false or misleading information on this form or who omits material or information requested on the form may be subject to criminal sanctions (including fines and imprisonment) and/or civil sanctions (including civil penalties).

Printed and bound by CPI Group (UK) Ltd, Croydon, CR0 4YY

03/10/2024

01040402-0007